Medical
Transcription
Guide *Do's and Dont's*

Medical Transcription Guide *Do's and Dont's*

MARCY OTIS DIEHL, **BVE, CMA-A, CMT, FAAMT**
Professor, Medical Transcription Specialist Curriculum,
Grossmont Community College,
El Cajon, California

THIRD EDITION

ELSEVIER
SAUNDERS

ELSEVIER
SAUNDERS

11830 Westline Industrial Drive
St. Louis, Missouri 63146

Previous editions copyrighted 1999, 1990

International Standard Book Number 0-7216-0684-9

Acquisitions Editor: Susan Cole
Associate Developmental Editor: Lisa M. Neumann
Publishing Services Manager: Pat Joiner
Project Manager: Gena Magouirk
Design Manager: Gail Morey Hudson

Printed in USA

Last digit is the print number: 9 8 7 6 5 4 3 2 1

To Paul
and
to Adrianna, Katelyn, Kirsten, Andrea, and Anthony
along with their uncle Kip and parents

Preface

Welcome to *Medical Transcription Guide: Do's and Don'ts*, third edition. This book is intended for anyone who writes, transcribes, or dictates in the medical or scientific fields. Technology is moving at such a rapid pace that many changes have occurred in grammar and typing. Basic rules, as well as current trends and formats, are presented throughout the book. Why pick up this book rather than a standard English reference? Because in this book most of the examples provided with the rules have been chosen from medical writing, and many of these will be familiar to you from your everyday transcription. How many times have you had a disagreement with someone you work with on a point of grammar or punctuation in medical phrases that does not appear in English nonmedical writing? You will discover how quick and easy it is to locate the section to solve your problem through the alphabetical sequencing arrangement or the comprehensive index. Examples of do's and don'ts allow you to see at a glance how to correct your difficulty. Rationales for specific rules are provided so you can manipulate the principles of style with knowledge and understanding.

Before you begin to use this reference, take a few minutes to glance through and see how it is organized. A detailed table of contents is provided at the beginning of the book, and each chapter begins with an outline for that chapter. Reference is made to other chapters and rules when pertinent to the rule you are investigating. The book is made up of many small chapters set up in alphabetical order and titled with the key word or words that will guide you to the specific area of your research. If you cannot locate a specific topic, the surest approach is to use the index. Another feature that will grow in appeal as you familiarize yourself with the contents is the organization by rule numbers. The current rule, its exceptions, and its variations are provided along with examples and, when necessary, the common contradictions of that rule, or the don'ts.

Very little narrative or explanatory material accompanies the rules, since it is assumed that the user of this book already has a working knowledge of medical transcription and is either searching for help with an obscure rule or looking for reinforcement of a common practice. Some chapters begin with an introduction to set the tone for that chapter or give you an overview of the material. It is important to read the introduction when it is provided.

Many authorities do not always agree on matters of style or grammar, so standard current practices that are generally accepted are shown as preferences, with exceptions and/or options appearing as notes following the rules. As with all exceptions or options, you have the latitude to choose what you or your employer, the author of the material, wishes.

The book is small and handy to pick off the shelf and clearly set up so you can find what you are looking for. Additional cross-reference guides have been placed within the book, leading directly to the proper chapter for reference. Many reference lists have been added to the appendixes, including an abbreviation and brief form minilist, French words used in medical documents, a genus and species list, plural forms, Latin phrases, English and Medical homonyms, and unusual and problem words encountered in transcription. We saved room for you at the back of the book for your own reference pages to add words or just page numbers of areas in the book to which you wish to quickly refer. This edition introduces a new chapter about working from home (Chapter 48), hints about using reference books (Chapter 37), and do's and don'ts on the HIPAA regulations (Chapter 18).

We are grateful to the users of this book for their suggestions to help make this handbook a more effective reference. Instructors, take note: The textbook *Medical Transcription: Techniques and Procedures* further explains and discusses many of the rules contained in this guide and provides many practical lessons for reinforcement. The fifth edition is available from Saunders. This text includes a study disc that provides computer exercises for student practice. Please write to the publisher, Saunders, 11830 Westline Industrial Drive, St. Louis, MO, 63146, with your comments and any constructive criticism so future editions may meet your needs.

Marcy O. Diehl, BVE, CMA-A, CMT, FAAMT

Acknowledgments

A number of individuals assisted in the production of the third edition of this book, including my family, friends, students, former students, medical transcriptionists, instructors, and reviewers. I am especially grateful for their encouragement and helpful suggestions.

I am most indebted to many on the staff at Saunders for the professional production of this handy reference. Special thanks to Susan Cole, Acquisitions Editor, and Barbara Halliburton, Ph.D., copy editor.

A word of thanks is also due to the reviewers. Their evaluation was invaluable in planning the revision of this reference.

Sharon B. Allred, BRE, CMT
Instructor, Guilford Technical Community College,
Jamestown, North Carolina

Celeste Harjehausen, BS
Director of Client Services, Career Step, LLC,
Springville, Utah

Carol Jones Scheer, CMT
Training Manager, InHealth Transcription Services,
Atlanta, Georgia

George Morton, CMT
QA Manager, All Type, Inc.,
North Brunswick, New Jersey

Cindy S. Seabright, RHIT
Owner, TransPro Medical Transcription Service,
Spring Valley, Minnesota

Millie Yates
Vice President of Operations, OAK Horizons, Inc.,
Thompson's Station, Tennessee;
Adjunct Instructor, Medical Transcription,
Columbia State Community College,
Columbia, Tennessee

Contents

Contents

Contents

Contents

Contents

Contents

Contents

Abbreviations and Symbols

INTRODUCTION

There are some abbreviations and symbols that we use so often that we no longer think of them as abbreviations but rather as complete words. We hear *percent,* and we see %. *Mister* and *Doctor* look a bit out of place because *Mr.* and *Dr.* are such familiar titles. Medicine, like other technical fields, involves the use of many abbreviations and symbols that are particularly familiar to the medical writer and reader; this section is a guide to their proper use.

Some abbreviations are typed in full capital letters, some in lower-case, and some in a combination. They are written with or without periods.

Symbols and abbreviations can save time, space, and energy and can prevent the needless duplication of repetitious words. The overuse of abbreviations is to be avoided, however, with only standard abbreviations appearing in the patient's record where permitted. Abbreviations are used freely in chart notes, medical history, physical examinations, and so on. When you are using an abbreviation that may not be readily understood, it is a good idea to spell out the word or phrase and place the abbreviation in parentheses after the spelled-out form. Thereafter, you may freely use the abbreviation. Be consistent in style. If you have decided to use STAT, for instance, to describe immediately, don't switch to stat or Stat. Furthermore, abbreviations of any type should never be used when there is a chance of misinterpretation. Facilities accredited by the Joint Commission on Accreditation of Healthcare Organizations (JCAHO) must abide by a new mandate prohibiting the use of certain abbreviations. In the interest of patient safety, there are many abbreviations in addition to JCAHO's minimum requirement that should be spelled out. (see Table 1–1 at the end of this chapter). It is a good idea to avoid these abbreviations, regardless of whether or not the institution for which you work is accredited by JCAHO. In addition to these problems, many reference books disagree on both the capitalization and the punctuation of abbreviations. When in doubt (and you know the meaning), spell out the abbreviation.

General guidelines are offered in this chapter to assist you. A brief list of common abbreviations used in records and notes is provided in Appendix A, starting on p. 533. You should have a complete abbreviation reference book available for thorough research when needed.

1–1 ACADEMIC DEGREES, LICENSURE, RELIGIOUS ORDERS

✓ **DO**   abbreviate and omit periods from academic degrees and religious orders.

         MD   PhD   DDS   BVE   MS   LLD   SJ   OSA

         NOTE: *It is still acceptable to punctuate these if that is preferred by the author or institution for whom you work.*

🚫 **DON'T**   punctuate certification, registration, and licensure abbreviations.

         CMT   RRA   ART   RN   LVN   MFCC

DO place abbreviations for honor after academic degrees and in ordor of inoroaoing dictinotion.

> Neal J. Kaufman, MD, FACCP
> Rachel L. Connors, MD, LLB

 DO conform always to the preference of the person as far as sequence and exactly what is listed.

1-2 ACCURACY WITH ABBREVIATIONS

See also 1-18 and 1-19 for rules concerning spelling out terms that are abbreviated and accurate use of abbreviations.

 DO check any unfamiliar abbreviations or those that seem inappropriate with your reference lists. Individual letters in spoken form can sound alike.

> I performed an IND . . . (or I&D or IMD or IMB or IMP or IME) (This list could go on and on.)

 DON'T use the abbreviation in formal documents when the dictator has used the full word or words. You may follow the spelled-out form with the abbreviation in parentheses.

Incorrect:
A representative from SADD was invited as a conference speaker.
Correct:
A representative from Students Against Drunk Drivers (SADD) was invited as a conference speaker.

> EXCEPTIONS: Use the abbreviation for standard expressions of units of measurements (mg, ft, lb, and so on) and titles (Mr., Mrs., Dr., Jr., and so on).

 DO spell out an abbreviation when you realize that there could be a misunderstanding in its interpretation. You must be positive, of course, that your interpretation is correct; otherwise, leave it alone or flag the transcript for the dictator to interpret. (See Flagging in Chapter 11, p. 117.)

> The patient had a history of CVRD.
> cardiovascular renal disease?
> or
> cardiovascular respiratory disease?

🚫 DON'T   spell out abbreviations that are commonly accepted, unless they have been prohibited by JCAHO or the facility for which you work.

He was treated with Stelazine 10 mg t.i.d. with considerable improvement.

1–3   ACRONYMS

An acronym is the name for an abbreviation that forms a pronounceable word.

 DO   write acronyms in full capital letters without punctuation.

AAMT	(*American A*ssociation for *M*edical *Transcription*)
ACE inhibitor	(*angiotensin-c*onverting *e*nzyme)
AIDS	(*a*cquired *i*mmuno*d*eficiency *s*yndrome)
ARC	(*AIDS-r*elated *c*omplex)
CABG	(*c*oronary *a*rtery *b*ypass *g*raft)
CARE	(*C*ooperative for *A*merican *R*emittance to *E*verywhere)
COBOL	(*Co*mmon *B*usiness-*O*riented *L*anguage)
EAST	(*e*xternal rotation, *a*bduction, *s*tress *t*est)
HOPE	(*H*ealth *O*pportunities for *P*eople *E*verywhere)
OSHA	(*O*ccupational *S*afety and *H*ealth *A*dministration)
PERRLA	(*p*upils *e*qual, *r*ound, *r*eactive to *l*ight and *a*ccommodation)
POMR	(*p*roblem-*o*riented *m*edical *r*ecord)
SADD	(*S*tudents *A*gainst *D*runk *D*rivers)
SOAP	(*s*ubjective, *o*bjective, *a*ssessment, *p*lan)
TENS unit	(*t*ranscutaneous *e*lectrical *n*erve *s*timulation)
TURP	(*t*rans*u*rethral *r*esection of the *p*rostate)
ZIP code	(*Z*one *I*mprovement *P*rogram)

Unfamiliar acronyms may be difficult to deal with, because when we hear a familiar word we do not know if we are, in fact, dealing with an abbreviation or a word. Sometimes the construction of the sentence will alert you to the possibility of an acronym.

Dictated:

The patient was given a cage screen.

Transcribed:

The patient was given a CAGE screen. (*CAGE is an acronym for questions about drinking alcohol: cutting, annoyance, guilt, eye-opener.*)

4

🚫 **DON'T** use capital letters to write acronyms that have become accepted as words in themselves.

laser   radar   scuba   sonar   modem

1–4 ADDRESS PARTS

✅ **DO** use the post office abbreviations for the state names *(see Table 1–2 at the end of this chapter)* on both the inside and outside addresses.

936 North Branch Street
Bay Village, OH 44140

🚫 **DON'T** abbreviate the words *street, road, avenue, boulevard, north, south, east, west* in an inside address. However, *southwest (SW)*, *northwest (NW)*, and so forth are abbreviated after the street name.

936 North Branch Street
1876 Washington Boulevard, NW

1–5 CHART NOTES AND PROGRESS NOTES

✅ **DO** use abbreviations freely in progress notes, emergency department notes, and office chart notes and reports. Use them infrequently, except as indicated in previous rules, in formal correspondence, legal reports, articles, and hospital reports.

Office note: The GU tract was clear.
Report to insurance examiner: The genitourinary tract was clear.
Emergency department note: pt had cysto on 7-1-0X
Formal report to another physician: The patient had cystoscopy performed on July 1, 200X.
Hospital history and physical report: Patient had cystoscopy (*or* cysto) on July 1, 200X *(Complete sentences are not necessary.)*

✅ **DO** use symbols and abbreviations in the medical record only when they have been approved by the medical staff and an explanatory legend is available to those authorized to make entries in the medical record and to those who must interpret the entries.

NOTE: *These lists will vary, of course, among institutions. If the institution is accredited by JCAHO, its "do not use" list will include*

5

abbreviations prohibited by this accrediting body. Obtain lists from the institutions for which you work and refer to them carefully. Many hospitals are choosing a published abbreviation handbook to serve as the facility's approved list. This practice makes choices easier for the transcriptionist and those reviewing the records.

1–6 CHEMICAL AND MATH ABBREVIATIONS

✔️ DO   write chemical and mathematical abbreviations in a combination of both uppercase and lowercase letters without periods.

CO_2 (CO2)	*(carbon dioxide)*
Hb	*(hemoglobin)*
Hg	*(mercury)*
Na	*(sodium)*
T_4 (T4)	*(thyroxine)*
O_2 (O2)	*(oxygen)*
Ca^{++}	*(calcium ion)*
NaCl	*(sodium chloride)*
pH	*(hydrogen ion concentration)*
DNA	*(deoxyribonucleic acid)*
HCl	*(hydrochloric acid)*
10^4	*(ten to the fourth)*
K	*(potassium)*

NOTE: *The pH of a substance is a measure of its acidity or alkalinity* (ranging from 0 to 14). *It is indicated with a whole number or a whole number and a decimal fraction. If there is no following fraction, this is indicated with a zero (0).*

Dictated:
pee h was seven.
Transcribed:
The pH was 7.0. *(not hydrogen ion concentration)*
Dictated:
The patient had a pee h of five point two.
Transcribed:
The patient had a pH of 5.2.
Dictated:
The dee en a is unavailable for further study.
Transcribed:
The DNA is unavailable for further study.
Dictated:
STAT report shows sodium one hundred thirty eight milliequivalents per liter potassium three point three milliequivalents per liter chloride ninety seven milliequivalents per liter and a total see oh two of five

milliequivalents per liter blood glucose is seven hundred milligrams percent.

Transcribed:

STAT (*or* Stat) report shows sodium 138 mEq/L, potassium 3.3 mEq/L, chloride 97 mEq/L, and a total carbon dioxide (CO_2 *or* CO2 *also correct*) of 5 mEq/L. Blood glucose is 700 mg% (*not* mg percent *or* milligrams percent).

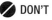 **DON'T** write these as abbreviations if the author has used the full word without a number in the expression or sentence

There was a high sodium level noted (*not* a high Na level).

NOTE: *See Appendix A, p. 533, for a list of common abbreviations.*

1–7 COMMON ABBREVIATIONS

 DO type familiar, frequently used common abbreviations, and words that can be readily understood as abbreviations, as abbreviations with no punctuation. These abbreviations usually apply to hospital departments and areas; time zones; business, educational, union, government, and military facilities; fraternal, service, professional, and religious organizations; and network and local broadcasting companies. They often represent long, complicated (sometimes forgotten) words or words that are seldom or never seen in any form other than an abbreviation.

DNA	ER	pH	Rh	PDR	CBS
FICA	TAC	AMA	ICU	TWA	NAACP

1–8 COURTESY TITLES

 DO abbreviate and punctuate *Mrs., Mr., Dr., Ms., Jr.,* and *Sr.* when used with a surname.

Dr. William A. Blake
Mrs. Frances Fishbein

NOTE: *There is a growing trend to eliminate the periods with these abbreviations.*

 DO drop the titles *Mr., Mrs., Ms.,* and *Dr.* if another title is used.

Correct:
Clifford Storey, MD

Incorrect:
Dr. Clifford Storey, MD
Incorrect:
Dr. William A. Blake, PhD

 DON'T   abbreviate courtesy titles when used alone.

The doctor was not in attendance at the time.

 DON'T   abbreviate titles, other than *Dr.*, *Mr.*, *Mrs.*, and *Ms.*, unless a first name or initial accompanies the last name.

Major Emery
Honorable Wilson
Right Reverend Turner *or* Rt. Rev. John J. Turner

1–9   DAYS OF THE WEEK AND MONTHS

 DON'T   abbreviate the days of the week and months of the year. In order to avoid confusion, numbers should not be substituted for the names of the months in correspondence; however, the use of six-digit dates is acceptable and often preferable in dating some records and reports.

Narrative copy: February 1, 200X
Not: Feb 1, XX *or* 2-1-XX *or* 2/1/XX *or* 02-01-XX *or* 1 Feb XX
Military documents only: 1 February 20XX
Charts and records: 02-01-XX   2-1-XX   February 1, XX
2/1/XX   2/1/200X

1–10   GENUS AND SPECIES

✔ **DO**   abbreviate the genus (but not the species) name *after* the genus has been used once in the text.

The test result was negative for Escherichia coli. We had expected to find E. coli . . .

 DON'T   abbreviate the genus name when used alone.

His Mycoplasma serology will not be repeated.

NOTE: *See Appendix E, p. 557, for a list of genus and species names used in medical reports.*

1–11   LATIN ABBREVIATIONS

✓ DO   write Latin abbreviations in lowercase letters with periods.

i.e.	a.c.
op. cit.	b.i.d.
et al.	t.i.d.
etc.	q.i.d.
e.g.	p.c.
a.m. (*also* AM)	
p.m. (*also* PM)	

EXCEPTION: *A.D.* (in the year of Our Lord)

🚫 DON'T   insert periods inaccurately in Latin abbreviations. Check the abbreviation when in doubt.

Incorrect:
et. al. (et *means* and *in Latin and requires no period*)
Correct:
et al.

✓ DO   avoid the overuse of Latin abbreviations as substitutes for Latin phrases; replace them with the English equivalent written out when possible.

Not: e.g. (*for* exempli gratia) *but* for example
Not: etc. (*for* et cetera) *but* and so forth

1–12   MEASUREMENTS, METRIC AND ENGLISH

✓ DO   use abbreviations for all metric measurements used *with* numbers.

You hear	You type
one millimeter	1 mm
five millimeters	5 mm (*not* mms)
ten centimeters	10 cm (*not* cms)
point five millimeters	0.5 mm
six cubic centimeters	6 cc (*not* ccs)
seven milliliters	7 mL *or* ml
twenty kilograms	20 kg (*not* kilos)
thirty-seven degrees Celsius	37°C

DO   place a zero (0) in front of a decimal point.

Dictated:
There remained a point four millimeter difference in the length of the two bones.
Transcribed:
There remained a 0.4-mm difference in the length of the two bones.

DON'T   add trailing zeros (0) after a number unless dictated.

Dictated:
three point five centimeters
Transcribed:
3.5 cm (*not* 3.50 cm)

EXCEPTION: *Specific gravity is typed with four digits with a decimal point between the first two.*

Dictated:
Specific gravity ten twenty
Transcribed:
Specific gravity 1.020

EXCEPTION: *The pH of a substance is indicated with a whole number and a decimal fraction. If there is no following fraction, you follow the number with a decimal point and a zero.*

Dictated:
pee h was seven
Transcribed:
The pH was 7.0.

NOTE: *Metric abbreviations are always written in lowercase letters, are typed with one space after the number, are not punctuated, and are not made plural. Exceptions are the capital* C *for* Celsius *and capital* L *for* liter. *In addition, some authors use the word* centigrade *rather than* Celsius. *Use the capital* C *as the abbreviation for both.*

DON'T   use an abbreviation for a unit of measurement when no number is given.

There was only a centimeter difference between the two.

DON'T separate the figure from the abbreviation that follows it. If the figure occurs at the end of a line, insert a space in front of the figure so that it will carry to the next line and appear with the abbreviation.

Correct:
....was 1400 mL
of serosanguineous fluid
Correct:
....was
1400 mL of serosanguineous fluid
Incorrect:
....was 1400
mL of serosanguineous fluid

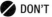 **DO** abbreviate all standard units of measurement used with numbers. Do not punctuate and do not make plural. It is the preferred practice, however, to spell out *inches* and *feet*.

She is 5 feet 6 inches tall and weighs 145 lb. (*not* lbs)

You hear	You type
thirty-five words per minute	35 wpm
two teaspoons every three hours	2 tsp every 3 hours
over eighty miles per hour	over 80 mph
there was three ounces left	there was 3 oz left

NOTE: *Notice the use of the singular form of the verb in the last example. The* three ounces *represents a single unit of measurement.*

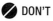 **DON'T** abbreviate *unit* or *grain*. The grain abbreviation *(gr)* can be mistaken for gram, and the unit abbreviation *(U)* can be misread, particularly when written by hand.

She had to be given 4 units of blood.
One unit of insulin was marked off.

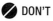 **DON'T** insert punctuation, such as a comma, between the individual parts of the same measurement. Also, measurement abbreviations do not require plural forms.

Preferred:
The birth weight was 9 pounds 6 ounces.
Also correct:
The birth weight was 9 lb 6 oz.
Incorrect:
The birth weight was 9 lbs, 6 ozs.

⊘ DON'T abbreviate these measurements when they are used without a number.

The cut was several centimeters long. (*not* cm)

NOTE: *See Chapter 26 for a complete guide on metric abbreviations.*

✓ DO use the following guidelines when typing drugs and dosages:

- *Metric units of measure are used in abbreviated form with numerals. They are not made plural.*
  25 mg   0.5 mg
- *Dosage instructions are preferably written in lowercase letters with periods separating the initials. It is suggested that you space between the number and the h in q.4 h. and so on, so that the number is more clearly seen.*
  q.4 h.   p.o.   t.i.d.   q.i.d.   b.i.d.   p.r.n.
- *Drugs in simple narration, especially without dosages given, are separated by commas.*

The patient was discharged home on Lanoxin, Calan, and Solu-Medrol.

- *In a more complex combination, when commas are needed within a string of information concerning a single drug, the units are separated by semicolons.*

MEDICATIONS: He will continue his 1800-calorie ADA diet and usual medicines, which include the following: estradiol, micronized, 2 mg/d for 25 of 30 days; propoxyphene HCl 65 mg q.i.d., which is an increase from his current t.i.d. regimen; flurazepam HCl 30 mg at bedtime; hydrocodone bitartrate 5 mg; ibuprofen 600 mg q.i.d.

- *A complex string can be typed in list format:*
  1. Continue his 1800-calorie ADA diet.
  2. Estradiol (micronized) 2 mg/d for 25 of 30 days.
  3. Flurazepam HCl 30 mg at bedtime
  4. Hydrocodone bitartrate 5 mg b.i.d
  5. Acetaminophen 500 mg b.i.d.
  6. Ibuprofen 600 mg q.i.d.
  7. Levothyroxine sodium 0.15 mg/d.
  8. Metoprolol tartrate 25 mg/d.
  9. Prednisone 5 mg/d.
  10. Propoxyphene HCl 65 mg q.i.d. (which is an increase from his current t.i.d. regimen).

DON'T separate the number at the end of the line from the symbols that may follow.

Correct

....25 mg

Incorrect

....25

mg

 DON'T use either the lowercase or capital "oh" on the keyboard for zero; use the zero symbol.

Correct:
50 mg
Incorrect:
5O mg *and* 5o mg

✓ **DO** see Chapter 10 for additional help with typing drugs.

1–13 NAMES

 DON'T abbreviate names unless the name is abbreviated in the correspondent's letterhead. Shortened forms of a person's name, such as a nickname, are allowed in the salutation.

Steven J. Clayborn *and* Dear Steve:

NOTE: *Some "nicknames" might not be a shortened form but rather the entire name.*

Ray	Gene	Will	Al	Alex	Ben	Ed
Fred	Sam	Pat	Beth	Hugh	Betty	

NOTE: *Do not use* Geo. *or* Chas. *with a last name unless it is abbreviated in the letterhead.*

Incorrect:
Chas. W. Ingles, MD
Judge Bea Murphy
Correct:
Judge Beatrice L. Murphy *(followed by an informal salutation:* Dear Bea,*)*

1–14 PLURAL FORMS WITH ABBREVIATIONS

✓ **DO** use an apostrophe to form the plurals of lowercase abbreviations and abbreviations that include periods.

Jr.'s   dsg's *(dressings)*   jt's *(joints)*

DON'T use an apostrophe with other plural abbreviations.

ECGs   BMRs   TMs   DTRs

1–15 PUNCTUATION WITH ABBREVIATIONS

DO use a period with single capitalized words and single-letter abbreviations.

Mr.   Jr.   Dr.   Inc.   Ltd.
Joseph P. Myers   E. coli

DO punctuate lowercase abbreviations made up of single letters.

a.m.   p.m.   e.g.   t.i.d.

DO use a period and space between the initial and the name following the initial.

William A. Knox Jr.

DON'T use a comma between *Jr.* or *Sr.* and the surname.

NOTE: *This style is the current trend. Always follow the dictates of the person if he prefers otherwise.*

DON'T use a comma between *II, III, 2d, 3d,* and so on and the surname.

William A. Knox II

NOTE: *This style is the current trend. Always follow the dictates of the person if he prefers otherwise.*

DON'T use a period in the following:

Units of measurement
wpm   mph   ft   oz
Certification, registration, and licensure abbreviations
CMA-A   CMT   RN   RRA   ART   LVN
Acronyms and metric abbreviations
CARE Project HOPE   AIDS   mg   mL   L   cm   km
Most abbreviations typed in full capital letters
UCLA   PKU   BUN   CBC   WBC   COPD
D&C   T&A   I&D   P&A
NBC   FICA   KEZL   TV   FM

Scientific abbreviations written in a combination of capital and lowercase letters

Rx   Dx   ACh   Ba   Hb   IgG   mEq   mOsm   Rh

Academic degrees and religious orders

MD   PhD   DDS   BVE   MS   SJ

NOTE: *It is still acceptable, however, to punctuate these when preferred.*

M.D.   Ph.D.   D.D.S.   M.A.   S.J.

1–16   SAINT, ABBREVIATED

✓ DO   abbreviate and punctuate *Saint (St.)* when it is the name of a place or part of the name of a person who prefers the abbreviation.

Margaret St. James
St. Paul, Minnesota

1–17   SENTENCE STRUCTURE

 DON'T   begin a sentence in formal writing with an abbreviation. Restructure the sentence or spell out the abbreviation. However, you may use an abbreviation as a sentence or phrase opening in informal chart notes, exams, operative reports, and so on.

CBC, urinalysis, and chest x-ray remain within normal limits.
or
A CBC, urinalysis, and chest x-ray . . .
Pt was seen for first time in ED on . . .
Preferred:
The patient was seen for the . . .

1–18   SHORT FORMS/BRIEF FORMS

✓ DO   type the short forms, or brief forms, when dictated if they do not violate any of the guidelines listed under 1–20 or as presented in the list of brief forms in Appendix C, p. 547.

Pap smear   *(Papanicolaou)*
exam   *(examination)*
sed rate   *(sedimentation rate)*
flu   *(influenza)*
phenobarb   *(phenobarbital)*

1–19 SPECIALIZED ABBREVIATIONS

✓ DO   use and follow the unique abbreviations used in the various medical specialty fields. These abbreviations are generally featured in the lists of spelling words for those specialties.

Genetics: R bands, cDNA, c-abl
Laboratory: Rh, HLA-A, ACC I, A+
Electrocardiography: aVR, V1, AE-60-I-2, d-TGA
Gynecology: G 2 P 1, D&C, AB
Ophthalmology: J1 reading
Orthopedics: DIP, MP, PIP

1–20 SPELLED-OUT ABBREVIATIONS

✓ DO   use an abbreviation to refer to a test, committee, drug, diagnosis, and so forth in a report or paper *after* the word or phrase has been used once in its completely spelled-out form.

All newborns are routinely tested for phenylketonuria (PKU). As a result, the incidence of PKU as a cause of infant . . .

NOTE: *Some abbreviations, particularly acronyms, become so common that it is no longer necessary to spell them out.*

Everyone involved with the patients' records has become familiar with HIPAA regulations.

✓ DO   spell out all abbreviations in the admission and discharge diagnoses, preoperative and postoperative diagnoses, impressions, assessments, and the names of surgical procedures.

Discharge diagnosis: Pelvic inflammatory disease (*not* PID)
Operation performed: Tonsillectomy and adenoidectomy (*not* T&A)

⊘ DON'T use symbols and abbreviations in the medical record when they have not been approved and listed by the medical staff. These lists will vary among institutions.

✓ DO   avoid using abbreviations in the titles of abstracts and papers or articles for publication.

1–21 STATE NAMES

 DO use the two-letter state abbreviations approved by the United States Postal Service for both inside and envelope addresses. *(See Table 1–2 at the end of the chapter.)*

 DO write out the name of the state in narrative copy.

She was born in New Hampshire and moved to Colorado when she was in college. (*Do not use* NH *and* CO.)

DON'T use the abbreviations without the city name and ZIP code.

1–22 SYMBOLS WITH ABBREVIATIONS
Symbols are just another form of abbreviation. Most standard symbols are available on the keyboard or specialized word processing font menus. *(See Chapter 44 for a complete discussion of symbols.)*

 DO use the ampersand symbol (&) with abbreviations. *(There is no space on either side of the &.)*

  I&D   P&A   L&W

 DO use symbols only when they occur in immediate association with a number or another abbreviation.

8×3	*(eight by three)*
4-5	*(four to five)*
#3-0	*(number three oh)*
2+	*(two plus)*
Vision: 20/20	*(Vision is twenty-twenty.)*
6/day	*(six per day)*
diluted 1:10	*(diluted one to ten)*
at −2	*(at minus two)*
60/40	*(sixty over forty)*
nocturia $\times$ 2	*(nocturia times two)*
T&A	*(tonsillectomy and adenoidectomy)*
25 mg/h	*(twenty-five milligrams per hour)*
limited by 45%	*(limited by forty-five percent)*
35 mg/dl	*(thirty-five milligrams per deciliter)*
30°C	*(thirty degrees Celsius)*
99°F	*(ninety-nine degrees Fahrenheit)*
BP: 100/80	*(Blood pressure is one hundred over eighty.)*
rSR′	*(RSR prime)*
$\times$ 3 days	*(times three days)*
3.5 cm	*(three point five centimeters)*
0.5 cm	*(point five centimeters)*

47% segs	*(forty-seven percent segs)*
Rh–	*(Rh negative)*
A Rh+	*(blood type A with positive Rh factor)*
#1 French	*(number one French)*

 DO   spell out the symbol abbreviation when it is used alone, not in association with a number.

What is the percentage of cure rates using this modality? (*not* %)

1–23   TITLES

 DO   use the abbreviation *Esq.* only when no other title is used.

Correct:
D. Kirk Knight, Esq.
Incorrect:
Mr. D. Kirk Knight, Esq.

NOTE: *The spelled-out* Esquire *is also correct.*

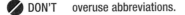 **DO**   drop the titles *Mr.*, *Mrs.*, *Ms.*, and *Dr.* if another title is used.

Correct:
Clifford Storey, MD
Incorrect:
Dr. Clifford Storey, MD

DO   use any required punctuation mark, except a period, after the period used with an abbreviation.

Are you sure his name is John R. Robertson Sr.?

1–24   WHEN NOT TO ABBREVIATE

DO   use standard abbreviations. However, be sure to confine office and emergency department "shorthand" to office and ED records.

DON'T   overuse abbreviations.

DON'T   use an abbreviation that logically may have more than one meaning.

DON'T   use any of the symbols or abbreviations that have been banned by JCAHO.

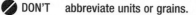
🚫 DON'T   abbreviate units or grains.

🚫 DON'T   use abbreviations in the following parts of the patient's medical record: admission and discharge diagnoses, preoperative and postoperative diagnoses, and the names of surgical or diagnostic procedures.

Operation performed: TURP *(incorrect)*
Operation performed: Transurethral resection of the prostate *(correct)*

🚫 DON'T   substitute an abbreviation such as q.i.d. when the author has said "every six hours" in narrative copy.

🚫 DON'T   abbreviate a unit of measurement that has no number accompanying it.

🚫 DON'T   abbreviate titles without a name.

🚫 DON'T   abbreviate a genus name when used alone (without the species name).

🚫 DON'T   abbreviate the names of states except in the address.

TABLE 1-1

ISMP LIST OF ERROR-PRONE ABBREVIATIONS, SYMBOLS, AND DOSE DESIGNATIONS

Abbreviations	Intended Meaning	Misinterpretation	Correction
μg[†]	Microgram	Mistaken as "mg"	Use "mcg"
AD, AS, AU[†]	Right ear, left ear, each ear	Mistaken as OD, OS, OU (right eye, left eye, each eye)	Use "right ear," "left ear," or "each ear"
OD, OS, OU	Right eye, left eye, each eye	Mistaken as AD, AS, AU (right ear, left ear, each ear)	Use "right eye," "left eye," or "each eye"
BT	Bedtime	Mistaken as "BID" (twice daily)	Use "bedtime"
cc[†]	Cubic centimeters	Mistaken as "u" (units)	Use "mL"
D/C[†]	Discharge or discontinue	Premature discontinuation of medications if D/C (intended to mean "discharge") has been misinterpreted as "discontinued" when followed by a list of discharge medications	Use "discharge" and "discontinue"
IJ	Injection	Mistaken as "IV" or "intrajugular"	Use "injection"
IN	Intranasal	Mistaken as "IM" or "IV"	Use "intranasal" or "NAS"
HS[†]	Half-strength	Mistaken as bedtime	Use "half-strength"
hs	At bedtime, hours of sleep	Mistaken as half-strength	Use "at bedtime"
IU**	International unit	Mistaken as IV (intravenous) or 10 (ten)	Use "units"
o.d. or OD	Once daily	Mistaken as "right eye" (OD-oculus dexter), leading to oral liquid medications administered in the eye	Use "daily"

OJ	Orange juice	Mistaken as OD or OS (right or left eye); drugs meant to be diluted in orange juice may be given in the eye	Use "orange juice"
Per os	By mouth, orally	The "os" can be mistaken as "left eye" (OS-oculus sinister)	Use "PO," "by mouth," or "orally"
q.d. or QD**	Every day	Mistaken as q.i.d., especially if the period after the "q" or the tail of the "q" is misunderstood as an "i"	Use "daily"
qhs	At bedtime	Mistaken as "qhr" or every hour	Use "at bedtime"
qn	Nightly	Mistaken as "qh" (every hour)	Use "nightly"
q.o.d. or QOD**	Every other day	Mistaken as "q.d." (daily) or "q.i.d. (four times daily) if the "o" is poorly written	Use "every other day"
q1d	Daily	Mistaken as q.i.d. (four times daily)	Use "daily"
q6PM, etc.	Every evening at 6 PM	Mistaken as every 6 hours	Use "6 PM nightly" or "6 PM daily"
SC, SQ, sub q†	Subcutaneous	SC mistaken as SL (sublingual); SQ mistaken as "5 every;" the "q" in "sub q" has been mistaken as "every" (e.g., a heparin dose ordered "sub q 2 hours before surgery" misunderstood as every 2 hours before surgery)	Use "subcut" or "subcutaneously"
ss	Sliding scale (insulin) or ½ (apothecary)	Mistaken as "55"	Spell out "sliding scale;" use "one-half" or "½"
SSRI	Sliding scale regular insulin	Mistaken as selective-serotonin reuptake inhibitor	Spell out "sliding scale (insulin)"
SSI	Sliding scale insulin	Mistaken as Strong Solution of Iodine (Lugol's)	Spell out "sliding scale (insulin)"
t/d	One daily	Mistaken as "tid"	Use "1 daily"

Continued

◆ **TABLE 1-1**

ISMP LIST OF ERROR-PRONE ABBREVIATIONS, SYMBOLS, AND DOSE DESIGNATIONS—Cont'd

Abbreviations	Intended Meaning	Misinterpretation	Correction
TIW or tiw[†]	3 times a week	Mistaken as "3 times a day" or "twice in a week"	Use "3 times weekly"
U or u**	Unit	Mistaken as the number 0 or 4, causing a 10-fold overdose or greater (e.g., 4U seen as "40" or 4u seen as "44"); mistaken as "cc" so dose given in volume instead of units (e.g., 4u seen as 4cc)	Use "unit"

Dose Designations and Other Information	Intended Meaning	Misinterpretation	Correction
Trailing zero after decimal point (e.g., 1.0 mg)**	1 mg	Mistaken as 10 mg if the decimal point is not seen	Do not use trailing zeros for doses expressed in whole numbers
No leading zero before a decimal dose (e.g., .5 mg)**	0.5 mg	Mistaken as 5 mg if the decimal point is not seen	Use zero before a decimal point when the dose is less than a whole unit
Drug name and dose run together (especially problematic for drug names that end in "L" such as Inderal 40 mg; Tegretol 300 mg)	Inderal 40 mg Tegretol 300 mg	Mistaken as Inderal 140 mg Mistaken as Tegretol 1300 mg	Place adequate space between the drug name, dose, and unit of measure
Numerical dose and unit of measure run together (e.g., 10 mg, 100 mL)	10 mg 100 mL	The "m" is sometimes mistaken as a zero or two zeros, risking a 10- to 100-fold overdose	Place adequate space between the dose and unit of measure

	Intended Meaning	Misinterpretation	Correction
Abbreviations such as mg. or mL. (with a period following the abbreviation)	mg	The period is unnecessary and could be mistaken as the number 1 if written poorly	Use mg, mL, etc. without a terminal period
	mL		
Large doses without properly placed commas (e.g., 100000 units; 1000000 units)	100,000 units	100000 has been mistaken as 10,000 or 1,000,000;	Use commas for dosing units at or above 1,000, or use words such as 100 "thousand" or 1 "million" to improve readability
	1,000,000 units	1000000 has been mistaken as 100,000	
Drug Name Abbreviations	**Intended Meaning**	**Misinterpretation**	**Correction**
ARA A	vidarabine	Mistaken as cytarabine (ARA C)	Use complete drug name
AZT	zidovudine (Retrovir)	Mistaken as azathioprine or aztreonam	Use complete drug name
CPZ	Compazine (prochlorperazine)	Mistaken as chlorpromazine	Use complete drug name
DPT	Demerol-Phenergan-Thorazine	Mistaken as diphtheria-pertussis-tetanus (vaccine)	Use complete drug name
DTO	Diluted tincture of opium, or deodorized tincture of opium (Paregoric)	Mistaken as tincture of opium	Use complete drug name
HCl	hydrochloric acid or hydrochloride	Mistaken as potassium chloride (The "H" is misinterpreted as "K")	Use complete drug name unless expressed as a salt of a drug

Continued

◆ TABLE 1-1

ISMP LIST OF ERROR-PRONE ABBREVIATIONS, SYMBOLS, AND DOSE DESIGNATIONS—Cont'd

Abbreviations	Intended Meaning	Misinterpretation	Correction
HCT	hydrocortisone	Mistaken as hydrochlorothiazide	Use complete drug name
HCTZ	hydrochlorothiazide	Mistaken as hydrocortisone (seen as HCT250 mg)	Use complete drug name
MgSO4''	magnesium sulfate	Mistaken as morphine sulfate	Use complete drug name
MS, MS04''	morphine sulfate	Mistaken as magnesium sulfate	Use complete drug name
MTX	methotrexate	Mistaken as mitoxantrone	Use complete drug name
PCA	procainamide	Mistaken as Patient Controlled Analgesia	Use complete drug name
PTU	propylthiouracil	Mistaken as mercaptopurine	Use complete drug name
T3	Tylenol with codeine No. 3	Mistaken as liothyronine	Use complete drug name
TAC	triamcinolone	Mistaken as tetracaine, Adrenalin, cocaine	Use complete drug name
TNK	TNKase	Mistaken as "TPA"	Use complete drug name
ZnSO4	zinc sulfate	Mistaken as morphine sulfate	Use complete drug name
Stemmed Drug Names	**Intended Meaning**	**Misinterpretation**	**Correction**
"Nitro" drip	nitroglycerin infusion	Mistaken as sodium nitroprusside infusion	Use complete drug name
"Norflox"	norfloxacin	Mistaken as Norflex	Use complete drug name
"IV Vanc"	intravenous vancomycin	Mistaken as Invanz	Use complete drug name

Symbols	Intended Meaning	Misinterpretation	Correction
ʒ	Dram	Symbol for dram mistaken as "3"	Use the metric system
ℳ	Minim	Symbol for minim mistaken as "mL"	
x3d	For three days	Mistaken as "3 doses"	Use "for three days"
> and <	Greater than and less than	Mistaken as opposite of intended; mistakenly use incorrect symbol; "< 10" mistaken as "40"	Use "greater than" or "less than"
/ (slash mark)	Separates two doses or indicates "per"	Mistaken as the number 1 (e.g., "25 units/10 units" misread as "25 units and 110" units)	Use "per" rather than a slash mark to separate doses
@	At	Mistaken as "2"	Use "at"
&	And	Mistaken as "2"	Use "and"
+	Plus or and	Mistaken as "4"	Use "and"
°	Hour	Mistaken as a zero (e.g., q2° seen as q 20)	Use "hr," "h," or "hour"

**Abbreviation is also included on JCAHO's "minimum list" of dangerous abbreviations, acronyms and symbols that must be included on an organization's "Do Not Use" list, effective January 1, 2004. An updated list of frequently asked questions about this JCAHO requirement can be found on their website at www.jcaho.org.
†Effective April 1, 2004, each organization accredited by JCAHO must include at least three items from this selection on their list.

◆ **TABLE 1-2**

STATE NAMES AND OTHER U.S. POSTAL SERVICE ABBREVIATIONS
Two-Letter State Abbreviations for the United States and Its Dependencies

Alabama	AL	Kansas	KS	Northern Mariana Islands	MP
Alaska	AK	Kentucky	KY	Ohio	OH
American Samoa	AS	Louisiana	LA	Oklahoma	OK
Arizona	AZ	Maine	ME	Oregon	OR
Arkansas	AR	Marshall Islands	MH	Palau	PW
California	CA	Maryland	MD	Pennsylvania	PA
Canal Zone	CZ	Massachusetts	MA	Puerto Rico	PR
Colorado	CO	Michigan	MI	Rhode Island	RI
Connecticut	CT	Minnesota	MN	South Carolina	SC
Delaware	DE	Mississippi	MS	South Dakota	SD
District of Columbia	DC	Missouri	MO	Tennessee	TN
Federated States of Micronesia	FM	Montana	MT	Texas	TX
Florida	FL	Nebraska	NE	Utah	UT
Georgia	GA	Nevada	NV	Vermont	VT
Guam	GU	New Hampshire	NH	Virgin Islands	VI
Hawaii	HI	New Jersey	NJ	Virginia	VA
Idaho	ID	New Mexico	NM	Washington	WA
Illinois	IL	New York	NY	West Virginia	WV
Indiana	IN	North Carolina	NC	Wisconsin	WI
Iowa	IA	North Dakota	ND	Wyoming	WY

Two-Letter Abbreviations for Canadian Provinces and Territories

Alberta	AB	Newfoundland	NF	Quebec	QC
British Columbia	BC	Northwest Territories	NT	Saskatchewan	SK
Labrador	LB	Nova Scotia	NS	Yukon Territory	YT
Manitoba	MB	Ontario	ON		
New Brunswick	NB	Prince Edward Island	PE		

2

Address Formats for Letters and Forms of Address

The topics in this chapter are not arranged alphabetically but rather in the progression of an address from top to bottom, that is, from name of addressee to salutation and on to the complete address.

ADDRESS FORMATS FOR LETTERS

The inside address is typed flush with the left margin and is begun on approximately the fifth line below the date of the letter. It may be moved up or down one or two lines depending on the length of the letter.

2–1 NAMES OF PERSONS AND FIRMS

A courtesy title *(Mr., Mrs., Ms.)* or professional title is added to a name. If you do not know whether the person is a man or a woman, omit using a title. The title *Ms.* may be used when you do not have a title for a woman. The degree is preferred over a title, and in no case should a title and a degree be used together. Use the middle initial when it is known.

DON'T use both title and degree with a name.

Incorrect:
Dr. Clifford F. Adolph, MD
Dr. Bertrum L. Storey, DDS
Mrs. Beatrice Wood, PhD
Correct:
Dr. Beatrice Wood
Beatrice Wood, PhD
Mrs. Beatrice Wood *(in a social setting)*

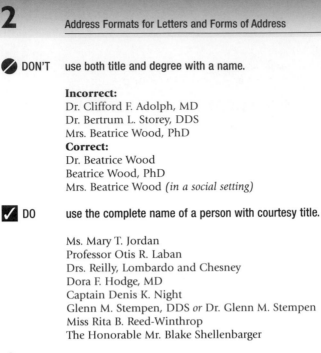 **DO** use the complete name of a person with courtesy title.

Ms. Mary T. Jordan
Professor Otis R. Laban
Drs. Reilly, Lombardo and Chesney
Dora F. Hodge, MD
Captain Denis K. Night
Glenn M. Stempen, DDS *or* Dr. Glenn M. Stempen
Miss Rita B. Reed-Winthrop
The Honorable Mr. Blake Shellenbarger

DON'T abbreviate any part of the name unless the person does so on the letterhead.

William A. Berry, MD *not* Wm. A. Berry, MD

DO copy the complete name of the firm exactly as it is printed on the letterhead or as printed in the telephone book or other professional directory. Always follow the firm's style for capitalization, abbreviations, and punctuation.

Palm Grove Medical Center Inc.
South Bay Medical Group Ltd.
Atlantic Shores 24-Hour Clinic
Valley Presbyterian Hospital
Maynard County Medical Supply
Kimbrell, Owen, Sweis & Schonbrun

NOTE: *In a series of names, no comma is placed in front of the ampersand (&).*

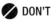 **DON'T** use a comma to set off *Inc., Ltd.,* and so forth from the company name unless the company does so.

DO place abbreviations for honorary and academic degrees after the name and in order of increasing distinction.

Neal J. Kaufman, MD, FACP
Rachel L. Connors, MD, LLB
Christine M. Braun, Esquire
Christine M. Braun, Esq.
Esquire (Esq.) is used by architects, engineers, attorneys, and justices of the peace. Do not use with a courtesy title.

 DO separate the parts of a name with a comma or commas when the name is given in inverted order.

Jacobs, Barney K.
Kaufman, Neal J., MD, FACP

2–2 TITLES

If a business title accompanies the name, it may follow the name on the same line, or, if lengthy, it may appear on the next line. When two lines are used, no punctuation is placed at the end of the first line, and the title is typed flush with the name above.

 DO use titles when and as appropriate.

F. E. Gidwani, MD, Medical Director

Ms. Catherine A. Wendall
Purchasing Agent

Adrian N. Abott, MD, LLB
Chief-of-Staff
Sinai-Lebanon Hospital

Dean Karl T. Brent, Chairman
Biology Department
International University

Christine M. Braun, Esq.
Sylvan, Beeds & Braun Inc.

2–3 ADDRESS

Following the name of the person or firm is the street or post office box address. *(If both are given, use the post office box address.)* Do not abbreviate *North, South, East, West, Road, Street, Avenue,* or *Boulevard. Apartment* is abbreviated only if the line is unusually long. The apartment, suite, or space number is typed on the same line with the street address, separated by a comma. The abbreviations *NW, NE, SW,* and so forth are used after the street name.

The name of the city is spelled out and separated from the state name with a comma. The state name may be spelled out or abbreviated and is separated from the ZIP code by one to three spaces. The United States postal abbreviations of state names are not used without the ZIP code *(see 1–21, State Names)*.

 DO   complete the address as approved by United States postal regulations, avoiding all unnecessary abbreviations. For ease of understanding, spell out the number *one* when it is the street, building, or apartment number.

One Cable Avenue
Little Creek, CA 94524

1731 North Branch Road, Suite B
Toledo, OH 43505

196 Blackmoor Road
Hatchend
Pinner, Middlesex
ENGLAND HA 5 4PF

PO Box 1966
Naples, FL 33940

Rural Route #3
Crow Poison, AK 99516

NOTE: *If the delivery address line information is too long to be typed in a single line above the city, state, and ZIP code, then place the secondary address information (e.g., suite, apartment, building, room, space numbers) on the line immediately above the delivery address line. This placement may seem awkward, but it is correct.*

Apartment 54   Building 4
845 Medford Circle   1951 52nd Street
Bearden, KS 66743   Tucson, AZ 85715

 DON'T   use post office abbreviations without the ZIP code.

 DO   spell out the street number for ease of reading.

1335 Ninth Street

FORMS OF ADDRESS/SALUTATIONS

The manner in which a person is addressed in a letter is determined by the relationship between the writer and the receiver of the document, if the receiver is known. If the receiver of the document is unknown, careful protocol must be observed and stereotypic language avoided.

The salutation is typed a double space after the last line of the address and is followed by a colon if mixed punctuation is used. If open punctuation is used, neither a colon nor a comma is used. Formality demands a courtesy title; first names are used when appropriate and if formality is unnecessary.

2–4 *SALUTATIONS USED FOR MEN*

 DO   follow these formats when addressing men:

> Gentlemen:
> Dear Mr. Sutherland:
> Dear Dr. Hon:
> *or*
> Dear Doctor Hon:
> Dear Doctors Blake and Fortuna:
> Dear Dr. Blake and Dr. Fortuna:
> Dear Doctors:
> Dear Paul and Josh:
> *or*
> Dear Paul and Josh,

> **NOTE:** *When only first names are used, a comma is also correct.*

> Dear Dr. Johnson and Mr. Lombardo:
> Gentlemen:
> Dear Chuck and Jay:
> Dear Chuck and Jay,
> Dear Professor Abbott:
> Dear Dr. Abbott:
> Dear Rabbi Ruderman:
> (*likewise* Father, Bishop, Reverend, Monsignor, Cardinal, Brother, Deacon, Chaplain, Dean)

> **Name:**
> The Honorable Mr. Blake R. Shellenbarger
> **Salutation:**
> Dear Mr. Shellenbarger:
> *or*
> Dear Judge Shellenbarger:

> **Name:**
> Tony Lamb and Peter Lamb
> **Salutation:**
> Dear Mr. Tony Lamb and Mr. Peter Lamb:
> Dear Messrs. Lamb:
> Gentlemen:
> Dear Tony and Pete:

2–5 SALUTATIONS USED FOR WOMEN

✓ **DO**   follow these formats when addressing women:

Ladies:
Mesdames:
Dear Dr. Martin:
Dear Doctor Martin:
Dear Mrs. Clayborne:
Dear Ms. Robinson:
Dear Miss Glenn:
Dear Judge Peterson:
Dear Rev. Schwartz:
(*likewise* Rabbi, Chaplain, Dean, Deacon, Bishop)
Dear Sister Rose Anthony:
Dear Reverend Mother Reilly:
Dear Reverend Mother:
Dear Captain Jenkins:
Dear Professor Mayz:

Name:
The Honorable Ms. Francine Shellenbarger
Salutation:
Dear Ms. *(Miss, Mrs.)* Shellenbarger
or
Dear Judge Shellenbarger

Dear Dr. Rose Martin and Dr. Lily Martin:
Dear Doctors Martin:
Dear Doctors:
Dear Rose and Lily:

Dear Doctors Person and Higgins:
Dear Dr. Person and Dr. Higgins:
Dear Doctors:
Dear Jeanette and Beverly:
Dear Jeanette and Beverly,

Dear Dr. Phillips and Ms. Cox:
Ladies:
Dear Bertha and Wanda:

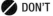 **DON'T**   use social titles in business correspondence.

Incorrect:
Dear Mrs. John Becker and Ms. Patty Becker:
Correct:
Dear Mrs. Sheila Becker and Ms. Patty Becker:
Ladies:

Dear Sheila and Patty:
Dear Sheila and Patty,

2–6 FORMATS FOR ADDRESSING A MAN AND A WOMAN AS A MARRIED COUPLE

 DO   follow these formats when addressing a man and a woman as a married couple:

Dear Mr. and Mrs. Knight:
Dear Dr. and Mrs. Wong:
Dear Professor and Mrs. Barnett:
Dear Professor Holloway and Ms. Blake:
Dear Professors Gonzales:
Dear Professor and Mr. Collings:
Dear Dr. Johnson and Ms. Lombardo:
Dear Professor Kala and Professor Barbaor:
Dear Rabbi Gold and Mr. Gold:

Dear Dr. Lois Candelaria and Dr. Fred Candelaria:
Dear Doctors Candelaria:
Dear Doctors:
Dear Lois and Fred:

Dear Captain and Mrs. Philips:
Dear Mr. Claborne and Mrs. Steen-Claborne:
Dear Mr. Mohrman and Captain Mohrman:

Dear Mr. Bailey and Dr. Bailey:
Dear Dr. and Mr. Bailey:

2–7 FORMATS FOR ADDRESSING A MAN AND A WOMAN NOT ASSOCIATED AS A MARRIED COUPLE

 DO   follow these formats when addressing men and women who are not associated as a married couple:

Dear Doctors DuPree and Ahrens:
Dear Dr. DuPree and Dr. Ahrens:
Dear Doctors:
Dear Nancy and Philip:

Dear Dr. Cleveland and Mrs. Easterly:
Dear Professor Garcia and Mr. Ireton:
Dear Professor Kimbrell and Ms. Knudsen:

Correct:
Dear Professors Wong and Shallie

Incorrect:
Dear Prof. Wong and Shallie

2–8 FORMATS FOR ADDRESSING LARGE GROUPS OF MEN AND/OR WOMEN

 DO follow this format when addressing a large group of men and/or women:

Gentlemen:
Ladies and Gentlemen:
Ladies:
Dear Doctors:
Dear Professor Bradley et al.:
Dear Dr. Mitchelson et al.: *(Use just the name of the senior person in the firm.)*

2–9 FORMATS FOR ADDRESSING PERSONS WHOSE SEX IS UNKNOWN OR UNKNOWN RECIPIENTS

 DON'T assign gender to the head of a firm.

✓ **DO** follow these formats when the sex is unknown:

Ladies and Gentlemen:
Dear Sir or Madam:
Dear Lane Wilkerson:

 DO follow this format when the recipient of the document is unknown:

To Whom It May Concern:
TO WHOM IT MAY CONCERN:

2–10 FORMATS FOR MILITARY ADDRESSES

✓ **DO** use the title and full name followed by the branch of service abbreviation.

Captain John P. Ligmahn, USN
or
Capt John P. Ligmahn, USMC/USCG
Incorrect:
Dear Capt Ligmahn:
Correct:
Dear Captain Ligmahn:
or
(for a physician) Dear Dr. Ligmahn:

Midshipman Francine R. Bodner
United States Naval Academy
Dear Midshipman Bodner:
or
Dear Ms. Bodner: (*A man would be addressed with the full title or* Dear Mr.)

Chief Warrant Officer Anthony d'Amato, USAF
Dear Chief Warrant Officer d'Amato:
or
Dear Mr. d'Amato: (*A woman would be addressed with the full title or* Dear Ms., Miss, *or* Mrs.)

A complete address:
Warrant Officer Phillip R. Wilson, USAF
Company B
2nd Helicopter Squad
APO New York, NY 09801

Dear Mr. Wilson:

2–11 ATTENTION LINE

The attention line is typed two spaces below the last line of the address. It is used so that the letter will receive attention by a specific person if he or she is available; if not, another member of the firm will take care of the matter.

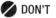 **DO**   type *attention* in full caps or with only the first letter capitalized.

ATTENTION Mr. Charles P. Trask, Buyer
or
Attention Mr. Charles P. Trask, Buyer

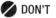 **DO**   use a second line if the title is very long.

Attention Mr. Charles P. Trask
Accounting Supervisor

DON'T   abbreviate *Attention* or use punctuation with it.

Incorrect:
ATTN: Mr. Charles P. Trask, Buyer

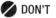 **DO**   type an appropriate salutation with an attention line. Since the first line of the address is the firm name, the salutation must agree with this line rather than with the attention line. These salutations are appropriate:

Dear Sir or Madam:
Gentlemen:
Ladies:
Ladies and Gentlemen:
Doctors:
Dear Doctors:

NOTE: *One often finds it awkward to follow an attention line that is obviously addressed to a specific person with a nonspecific salutation. For example:*

Engraved Letterhead Company
2171 Lincoln Boulevard
Philadelphia, PA 19105

ATTENTION Pauline Flinn, Buyer

Dear Sir or Madam:
However, this example is correct. It is suggested that one might address this document instead directly to Ms. Flinn and omit the attention line, so that the salutation then would read Dear Ms. Flinn.

Ms. Pauline Flinn, Buyer
c/o Engraved Letterhead Company
2171 Lincoln Boulevard
Philadelphia, PA 19105

Dear Ms. Flinn:

2–12 COMPLETE ADDRESS APPEARANCE

✓ DO   strive to prepare an attractive, balanced inside address. If one line is significantly longer than the rest, find an appropriate dividing point on the long line.

Victor R. Langworthy, MD
Medical Director
West View Community Hospital and Inland
Medical Center, Inc.
321 Roseview Drive
St. Louis, MO 63139

Better arrangement

Victor R. Langworthy, MD, Medical Director
West View Community Hospital and
Inland Medical Center, Inc.
321 Roseview Drive
St. Louis, MO 63139

Miss Josie M. Brooks
1879 Westchester Boulevard, Apartment 170-B
Normal Heights, SD 57701

Better arrangement

Miss Josie M. Brooks
Apartment 170-B
1879 Westchester Boulevard
Normal Heights, SD 57701

NOTE: *Please notice the correct placement of the apartment number, leaving the final two lines of the address with the primary delivery information.*

✓ **DO** type each name on a separate line when you are preparing a letter to more than one person.

Peter L. Johnson, DDS
Mr. Frank R. Lombardo
Street address
City, State + ZIP

Mr. Tony Lamb
Mr. Peter Lamb
Street address
City, State + ZIP

Renee L. Phillips, DO
Ms. Francine T. Cox
Street address
City, State + ZIP

Mrs. Glendora Robinson
c/o Steven Santiago
Street address
City, State + ZIP

Drs. Mitchelson, Francois, Peters, Moore, & Davis
Street address
City, State + ZIP
Dear Dr. Mitchelson et al.:

3

Apostrophe

3–1 ABBREVIATIONS AND PLURAL FORMS OF NUMBERS AND LETTERS

✓ DO   use an apostrophe to form the plural of the capital letters *A,*
I, O, M, and *U;* of all lowercase letters; and after a lowercase
letter in an abbreviation for the sake of clarity.

NOTE: *The reason for this rule is to avoid making what might
appear to be a word with the combination of some letters and s,
such as* Is, Ms, Us, is, *and* as. *It is not necessary to use the
apostrophe to form the plural of numbers or capital-letter
abbreviations.*

When you make an entry in a chart, be careful that your
2s don't look like z's.
You used four I's in that first paragraph.
He has a note for three Rx's on his desk.
There were elevated wbc's.
Accommodate is spelled with two c's, two m's, and two o's.

DON'T   use the apostrophe to form the plural of numbers or capital-letter abbreviations.

> The TMs were intact.
> There were no 4 × 4s left in the box.
> The DTRs were normal.
> He had repeat RBCs in our lab.

3–2   COMPOUND NOUNS

 DO   add an apostrophe plus *s* to the last element of the possessive compound.

> the chief-of-staff's decision
> my brother-in-law's book
> my brothers-in-law's book *(one book, two owners)*
> her daughters-in-law's visit

3–3   CONTRACTIONS

 DO   use an apostrophe in contractions of words or figures.

> it's   *(it is* or *it has)*
> he'll   *(he will)*
> won't   *(will not)*
> class of '91   *(1991)*
> o'clock   *(of the clock)*
> I'm   *(I am)*

 DO   *avoid* the use of contractions of words or figures except for *o'clock* in all medical reports and formal business letters.

You hear	You type
she'll	she will
doesn't	does not
'03	2003
nine o'clock	9 o'clock

3–4   EPONYMS

Many eponyms (adjectives derived from proper nouns) are used in medical writing. Most of these are not written as possessives. However, some authors prefer the possessive style and wish to have it expressed. It would be nice *(not to mention easier)* if everyone would agree. You will often find both styles in reference books. When eponyms are used to describe parts of the anatomy, disease, signs, or syndromes, they *may* show possession. However, for names of places, patients, or surgical instruments, the possessive is not used, nor is it used in a compound eponym. This practice is often confusing—how does one recognize the name of a place or patient in contrast to that of a researcher or physician? In addition, if the eponym is preceded by the article *an, a,* or *the,* one can eliminate the possessive as well. In the meantime, follow the guidelines and consult your reference books. If you hear the possessive dictated, use it *(and use it correctly).* If it is not dictated, do not use it. Eventually the use of these particular possessive eponyms will most likely be eliminated.

 DO use an apostrophe when the possessive is dictated in the following:

Signs and tests
Bell's phenomenon   *or* Bell phenomenon
Hoffmann's reflex   *or* Hoffman reflex
Babinski's phenomenon   *or* Babinski phenomenon
Ayer's test   *or* Ayer test
Anatomy
Bartholin's glands   *or* Bartholin glands
Beale's ganglion   *or* Beale ganglion
Mauthner's membrane   *or* Mauthner membrane

EXCEPTIONS *(always use possessive):*
Ringer's lactate
Taber's Cyclopedic Medical Dictionary

Diseases and syndromes
Fallot's tetralogy   *or* Fallot tetralogy
Tietze's syndrome   *or* Tietze syndrome
Hirschsprung's disease   *or* Hirschsprung disease

 DO use the possessive when the eponym closes the sentence.

The infant shows early signs of Reye's. *(syndrome is understood)*

 DON'T use the apostrophe if the word following begins with the sound of *s, z,* or *c.*

Hicks sign   Golgi zones   Langerhans cells

 DON'T show possession for eponyms that describe surgical instruments, are compounds, or represent the names of places or patients.

Surgical instruments
Mayo scissors   Richard retractors
Foley catheter   Liston-Stille forceps

Names of places or patients

Christmas factor   Lyme disease
Chicago disease

Compounds

Stein-Leventhal syndrome   Adams-Stokes disease
Leser-Trélat sign   Bass-Watkins test
Gruber-Widal reaction
But the following is not a compound: Blackberg and
Wanger's test *or* Blackberg and Wanger test

NOTE: *Be careful to check the correct spelling of the name. Is it* Water's *view or* Waters' *view? (The second choice is correct.)*

 **DON'T** use the apostrophe with an eponym if it is preceded by an article.

a Pfannenstiel incision   the Babinski sign
the Horner syndrome

DO when writing for publication, substitute the specific descriptive term for a disease for the equivalent eponymic term. Further, if the author prefers the eponym, *avoid* using the possessive form. Different rules apply when writing for publication.

Preferred:
alopecia parvimaculata syndrome
Second choice:
Dreuw syndrome
Avoid:
Dreuw's syndrome
Preferred:
pancreatic exocrine insufficiency syndrome
Second choice:
Clarke-Hadfield syndrome

3–5 GERUNDS

DO use an apostrophe to show possession when a noun modifies a gerund. (A gerund is a verb form that ends in *ing* and is used as a noun.)

Dr. Verbaron did not approve the cassette's leaving his office.
The safety committee members realized the meeting's being delayed was unavoidable.

3–6 JOINT POSSESSION

✓ DO show possession with the last noun when two or more nouns share possession.

Clark and Clark's new reference book is in.
Dr. Franklin and Dr. Meadow's patient was just admitted.
Dr. Pate and Dr. Frank's office *(one office)*
Dr. Pate's and Dr. Frank's offices *(two offices)*
Dr. Thomas's associate's diagnosis

🚫 DON'T use this rule when possession is not shared.

Dr. Franklin's and Dr. Meadow's patients were just admitted.

3–7 MISCELLANEOUS APOSTROPHE USE

✓ DO use an apostrophe when necessary to help clarify meaning.

The long convalescence was a result of Ron's falling.
She was in no mood for "what for's."
She OK'd my vacation.
He is a patient of Bob's.

✓ DO use the apostrophe as the symbol for the word *prime* in completing the description of an ECG's smaller R wave component rSR' *(pronounced RSR prime). (The lowercase* r *refers to the smaller R wave component.)*

3–8 PLURAL POSSESSIVE NOUNS

✓ DO add an apostrophe plus *s* to plural nouns that do not end in *s*.

women's studies
children's ward
mice's tracks

Singular	Plural
woman's watch	women's watches
child's toy	children's toys
man's shoe	men's shoes

✓ DO use an apostrophe after the *s* in plural nouns that end in *s*.

the typists' responsibility *(more than one typist)*
the Joneses' records *(more than one Jones)*
the heroes' methods
the berries' ripeness
the employees' records

DON'T   use an apostrophe to show possession of institutions or organizations *unless they elect to do so.*

Veterans Administration Hospital *(and certainly not Veteran's Hospital!)*
Childrens Hospital
St. Josephs Infirmary
Boys Club

3–9   PRONOUNS

✔ **DO**   form the possessive of relative pronouns such as *everyone, nobody, someone, anyone,* and *anybody* just as you would with possessive nouns.

It is nobody's fault.
That is anyone's guess.
It is somebody else's responsibility.

 DON'T   use an apostrophe with personal pronouns such as *its, hers, yours, his, theirs, ours, whose,* or *yours.*

Incorrect:
The next appointment is her's.
Correct:
The next appointment is hers.
Incorrect:
The dog injured it's foot.
Correct:
The dog injured its foot.
Incorrect:
You're lab coat is soiled.
Correct:
Your lab coat is soiled.

NOTE: *Notice the following contractions, however:*

It's time for your next appointment.
Who's going to clean the operatory?

COMMENT: *Probably one of the most common errors made concerns the misuse of the apostrophe with it. Both its and it's are correct when used in the proper context.*

3–10 SINGULAR POSSESSIVE NOUNS

☑ DO   use an apostrophe plus *s* with a singular noun not ending in
         s to show possession.

> the typist's responsibility *(one typist)*
> Bob's doctor
> Dr. Mitch's office

☑ DO   use an apostrophe only (no *s*) to show possession of singular
         nouns that end in *s* or in a strong *s* sound.

> the waitress' table
> for appearance' sake
> Mr. Gomez' surgery

☑ DO   use an apostrophe only after the *s* in two-syllable singular
         proper nouns ending in *s*.

> Dr. Harris' diagnosis
> Frances' report
> Mr. Walters' point of view

🚫 DON'T break up a proper noun that ends in an *s* by placing the
         apostrophe in front of the *s*.

> **Concerning Mr. Walters**
> **Incorrect:**
> Mr. Walter's point of view
> **Correct:**
> Mr. Walters' point of view

☑ DO   add an apostrophe plus *s* to singular nouns ending in *s* or an
         s sound when they are of a single syllable.

> Mr. Jones's medical record
> James Rose's appointment

3–11 TIME, DISTANCE, VALUE, AND SOURCE

☑ DO   use an apostrophe to show possession of time, distance,
         value, and source.

> return in one month's time
> at 10 weeks' gestation
> get your money's worth
> too much exposure to the sun's rays
> two days' convalescence

NOTE: *Notice the following expressions:*

a 10-week gestation
a 2-day convalescence
a one-year history *or* a 1-year history

🚫 **DON'T**   **show possession of inanimate things:**

the roof of the car *rather than* the car's roof
the color of the bruise *rather than* the bruise's color
the cover of the book *rather than* the book's cover

3–12   UNDERSTOOD NOUNS

✅ **DO**   **follow the same rules for showing possession when the noun is understood.**

That stethoscope is Dr. Green's. *(stethoscope)*
He bought that at William's. *(store)*
I consulted Dorland's. *(dictionary)*
That is where he earned his master's. *(degree)*
I believe this copy is yours. *(your copy)*
The infant shows early signs of Reye's. *(syndrome)*

Brief Forms, Short Forms, and Medical Slang

INTRODUCTION

Sometimes an author will say an unusual medical or English word or phrase that may puzzle you. It may be a brief form, which is also referred to as a short form, or a slang expression. You may try to find it in medical or English reference books with no success. Then you will resort to keyboarding the phrase the way you heard it and flag it for the physician to double-check. *(See also Chapter 11, Editing, in regard to inflammatory expressions.)*

 DO   contact the author and diplomatically and tactfully question his or her use of the slang expression before the expression becomes a permanent part of the patient's medical record.

 DO   translate brief forms in full when dictated.

Appy should be typed as appendectomy.
Cathed should be typed as catheterized.
Dex should be typed as dexamethasone.
Lab may be typed as laboratory.
Lytes should be typed as electrolytes.

EXCEPTIONS: *See forms shown without asterisks in Appendix C, Brief Forms, Short Forms, and Medical Slang. Those forms may be used as such unless they might be misread or misinterpreted in the medical report or chart note.*

4–1 ABBREVIATED FORMS

 DO keyboard commonly used and widely recognized brief forms, when dictated, except in headings, diagnoses, or operative titles. If the term does not violate any of the guidelines listed under 1–20, Spelled-Out Abbreviations, and 21–1, Abbreviations, it may be typed as a brief form.

alk. phos.   *(alkaline phosphatase)*
basos   *(basophils)*
chem profile   *(chemistry profile)*
eos   *(eosinophils)*
exam   *(examination)*
lymphs   *(lymphocytes)*
monos   *(monocytes)*
Pap smear/test   *(Papanicolaou smear or test)*
phenobarb   *(phenobarbital)*
sed rate   *(sedimentation rate)*

4–2 CAPITALIZATION

 DO lowercase a brief form unless the unabbreviated form is capitalized.

flu *(influenza)*
Pap smear *(Papanicolaou smear)*

4–3 EDITING

 DO edit brief forms of words and phrases.

Incorrect:
The patient had a right thoracotomy for removal of cocci nodules.
Correct:
The patient had a right thoracotomy for removal of coccidiomas.
Incorrect:
She failed to hand me the Mets (*or* Metz) scissors.
Correct:
She failed to hand me the Metzenbaum scissors.
Incorrect:
Mrs. Becker's temp was 102°.
Correct:
Mrs. Becker's temperature was 102°.
Incorrect:
At the end of surgery, I introduced an intracath.

Correct:
At the end of surgery, I introduced an intravenous catheter.
Incorrect:
The sputum culture grew out H. flu.
Correct:
The sputum culture grew out Hemophilus influenzae.

4–4 FLAGGING, CARDING, TAGGING, OR MARKING

✓ DO leave a blank and query a slang expression if you cannot translate the brief form in full. Attach a note to the transcript with a short description of where the blank is located. *(See Figure 11–1 at the end of Chapter 11 for an example of a flagging note.)*

4–5 LABORATORY TERMS

✓ DO add an *s* to a brief form for a plural laboratory term.

bands	lymphs	segs
basos	monos	stabs
eos	polys	

4–6 PLURAL FORMS

✓ DO add an *s* to the brief form when the form is used as a plural noun.

exams	Pap smears	quads

5

Capitalization

INTRODUCTION

The purpose of capitalizing a word is to give it emphasis, distinction, authority, or importance. Avoid unnecessary capitalization, and do not use capital letters to highlight something unnecessarily (e.g., a person's name on a document). Words completely composed of capital letters often are more difficult to read because there is not as much "white space" around them.

Correct:
Frank Flexner, CMT
Incorrect:
FRANK FLEXNER, CMT

Like rules regarding punctuation, rules regarding capitalization can differ. The current trend is toward less, rather than more, capitalization. Consequently, as with a punctuation mark, be sure you have a reason for using a capital letter, and when in doubt, check your references.

5–1 ABBREVIATIONS

✅ **DO**   capitalize abbreviations when the words they represent are capitalized. Capitalize most abbreviations of English words. *(See Chapter 1 for specific capitalization of abbreviations.)*

Ronda A. Drake, MD, graduated from UCSD.
Dr. Bowman is working with Project HOPE and UNICEF.
Our patient JB has converted from being HIV positive and now has AIDS.
Dr. Ashamed is scheduled to assist with the T&A.
The DTRs are intact.

✅ **DO**   capitalize the first letter in the abbreviation of chemical elements.

Hg   Na   K

🚫 **DON'T**   capitalize the spelled-out names of the chemical elements and chemical compounds.

oxygen   sodium chloride
hydrochloric acid   carbon dioxide

✅ **DO**   capitalize each letter in an acronym.

Dr. Bowman is working with Project HOPE and UNICEF.

🚫 **DON'T**   capitalize most brief forms.

amt   cysto   eos   hypo

EXCEPTION: Pap *(smear or test)*

🚫 **DON'T**   generally capitalize metric and English forms of measurement or Latin abbreviations. *(See also 1–11 and 1–12.)*

e.g.   t.i.d.   ft   cm   oz   mph

EXCEPTIONS: C *(Celsius)*   F *(Fahrenheit)*   L *(liter)*

NOTE: *The abbreviations* a.m. *and* p.m. *may also be capitalized.*

AM   PM

✓ DO   capitalize the abbreviation of academic degrees and religious orders.

MD   PhD   DDS   MS   SJ
BVE   DPM   LLB   AS   AA

✓ DO   capitalize cardiologic symbols and abbreviations that are used to express electrocardiographic results.

The P waves are slightly prominent in V_1 to V_3.
or V_1-V_3 *or* V1-V3
It is not clear whether it contains a U wave.
The QRS complexes are normal, as are the ST segments.
There are T-wave inversions in LI, aVL, and V1-V4.

5–2   *ACADEMIC COURSE NAMES*

✓ DO   capitalize the names of specific academic courses when used with a numeral.

DON'T   capitalize academic subject areas unless they contain a proper noun.

I am enrolled in Medical Transcription 103; I am also taking anatomy and business English.

5–3   *ALLERGIES AND OTHER WARNINGS*

✓ DO   capitalize each letter in the name of a drug, use bold print, or use underscoring when reporting drug allergies in a *chart note* or in a patient's *history*.

The patient has a history of an ALLERGY TO PENICILLIN AND CODEINE PRODUCTS. *(chart note)*

The patient has a history of an allergy to penicillin and codeine products. *(written in a letter)*

ALLERGIES: <u>PENICILLIN AND CODEINE PRODUCTS</u>. *(an entry under "History" in the medical report)*

The patient denied having any food, environmental, or drug allergies.

NOTE: *Some facilities also use bright adhesive labels placed on patients' file folders to draw attention to allergies.*

 DO   use full capital letters to write such warnings as DO NOT RESUSCITATE and COMFORT CARE ONLY when they are dictated so that the warnings will stand out in the record.

5–4   BUSINESS AND ORGANIZATION NAMES

 DO   capitalize the official names of businesses, organizations, publications, conferences, government agencies, symposia, buildings, structures, postgraduate courses, and so forth.

National Broadcasting Company
American Association for Medical Transcription
Risk Management Symposium
Utilization Review Board
Library of Congress
American College of Chest Physicians
Pima County Medical Society
Sports Medicine and Rehabilitation Conference
Medical Political Action Committee
United States Navy

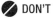 **DON'T**   capitalize the article *the* in referring to names of newspapers and magazines unless the word is part of the title.

The New York Times   the Wall Street Journal

5–5   CALENDAR AND DATES

 DO   capitalize the names of the days of the week, months of the year, holidays, historic events, and religious festivals.

Holy Week   Lent   Passover   Yom Kippur   Yuletide

There will be no class on Friday, November 11, because it is Veterans' Day.

We plan to celebrate Medical Transcriptionist Week.

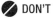 **DON'T**   capitalize the four seasons of the year.

I am taking an advanced terminology class in the spring semester; I wish I had taken it this fall.

5–6   COLONS WITH CAPITAL LETTERS

 DO capitalize the first word following a colon if it begins a complete sentence, requires special emphasis, or is part of an outline entry.

Now for some brighter views: The new equipment will be installed over the three-day weekend.

Impression: Chronic hypertrophic tonsils and adenoids.

Mouth: The teeth are in poor repair.

The patient was treated for the following problems: insomnia, malaise, depression, substance abuse.

I see only one alternative: Chemotherapy. *(Notice the use of the capital letter in this example.)*

5–7   DEPARTMENTS AND SECTIONS IN INSTITUTIONS

 DO capitalize the names of *specific* departments, sections, or campus outbuildings in the hospital or institution.

NOTE: *Some teaching hospitals and military hospitals prefer capitalization for individual departments within their facility. Many large hospitals have a variety of named outbuildings: The Eye Center, Imaging, The Women's Center, Rehabilitation, and so on. They refer to this entire entity as "the campus."*

Please see that the records are sent to St. Joseph's Hospital Admitting Department.
The admitting department was overwhelmed with 45 new admissions yesterday.

Albertson City Hospital Pathology Department received an award from the Greater Albertson County Industrial Council.
The specimen was sent to pathology.
All pathology departments should have this notice posted.

The Emergency Department at Westside General Hospital has just received a new hyperbaric unit.
Some emergency departments are sending patients to acute care centers after triage.

The baby was born in the hallway somewhere between the pharmacy and The Women's Center.

The patient was sent to the recovery room in good condition.

The patient was admitted to 4-North for observation; he is scheduled for an appointment at 1 p.m. in the Advanced-Imaging Center.

☑ DO **capitalize the names of departments when they are referred to as the people who represent them.**

I asked Pathology to send the report to me stat.

He said Oncology called again about the change in their extension.

Dr. Wood notified Admitting to expect an audit.

5–8 DISEASES AND SYNDROMES

☑ DO **capitalize the names of diseases that include proper nouns, eponyms, or genus names.**

⊘ DON'T **capitalize the common names of diseases.**

⊘ DON'T **capitalize the names of viruses unless they include a proper noun.**

The patient tested positive for Rocky Mountain spotted fever. *(proper noun)*

She was given the final series of diphtheria, pertussis, and tetanus. *(common diseases)*

She is now suffering from postpoliomyelitis syndrome and is unable to breathe without the use of her respirator. *(virus name)*

There has been an increase in Chlamydia infections in this age group. *(genus)*

We have had the usual problems with rubella, rubeola, and chickenpox in the kindergarten population. *(common diseases)*

We do not know if he should be designated as showing signs of early senility or Alzheimer disease. *(eponym)*

herpesvirus	varicella
Lassa arenavirus	German measles
Hansen disease	myasthenia gravis
San Joaquin Valley fever	
Mycobacterium tuberculosis (*also* M. tuberculosis)	
tuberculosis	Parkinson's
Spanish influenza	Hemophilus influenzae

5–9   DRUG NAMES AND COMMERCIAL PRODUCTS

 DO   capitalize the trade names and brand names of drugs and other trademarked materials. You may maintain any idiosyncratic capitalization used by the proprietor of the brand name or just capitalize it.

Ace bandage	Xerox	Dictaphone

DON'T   capitalize generic names.

Trade names of drugs

Fiorinal	Darvon	Cortisporin
Theokin	pHisoHex	Gelfoam
GoLYTELY	HydroDIURIL	
(*also* Golytely)	(*also* Hydrodiuril)	

Generic names of drugs and other substances

nitroglycerin	analgesic	hydrocortisone
potassium iodide	oxytocin	alcohol
ether	epinephrine	

DO   capitalize the trademarked forms for packaging and delivery systems of drugs.

Dropperettes	Dura-Tab	Secule
Dispenserpak	Unisert	Tamp-R-Tel

DON'T   capitalize the common noun following the brand name of a drug.

Tylenol tablets	Neosporin ointment

DO   be alert to the internal caps and spacing in commercial products.

PowerPoint	DuraSoft lenses	NeXT	
Post-it notes	iMac	StairMaster	Q-tips

5–10   GENUS AND SPECIES

NOTE: *See Appendix E, p. 557, for a general list of genus and species names.*

DO capitalize the name of the genus but not the name of the species that follows it. Capitalize the name of the genus when it is written alone.

The patient was admitted by the ophthalmologist because of infection with Onchocerca volvulus.

Ralph saw the doctor because he had a bad reaction to Cannabis.

NOTE: *The genus may be referred to by its first initial only; the initial is capitalized with a period and followed by the species name. (See 1–10.)*

E. coli *(Escherichia coli)*
M. tuberculosis *(Mycobacterium tuberculosis)*
H. influenzae *(Hemophilus influenzae)*

 DON'T capitalize the plural or adjectival form of a genus name.

Giardia lamblia *but* giardiasis
Diplococcus *but* diplococci *and* diplococcal
Streptococcus *but* streptococci *and* streptococcal

5–11 GEOGRAPHIC LOCATIONS

 DO capitalize both the noun and the adjective when they make reference to a specific geographic location.

The patient was born and raised in the Southwest; he has lived in the Deep South only a short while.

the Great Lakes   Apache Reservation
Cape of Good Hope   Crow Poison Crossing

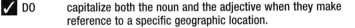 **DON'T** capitalize the names of places when they appear before the names of a specific place or are general directions.

We plan to stay at a resort by the Atlantic Ocean when we go east for the medical meeting this fall.

Travel west on Highway 10.

the state of New York *but* New York State

 DO capitalize *boulevard, street, avenue, drive, way,* and so on when used with a proper noun.

321 Westvillage Drive

One of the most attractive streets in Naples is Palm Avenue.

5–12 LETTER PARTS

 DO capitalize the first word of the salutation and the complimentary close.

Dear Dr. Reynolds:
Sincerely yours,
Yours very truly,

 DO capitalize the first letter or all the letters in the word *attention* when it is part of an address; capitalize the first letter of each word or all the letters in the title *To Whom It May Concern. (See 2–11.)*

ATTENTION Reservation Clerk
or
Attention Reservation Clerk

TO WHOM IT MAY CONCERN:
or
To Whom It May Concern:

 DO capitalize a person's title in business correspondence when it appears in the inside address, typed signature line, or envelope address.

Ms. Marilyn Alan, President
W. Raul Deal, MD, Director
ATTENTION Ralph Cavanaugh, Buyer

 DO capitalize both letters of the state abbreviation when it is part of the address and precedes the ZIP code. *(See Table 1–2.)*

District Heights, MD 20028
San Diego, CA 92119

5–13 *MEDICAL SPECIALTIES*

 DON'T capitalize the names of medical or surgical specialties or the type of specialist.

The internist referred him to a thoracic and cardiovascular surgeon.

She is studying to be an emergency room specialist.

We asked for a second opinion from the cardiologist.

Her initial desire had been to practice anesthesiology, so we were surprised when she elected to be a trauma surgeon.

Specialty	Practitioner
allergy and immunology	allergist
anesthesia	anesthesiologist
dentistry	dentist
gastroenterology	gastroenterologist
gerontology	gerontologist
gynecology	gynecologist
internal medicine	internist
kidney diseases	nephrologist
neonatology	neonatologist
neurology	neurologist
neurosurgery	neurosurgeon
obstetrics	obstetrician
ophthalmology	ophthalmologist
orthopedics	orthopedic surgeon
otolaryngology	otolaryngologist *(head and neck surgeon)*
pathology	pathologist
pediatrics	pediatrician
physical medicine	physiatrist
plastic surgery	plastic surgeon
podiatry	podiatrist
proctology	proctologist
psychiatry	psychiatrist
psychology	psychologist
radiology	radiologist
urology	urologist

5–14 NAMES, NOUNS, AND EPONYMS

✓ **DO**   capitalize proper nouns, well-known nicknames for proper nouns, and eponyms.

Proper nouns
Dr. Watson was a fictional hero in Sherlock Holmes's classics.

Do you realize that Mother will have to be placed in a nursing facility if she is unable to care for herself?

COMPARE WITH: *Our mother will have to be placed in a nursing home.*

Proper nouns and well-known nicknames for proper nouns

Josephine Holman just moved here from the Rockies and is looking for a job as a medical assistant.

We learned that valley fever is endemic to Imperial Valley, San Joaquin Valley, and the Sonoran deserts.

She moved to the Bay Area after winning the Nobel Prize.

Ellen wanted to return to the Deep South after working in California for just a few years.

Eponyms

We need a #15 Foley catheter.

The diagnosis proved to be Hodgkin's.

It is interesting that Christmas disease was named for a family with a particular type of hereditary condition.

The procedure was performed through a McBurney incision.

Some interesting names from mythology are used to describe parts of the anatomy, such as Achilles tendon, or conditions, such as Oedipus complex.

Newcomers to medicine often misspell Burow solution and think that the Sippy diet is one you sip!

NOTE: *See Chapter 14, Eponyms, for complete use of eponyms.*

NOTE: *Words derived from eponyms are not capitalized, nor are those that have acquired independent common meaning. When in doubt, check the dictionary.*

Nouns derived from eponyms

Parkinson disease *but* parkinsonism
Cushing syndrome *but* cushingoid facies
Gram stain *but* gram-positive results
Addison disease *but* addisonian crisis

Common nouns and adjectives formed from proper nouns

arabic number	klieg light
atlas	kocherize
braille symbol	koebnerization
brussels sprouts	manila folder
cesarean section	mendelian genetics

chinese blue	mullerian duct
curie unit	paris green
epsom salt	pasteurized milk
eustachian tube	petri dish
french fries	plaster of paris
freudian slip	politzerize
graafian follicle	portland cement
haversian system	roentgen unit
hippocratic clubbing	roman numeral
india ink	siamese twins
joule	watt

EXCEPTION: *Americanization*

🚫 **DON'T**   capitalize the prefixes and particles *de, de la, du, van, von, von der,* and so on when used with names unless so used by the individual.

Ronald J. von der Mehden
von Willebrand disease
Michel de la Vera, MD
Van Bogaert disease
de Quervain thyroiditis
duBois formula

✔️ **DO**   verify the sequence with unusual names.

Morgan Joyce *or* Joyce Morgan

Robertson Jayne *(the family name is Jayne)*

✔️ **DO**   verify the spelling of patients' names. When there is any doubt, contact whomever has a social document sheet (name, address, telephone number, place of employment, and so on) from the patient. This document could be with the referring physician, primary care physician, clinic, nursing home, insurance company, workers' compensation carrier, emergency department, medical records department, the unit where the patient is confined, and so on.

Mary Jane *or* Marijane *or* Mari Jane *or* Mary-Jane *or* Merry Jane *(and on and on)*

🚫 **DON'T**   capitalize the prefix in hyphenated proper nouns, but do capitalize the proper noun that follows it.

non-Hodgkin	mid-May
anti-Semitic	pseudo-Christian
anti-American	

EXCEPTION: *Pre-Raphaelite*

 DO   capitalize all references to a Supreme Being.

God	Messiah	Holy Spirit
Allah	Lord of All	Son of God
Mother Nature		The Almighty

5–15 NUMBERS WITH NOUNS

 DON'T   capitalize nouns used with numbers.

case	group	patient
chapter	lead	phase
chromosome	level	section
column	line	sentence
control	method	series
experiment	note	size
factor	page	stage
fraction	para	type
grade	paragraph	volume
gravida	part	wave
grant		

There is an error in your copy on page 27, paragraph 2, line 3.

 DO   capitalize *specific* designations used with numbers.

Axis III: No somatic disorder.
We found a deficiency in Complex I.
Kennedy Class II
Model 14 Medtronic pacemaker
Flight 717 from San Diego International

5–16 OUTLINES AND LISTS

 DO   capitalize the first word of each line in an outline or subheading of a report and the entire main heading of a formal report.

NOTE: *Often the fully capitalized main heading is also underlined; the topic is fully capitalized and not underlined; and the subtopic begins with a single capital letter.*

Diagnoses
1. Stress incontinence of urine.
2. Monilial vaginitis.

HEENT
HEAD: Normal.
EYES: Pupils round and equal, react to L&A.
EARS: Hearing normal, TMs intact, canals patent.

PHYSICAL EXAMINATION
HEENT
Head: Normal.
Eyes: Pupils round and equal, react to L&A.
Ears: Hearing normal, TMs intact, canals patent.
Nose: Canals patent.
Throat: Trachea in the midline.

OPERATIVE REPORT
PREOPERATIVE DIAGNOSIS: Glaucoma, chronic, simple, bilateral.
POSTOPERATIVE DIAGNOSIS: Glaucoma, chronic, simple, bilateral.
OPERATION PERFORMED: Iridencleisis, right eye.

 DO   capitalize each part of the outline and the first word following the colon in narrative copy.

Physical examination revealed the following: Thyroid: Normal to palpation with no cervical adenopathy. Breasts: No masses, tenderness, or axillary adenopathy. Abdomen: Flat, nontender. Liver, kidneys, and spleen not felt. There is a well-healed McBurney scar present. No masses, tenderness, or . . .

5–17 QUOTATIONS

 DO   capitalize a complete quotation when it is a complete sentence.

He said, and I quote, "This must be reported to risk management at once."

The instructor said, "Strive for mailable copy even when you are practice-typing."

DON'T   capitalize a complete quote when it expresses only part of a sentence.

The patient said that he feels like "something's hung up in there."
She told him to "strive for perfection."

NOTE: *See Chapter 36 for more information on quotation marks.*

5–18 RACES AND PEOPLES

 DO   capitalize the names of races, peoples, religions, and languages.

He is a well-developed, well-nourished Asian businessman in no acute distress.

The patient is a 59-year-old Caucasian female oriented to time, place, and person.

She is a Catholic, but they decided to be married in the Jewish temple.

We are taking an evening course in medical Spanish because we have many Hispanic patients who do not speak English.

DON'T   capitalize designations based on skin color.

She is a well-developed, well-nourished black female student.

This 43-year-old white farm worker fell from the back of a truck at 3:55 a.m.

5–19 SUTURE MATERIALS

DO   capitalize the brand name of suture materials.

Dexon	Dermalene	Dermalon
Surgicel	Vicryl	Prolene
Nurolon	Purlon	Surgilon
Tevdek	Tycron	Dacron

DON'T   capitalize the generic names of suture materials.

catgut	silk	nylon	chromic
cotton	elastic	linen	

DO   capitalize proper nouns associated with sutures and suture material.

Wysler	Taylor	Richardson
Emmet	Bell	Chinese silk
Barraquer silk	Bonney-type	Gaillard-Arlt

5–20 TITLES, FAMILY

 DO   capitalize a title that designates a member of a family *unless* it is preceded by a possessive noun or pronoun.

My father is bringing Aunt Mary here this afternoon for her flu shot.

The patient's mother died of carcinoma of the breast at age 56, and his father is living and well.

I saw Dad only last week.
I saw my dad last week.

 DON'T   capitalize a title when it is followed by an appositive.

My uncle, William Peters, moved here recently from Cleveland.

5–21 TITLES, LITERARY

 DO   capitalize all words in the titles of articles, books, and periodicals, with the exception of conjunctions, prepositions, and articles.

 DON'T   capitalize locants or other chemical prefixes and uncapitalized taxonomic names in a title.

The title of the film is "Unusual Reactions to the Use of Cannabis sativa."

The working title of the paper is "Isomer 11-cis-Retinal Rod Combination Factors."

NOTE: *Book titles are also underlined, journal titles are written in italics, and article titles are enclosed in quotation marks.*

The fall issue of *Perspectives on the Medical Transcription Profession* has an excellent article about job satisfaction written by Sidney Moormeister, PhD.

I just purchased the latest edition of the Pharmaceutical Word Book by Drake and Drake.

5–22 TITLES, ORGANIZATIONAL

 DO   capitalize the titles of organizations and the titles of officers in an organization's minutes, bylaws, or rules.

The Secretary read the minutes, and they were approved as read.

Dr. Sanderson has recently retired from the Navy.

The President proposed that the Board of Directors be polled.

American Cancer Society
Utilization Committee
Mortality and Morbidity Conference
the Internet
World Wide Web

 DON'T   confuse a general term for a formal name.

US Postal Service *but* the post office
Beta tests *but* beta cells
Eastridge Clinic *but* the clinic

5–23   TITLES, PERSONAL AND PROFESSIONAL

✅ **DO**   capitalize a person's title in business correspondence when it appears in the inside address, typed signature line, or envelope address.

Jean Lusk, M.D., Chief-of-Staff
Rhonda Williams, Dean
Charles Bruno, CMT, Secretary

Parkland Community College
3261 Parkview Drive
Boise, ID 83702

ATTENTION Ms. P. Lombardo, Administrator

✅ **DO**   capitalize professional titles, political titles, and military ranks when they immediately *precede* the name.

Military and professional titles
Capt. Max Draper, USN Medical Corps, will be the guest speaker at the annual meeting of the AMA.

Dr. Smith, the president, plans to meet his plane. The doctor will leave for the airport at four o'clock. We will meet with President Austin at the university this evening. Dean Caldwell may not be able to join us, however.

Professional and political titles

Dr. Randolph, the president of the medical society, was invited to speak at the joint meeting with the local bar association. Rev. John Hughes will give the invocation. The attorney will be here at 9:30 a.m. to meet with the doctor about his testimony.

She is taking the examination to become a certified medical transcriptionist.

NOTE: *Only titles of* high distinction *are capitalized following a person's name, except in the address and typed signature line. High distinction can be very subjective, depending upon who is doing the writing. High distinction often refers to persons of rank in one's own firm and to high government officials.*

Abraham Lincoln, President of the United States

6

The Colon

INTRODUCTION

Think of the colon as a pointer, drawing your attention to an important and concluding part. It is a strong mark of anticipation. The colon emphasizes the relationship between the elements it separates. Often the material to the right of the colon means the same as the material to the left of the colon. In the past, a double space was inserted after the colon in narrative copy. Today a single space is acceptable as well.

6–1 EXAMPLES AND CLARIFICATION

 DO use a colon followed by one or two spaces to introduce an example or to clarify an idea.

NOTE: *These ideas or examples are often introduced by the expressions* thus *or that* is, *or the expression could be supplied mentally.*

I see only one alternative: chemotherapy.
You have only one goal here: accuracy.

DO   use a colon to separate two independent clauses when the second illustrates, amplifies, or clarifies the first.

The patient is a terrible driver: He speeds, cuts in and out of traffic, and refuses to use the turn indicator.

In the ED we have an important saying: If you didn't write it in the chart, you didn't do it.

 DO   capitalize the first word after the colon if the word is a proper noun or begins a complete sentence.

Notice please: There will be no further parking allowed in the staff lot without a valid parking sticker.

Please place the following warning on the door to Room 16: "Caution: Radioactive materials in use."

There is one major problem with surgery in this young man: his fear of being anesthetized.

6–2   FOOTNOTES, REFERENCES, AND BIBLIOGRAPHIES

 DO   use a colon and one or two spaces between the title and subtitle and between the place of publication and the name of the publisher. Use a colon and no extra space between the volume number and the page number. Use a period and a double space between the name of the author and the title and between the title and publication data.

Dorland's Illustrated Medical Dictionary, 30th ed. Philadelphia: WB Saunders Company; 2003.

Pyle, V. Current Medical Terminology, 9th ed. Modesto: Health Professions Institute; 2003.

Strickland, Debbie. Two New Transcription Tools: The 5-Word Proofread and Shadowing for QA. JAAMT. Modesto, California: American Assn. for Medical Transcription: January-February 2003.

6–3   LISTS

 DO   use a colon followed by one or two spaces to introduce a list preceded by a complete sentence. These lists are often introduced by the following expressed or implied words: *as follows, such as, namely, the following.*

Please bring the following items with you to the hospital: robe, slippers, toilet articles, and two pairs of pajamas.

The patient was treated for the following problems: insomnia, malaise, depression.

⊘ **DON'T**   use a colon when the items of the list come immediately after a verb or preposition or after the words *because* or *that.*

Incorrect:
The patient had: a history of chronic obstructive lung disease and congestive heart failure. *(Notice that this list is not introduced by a complete sentence; furthermore, the colon follows a verb.)*
Correct:
The patient had a history of chronic obstructive lung disease and congestive heart failure.

⊘ **DON'T**   use a colon when the sentence is continuous without it.

6–4   *OUTLINES*

☑ **DO**   use a colon followed by one or two spaces after the introductory word or words in an outline, after the introductory word or words in a written history and physical, and in listing the patient's vital signs.

CHIEF COMPLAINT: Hyperemesis.
HISTORY: Usual childhood diseases; no sequelae.
ALLERGY: Patient denies any drug or food sensitivity.

VITAL SIGNS
Temperature: 101°.
Pulse: 58.
BP: 130/90.
Respirations: 18.

DIAGNOSES
1. Gastritis.
2. Pancreatitis.
3. Rule out cholecystitis.

☑ **DO**   capitalize the first word after the colon when using outline format. Use open punctuation (no colon) when using the dropped outline format.

DIAGNOSES
1. Gastritis.
2. Pancreatitis.
3. Rule out cholecystitis.

CHIEF COMPLAINT
The patient is an engaging 42-year-old male who works as an air conditioning support technician at the convention center, who noted the insidious onset of painful swelling involving the prepatellar region of the left knee.

6–5 RATIOS

✓ DO   use a colon with no space on either side to express dilute solutions and ratios. The colon takes the place of the word *to*.

The solution was diluted 1:100.
We had a 2:1 mix.

6–6 SALUTATION

✓ DO   place a colon after the salutation in a business letter when "mixed" punctuation is used.

OPTIONAL: *When the salutation is informal and persons are addressed by their first names, you may use a comma.*

Dear Sir or Madam:
To Whom It May Concern:
Gentlemen:
Dear Dr. Berry:
Dear Bill: *or* Dear Bill,

6–7 SUBJECT AND REFERENCE NOTATION

✓ DO   use a colon followed by one or two spaces to separate the components of a document such as subject line, reference notations, enclosures, and so on.

Reference: #306-A
RE: Mary Ellen Wood
Re: Mary Ellen Wood
Subject: Soft-diet menus
Attention: Adrianna Brown
Enclosure: Pathology report
PS: Please note our new area code
Subject: Stress test

6–8 TIME OF DAY
See also 27–27, Time, in Chapter 27.

✓ DO   place a colon with no space on either side between the hours and minutes indicating the time of day in figures.

Her appointment is for 10:30 a.m.

🚫 DON'T   use a colon and double zeros with the even time of day.

10 a.m. *not* 10:00 a.m.
12 noon
3 p.m. *not* 3:00 p.m.

🚫 DON'T   use a colon in expressions of military time.

She had an appointment at 1200 hours.
Patient was admitted at 1430.

6–9 TITLES AND SUBTITLES

✓ DO   use a colon followed by a double space to separate titles from subtitles.

Medical Transcription: Techniques and Procedures

Chapter 8: Using Reference Books: Learn How to Get Help From the Experts

7

The Comma

INTRODUCTION

The comma is the most frequently used mark of punctuation and often causes the most problems for writers. At the same time, it is a very important aid in clarifying the meaning for a reader.

 DO   use commas appropriately and sparingly.

 DO   be able to justify your use of a comma or don't use it.

⊘ DON'T create a comma fault by using only one of a pair of commas or by using a comma to do the work of a semicolon or colon.

✓ DO remember that commas are placed *inside* quotation marks and *outside* parentheses.

7-1 ABBREVIATIONS

✓ DO use a comma or pair of commas to set off degrees and titles after a person's name. If there are multiple degrees or professional credentials after the person's name, place them in the order in which they were awarded or in order of increasing distinction and separate them with commas.

Neal J. Kaufman, MD, FACP

John A. Meadows, MD, saw the patient in consultation.

Mail this to John Vogt, Esq.

Frances Knight, LLB, MD, will be the first speaker about risk management.

NOTE: *The current trend is to eliminate commas, particularly when meaning is not sacrificed. Some writers are not using commas to separate degrees and titles after a person's name. As always, follow the wishes of the bearer of the name.*

⊘ DON'T place a comma before roman numerals indicating first, second, third, and so forth or *Jr.* or *Sr.* after a name unless the bearer of the name prefers that usage.

Howard J. Matlock III
Carl A. Nichols Jr. was admitted to Ward B.
A Billroth I anastomosis was performed.

⊘ DON'T use a comma or pair of commas to set off *Inc.* and *Ltd.* after the name of a company *unless the firm follows that practice.*

He was covered by Bowen Myers Insurance Ltd.

I was employed by Peach Valley Medical Group Inc. for three years.

Headquarters for The Reader's Digest Association, Inc., is Pleasantville, New York.

✓ **DO**   separate the parts of a name with a comma or commas when the name is given in inverted order.

> Jacobs, Barney K.
> Kaufman, Neal J., MD, FACP

✓ **DO**   use a comma or a pair of commas to set off Latin abbreviations *(e.g., i.e., viz.)* and the spelled-out English versions *(for example, that is, namely)* when the abbreviation or the spelled-out version is used at the end of a series or as a parenthetical expression. *(See also Rule 1-11 concerning Latin abbreviations.)*

> He was allergic to most pet dander, e.g., that of dogs, cats, and rabbits.

7–2   ADDRESSES
See also 7-18, Place Names.

✓ **DO**   use a comma to separate two different parts of a street address.

> 1335 11th Street, Apartment 3B

✓ **DO**   use commas to separate all the elements of a complete address when it is written in narrative form.

> Please mail this to my home address: 132 Winston Street, Park Village, IL 60612.

7–3   APPOSITIVES
An appositive is a noun or pronoun that renames the noun or pronoun that precedes it.

✓ **DO**   separate nonessential appositives from the rest of the sentence with a pair of commas.

> John Munor, your patient, was admitted to Centre City Hospital today.
>
> Laralyn Abbott, the head nurse, summoned me to the phone.

⊘ **DON'T**   separate an essential appositive in error. It is essential if you need to know *which one.*

> **Incorrect:**
> Your patient, Ralph Swansdown, died at 3:45 a.m. *(You need to know which patient.)*

77

NOTE: *Notice that if Ralph Swansdown is separated from the rest of the sentence with a pair of commas, it appears that the person being addressed by this remark had only one patient, the lately deceased Mr. Swansdown. It is essential to know which patient.*

Correct:
Your patient Ralph Swansdown died at 3:45 a.m.

NOTE: *One-word appositives do not require commas.*

I myself will stay late and finish the report.

My cousin Pat just arrived in Spring Valley.

7–4   CLARITY

✔ DO   use a comma or a pair of commas to avoid misleading or confusing the reader and to set off contrasts.

He demanded, rather hastily, that she be released from further care.

In 200X, 461 babies were delivered in our new obstetrics wing.

It is one thing to be assertive, another to be rigid.

We are here to work, not visit.

Soon after, he got up and discharged himself from the hospital.

The day before, I had seen her in the emergency department.

Diagnosis: Fracture, third and fourth ribs on right.

Operation performed: Hemorrhoidectomy, radical.

Impression: Diverticulosis, moderate.

As demonstrated earlier, chemotherapy had little effect on the rate of tumor growth.

Dr. Powell, not Dr. Franklyn, delivered the infant.

After three, surgeries are not scheduled.

Subcutaneous tissue was closed by using interrupted #4-0 Dexon, skin with the same material.

She was caught in that trap called last hired, first fired.

✓ **DO** **use a comma to separate repeated adjectives and adverbs.**

He was very, very anxious to avoid any potentially claustrophobic encounters.

NOTE: *Not used for past perfect verb form.*

He had had an automobile accident the previous week.

✓ **DO** **break up sets of words logically.**

Incorrect:
The father is living with cancer of the thyroid.
Correct:
The father is living, with cancer of the thyroid.
Incorrect:
There was no change in the cervix with that structure continuing to be long closed and posterior.
Correct:
There was no change in the cervix with that structure continuing to be long, closed, and posterior.

NOTE: *A comma is required after* long, *because the cervix is not* long closed *but* long *and* closed.

Incorrect:
The infant displayed normal reflexes of suck root and startle.
Correct:
The infant displayed normal reflexes of suck, root, and startle.
Incorrect:
Serum, electrolytes, alkaline, phosphatase, BUN, creatinine, glucose, and calcium will be checked.
Correct:
Serum electrolytes, alkaline phosphatase, BUN, creatinine, glucose, and calcium will be checked.
Incorrect:
Mouth, teeth in poor repair.
Correct:
Mouth: Teeth in poor repair.
Incorrect:
This 51-year-old alcoholic male was found in a confused and disoriented state, lying on the floor by his girlfriend.

Correct:
This 51-year-old alcoholic male was found in a confused and disoriented state, lying on the floor, by his girlfriend.

NOTE: *In the first statement it appears as if the man was lying on the floor next to his girlfriend. The second comma makes it clear that his girlfriend found him lying on the floor.*

Incorrect:
Air was aspirated from the left ventricle, and the aorta and the cross-clamp removed.
Correct:
Air was aspirated from the left ventricle and the aorta, and the cross-clamp removed.

NOTE: *In the first sentence it incorrectly states that the aorta was removed.*

7–5 COMPLIMENTARY CLOSE

✅ **DO**   use a comma after the complimentary close when "mixed" punctuation is used in a letter.

Sincerely yours,

7–6 COMPOUND SENTENCE
See 7-13, Independent Clause.

7–7 CONJUNCTIONS
See 7-13, Independent Clause.

7–8 COORDINATE WORDS

✅ **DO**   use a comma when two consecutive adjectives independently modify the same noun. Separate them with a comma if a mental *and* can be placed between them or if the order in which they are used can be reversed.

She is a spastic, retarded child.
It was a wide, deep wound.
He was left with windblown, contracted lips.

🚫 **DON'T**   use a comma when the first adjective modifies the next adjective-noun combination.

Incorrect:
He is an efficient, medical transcriptionist.

Incorrect:
He had crystal, clear urine.

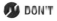 **DON'T** place a comma after the last modifier in front of the noun. In the following sentence, we would not place a comma in front of *memo.*

We received a poorly punctuated, rude memo from your department.

NOTE: *See 7-19, Series of Words, Tests, Studies, Vitals, Values, and So Forth.*

7–9   DATES

✓ **DO** use a comma to set off a year date that is used to explain a preceding date of the month.

He was born on March 3, 1933, in Reno, Nevada.
Make her an appointment for Wednesday, July 6, 200X.

🚫 **DON'T** use a comma when the complete date is not given.

He had surgery in April 200X in Arizona.
She is to be seen again on February 3 at 10:30.

✓ **DO** attempt to use a complete date when an incomplete date is dictated.

Incorrect: The patient was seen by me for the first time in December last year. *(When was that?)*

✓ **DO** use a comma to separate the parts of a date in the date line of a letter.

November 11, 200X

🚫 **DON'T** use a comma with the military date sequence.

11 November 200X

7–10   DIAGNOSIS

✓ **DO** use a comma to separate the parts of an inverted diagnosis. The correct inversion consists of what the problem is (comma) followed by where it is.

Atelectasis, left lower lobe.
Cataract, right eye.

Open fracture, tibiofibular, left lower extremity.

Serous otitis media, bilateral.

7–11   DIRECT ADDRESS

 DO   use a comma or pair of commas to enclose a name used in direct address and to set off the words *yes* and *no*.

My thanks, Paul, for agreeing to speak at the medical-legal conference.

No, it is not our policy to release that information.

Now is the time, medical language specialists, to make your voices heard.

7–12   ESSENTIAL AND NONESSENTIAL WORDS, PHRASES, EXPRESSIONS, AND CLAUSES

Nonessential or nonrestrictive descriptive phrases or clauses add information that is *not* essential to the meaning of the sentence.

 DO   use a comma or pair of commas to set off *nonessential* words, phrases, or clauses from the rest of the sentence.

Please notice, if you will, the depth of the incision.

She should have, in my opinion, immediate surgery.

Fred Barth, who had surgery last month, came in for his final examination today.

He recovered well after his surgery, except for one episode of postsurgical hemorrhage.

The amniotic fluid had become brownish green, suggesting some degree of fetal distress.

He is an excellent surgeon, whether or not you care for my opinion, and I feel that you must trust his judgment.

I would like her to be, and she probably will be, a candidate for coronary artery bypass surgery.

She required trifocal, not bifocal, lenses at this time.

Dr. Mitchell, having been in surgery since two this morning, collapsed on the day bed.

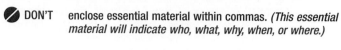

DON'T enclose essential material within commas. *(This essential material will indicate who, what, why, when, or where.)*

There is no doubt that she transcribed that report. *(In this instance, the expression* no doubt *is essential because it adds emphasis to the statement. Commas would be incorrect.)*

Incorrect:
I want to examine all the children, when they have been prepared.
Incorrect:
Medical staff members, who fail to attend the meeting, will lose their consulting privileges.
Incorrect:
Your patient, Ethel Clifford, saw me in consultation.

DON'T create a comma fault by leaving out one of the commas when a pair is required.

Incorrect:
Her temperature, which has been high fell suddenly.

DON'T create a comma fault by inserting a comma where none belongs.

Incorrect:
He had, had an automobile accident the previous week.

7–13 INDEPENDENT CLAUSE

DO use a comma to separate two or more independent clauses when they are joined by the conjunctions *and, or, nor, but, for, yet,* or *so.* Place the comma in front of the conjunction.

The diagnosis of urinary tract infection was made, and he was treated with Septra.

She used a cane in her right hand, but now she cannot use a cane at all because of pain in her right shoulder.

The condition is now stationary and permanent, and he should be able to resume his normal work load.

Your appendix appears to be inflamed, but I do not believe that you need surgery at this time.
Incorrect:
Your appendix appears to be inflamed, but not acutely. *(The second phrase is dependent and must not be separated with a comma.)*

OPTIONAL: *Many modern writers are no longer using this comma when the clauses are brief and closely related. You may ask the author of your documents about their preferences concerning this usage.*

 DON'T   take this option when it makes the initial impression unclear.

I kicked the ball, and John accidentally slipped reaching for it. *(A comma is needed in this sentence, or it might appear that you also kicked John when kicking the ball!)*

 DON'T   separate the parts of a compound from the main clause with a comma simply because a familiar conjunction is used.

Incorrect:
He has no other current skin complaints, and no history of skin cancer.
Incorrect:
The child weighed 7 pounds at birth, and was the result of an uncomplicated pregnancy and delivery.

7–14   INTRODUCTORY ELEMENTS

You will recall that an introductory element can be thought of as being out of place in the sentence; it is at the beginning rather than at the end where it would be in simple sentence order. Many of these introductory dependent phrases or clauses begin with words such as *since, because, after, about, during, by, if, when, while, although, unless, between, until, whenever, as,* and *before* and with verb forms such as *hoping, believing, allowing, helping,* and *working.*

✔ **DO**   use a comma to set off an introductory dependent phrase or clause.

After you have an x-ray, I will examine you. *(simple introductory clause)*

Dr. Chriswell was having difficulty dictating; however, after the equipment was adjusted, she was able to finish her reports. *(part of the second independent clause)*

Fully aware of his budget restrictions and with concern for the high cost of the equipment, Dr. Jellison approved the purchase of the word processor. *(compound introductory phrase)*

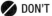 **DON'T**   separate the subject from the rest of the sentence in error.

Incorrect:
To transcribe this accurately the first time, is the main goal. *(not an introductory phrase)*

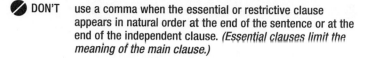

⊘ DON'T use a comma when the essential or restrictive clause appears in natural order at the end of the sentence or at the end of the independent clause. *(Essential clauses limit the meaning of the main clause.)*

> I will examine you after you have an x-ray. *(tells when the patient will be examined)*

> During the course of the procedure, a power failure occurred. *(introductory)*

> A power failure occurred during the course of the procedure. *(natural order)*

✓ DO omit the comma after a brief (fewer than five words) introductory element if clarity is not sacrificed.

> In the meantime he was discharged to his home.

> If possible schedule the thoracotomy to follow the bronchoscopy.

7–15 NAMES

✓ DO use commas to separate the first name from the last name when they are expressed in reverse order.

> RE: Lombardo, Vito
> Falsworth, Marianne P. (Mrs. John R.)

7–16 NUMBERS
See 7-9 for numbers in dates.

✓ DO use commas to group large numbers in units of three.

> platelets 250,000; wbc 15,000

⊘ DON'T use commas in four-digit numbers, street numbers, dates, ZIP codes, and some ID and technical numbers.

> My bill to Medicare was $1250.

⊘ DON'T use commas with the metric system or with decimals.

> **Correct:**
> 1000 ml
> **Incorrect:**
> 1,000 ml

DON'T use commas to separate two units of the same dimension.

The patient's height is 6 ft 3 in.
The infant was 3 days 4 hours old.
The surgery was completed in 2 hours 40 minutes.
The infant weighed 4 lb 15 oz on delivery.
The patient is a 24-year-old, unemployed, gravida 2
para 1 white female in no acute distress. *(To place a
comma after* gravida 2 *would be incorrect.)*

 DON'T separate the units at the end of a line with the first part on
one line and the second and/or third part at the beginning of
the next line.

Incorrect:
The infant weighed 4 lb
15 oz on delivery.

7–17 PARENTHETICAL EXPRESSIONS

✅ **DO** use a comma or a pair of commas to set off a parenthetical
expression from the rest of the sentence. These expressions
may begin, interrupt, or end a sentence and are always
nonessential. *(See also 7–12, Essential and Nonessential
Words, Phrases, Epressions, and Clauses.)*

She said, if my memory serves me right, that she had
graduated from medical school in 2001.

This burn needs immediate attention, in my opinion.

✅ **DO** use a comma to set off a one-word parenthetical expression
if you wish to indicate a pause.

Furthermore, she was to be seen by Dr. Sumners in
surgical consultation.

He was indeed concerned about her progress. *(comma not
needed for pause or emphasis here)*

 DON'T use a comma to separate a parenthetical expression used as
an adverb.

However sick he may be, it is not wise to intubate him at
this time.

NOTE: *The following are some commonly used parenthetical expressions:* as already stated, in my opinion, as you probably know, without a doubt, nevertheless, as a matter of fact, between you and me, consequently, in the meantime, needless to say, therefore, by the way, for example, however, furthermore, to be sure.

Finally, the author often gives a vocal clue indicating if something is nonessential by dropping his or her voice. The voice goes up when something is emphasized.

Examine these two sentences by reading them aloud.
We were determined, nevertheless, to proceed with the surgery.
We were nevertheless determined to go ahead with the surgery.

Listen for these vocal hints and also observe the position of *nevertheless* in the sentence.

7–18 PLACE NAMES

✓ **DO**   use commas to separate all the elements of a complete address.

Please mail this to my home address: 132 Winston Street, Park Village, IL 60612.

✓ **DO**   use a comma to set off the name of the state when the city precedes it.

The pacemaker was shipped to you from Syracuse, New York, by Federal Express.

🚫 **DON'T**   place a comma between the state name and the ZIP code. The ZIP code is considered part of the state name.

His address is 721 Thunderbird Drive, Tucson, Arizona 85719.

7–19 SERIES OF WORDS, TESTS, STUDIES, VITALS, VALUES, AND SO FORTH

✓ **DO**   use a comma after each element or each pair of elements in a series of coordinate nouns, adjectives, verbs, or adverbs.

Please make a copy of the patient's operative report, pathology report, and consultation report for Dr. Reilly.

The patient underwent daily group, milieu, and individual psychotherapy.

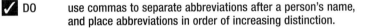 **DON'T** use a comma between the last adjective and the noun phrase it modifies.

The patient is a well-developed, well-nourished, elderly, white female telephone operator. (*The noun phrase is* female telephone operator, *and the adjective immediately preceding the noun phrase is* white. *A test of whether commas are needed is to transpose the two modifiers. For example, one would not say* female white telephone operator.)

OPTIONAL: *You may omit the comma before the conjunction if clarity is not sacrificed.*

NOTE: *The option is not to be taken in the following example because the color scheme would be unclear:*

The various hospital departments were decorated in green and yellow, blue and brown, and green and white.

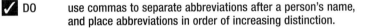 **DON'T** use a comma before the ampersand (&).

He is now employed as a transcriptionist for Chandor, Kerry & Pemsel.

✓ DO use commas to separate abbreviations after a person's name, and place abbreviations in order of increasing distinction.

Neal J. Kaufman, MD, FACCP
Rachel L. Connors Jr., MD, LLB

✓ DO use commas to separate groups of tests, studies, values, laboratory data, and so forth.

Speech, gag, jaw jerk, corneals, facial sensation are all intact.

Weight 83.5 kg, height 166 cm, temperature 98°, pulse 80, respirations 20, blood pressure 120/86.

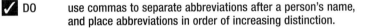 **DON'T** use commas to separate more complex value groups or groups with internal punctuation. *(See Chapter 39, Semicolon, and Chapter 6, The Colon.)*

Blood pressure 194/97; pulse 127; respirations 32, regular, and gasping.

Also correct
Blood pressure: 194/97
Pulse: 127
Respirations. 32, regular, and gasping

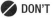 **DON'T** use commas to separate two units of the same dimension.

The patient's height was 6 ft 3 in.
The infant was 3 days 4 hours old.
The surgery was completed in 2 hours 40 minutes.
She was a gravida 3 para 2 white female.

✅ **DO** use commas to separate a series of short independent clauses. *(See Chapter 39, Semicolon, concerning the usual punctuation used to separate a series of independent clauses.)*

She was upset about being seen, she resented my intrusion, and she said so.

7–20 TITLES AND DEGREES

✅ **DO** use a comma or pair of commas to set off titles and degrees after a person's name.

John A. Meadows, MD, saw the patient in consultation.
Ms. Nancy Bishop, administrator, gave him ten days to bring his incomplete charts up to date.

NOTE: *If there are multiple degrees or professional credentials after a person's name, place them in the order in which they were awarded or in order of increasing distinction and separate them with commas.*

Mary Watkins, BS, MS, JD

Nancy Casales, CMA, CMT, president of AAMT, Mountain Meadows Chapter, was the keynote speaker for our MT Week banquet.

7–21 WRONG USE REVIEW

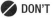 **DON'T** use a comma to separate an independent clause from a dependent clause.

Incorrect:
The child weighed 7 pounds at birth, and was the product of an uncomplicated pregnancy and delivery.

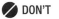 **DON'T** separate restrictive modifiers.

Incorrect:
Please telephone the unit, if you are agreeable to postponing the surgery.

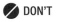 **DON'T** enclose essential appositives.

Incorrect:
My patient, James Edney, was admitted through the emergency department.

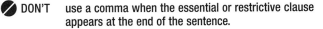 **DON'T** separate two adjectives with a comma when the second adjective forms a single unit with the noun.

Incorrect:
The patient is a 36-year-old, 175 lb, married, police, motorcycle operator who . . .

DON'T use a comma before an adjective that modifies another adjective in the series.

Incorrect:
He came into the ER with a copiously, bleeding gunshot wound.

DON'T use a comma when the complete date is not given.

Incorrect:
He was last seen in March, 200X, by the physician's assistant.

DON'T create a comma fault by leaving out one of the commas when a pair is required.

Incorrect:
She should have, I understand immediate surgery.

DON'T use a comma when the essential or restrictive clause appears at the end of the sentence.

Incorrect:
I will contact the anesthesiologist, as soon as the OR is free.

🚫 DON'T use commas in four-digit numbers.

Incorrect:
We removed 1,200 ml of serosanguineous fluid from the abdomen.

🚫 DON'T use a comma to separate two units of the same dimension.

Incorrect:
The child had a very low birth weight of 2 lb, 4 oz.

🚫 DON'T separate sets of words incorrectly.

Incorrect:
The stomach and duodenum which usually lie in the left upper abdomen, and epigastrium are rarely felt, unless they are involved with large tumors.
Correct:
The stomach and duodenum, which usually lie in the left upper abdomen and epigastrium, are rarely felt, unless they are involved with large tumors.
See also 7–4, Clarity.

8

Compounds

INTRODUCTION

Compounds consist of two or more separate words or phrases that are used as a single word, often joined by a hyphen. It can be difficult to know if a compound should be typed as one word, two or more separate words, or as a compound hyphenated word. Often there are no specific rules to follow for these compound words or modifiers. (Consider *chin bone* and *cheekbone.*) The general rules in this chapter will assist you with most words. Many of the "rules" are actually suggestions and have long lists of exceptions, and even some rule books and reference books differ on both rules and exceptions. Because compound words are also a spelling problem, consult the dictionary for help with specific compounds. *(See also Chapter 20, Hyphen Use and Word Division; and 43–11, One Word, Two Words, or Hyphenated, in Chapter 43. Finally, check Appendix F, Homonyms and Sound-alike Words.)*

8 Compounds

8–1 CHEMICAL COMPOUNDS AND FORMULAS

 DO join prefixed locants *(the chemical location in the molecule)* and descriptors to the name of the organic compound with a hyphen.

> beta-sitosterol   cis-dichloroethene   2-hexanone

 DO use a hyphen to separate the abbreviations for known amino acid sequences.

> Lys-Asp-Gly

> **NOTE:** *Unknown sequences are enclosed in parentheses and separated by commas.*

DO join chemical compounds and formulas with hyphens and close up punctuation.

> 9-nitroanthra(1,9,4,10)bis(1)oxathiazone-2,7-bisdioxide
> Leu-Glu-Pro-Ser-Thr-Ala

8–2 COINED COMPOUNDS

 DO join a single letter to a word to form a coined compound.

T-shirt	V-neck
non-Q-wave myocardial infarction	X-Acto
S-shaped	X-rated
T-span	x-ray
U-bag	Z-plasty

EXCEPTIONS

3M	*B cell*
R wave	*T square*

DO join a number to a word to form a coined compound phrase.

> SMA-1   alpha-1   profile-1   OM-2

8–3 COMPOUND MODIFIER BEFORE A NOUN

 DO hyphenate phrases used as compound adjectives before a noun.

> diagnosis-related groups
> figure-of-eight sutures
> happy-go-lucky personality

ill-defined tumor mass
large-for-date fetus
mouth-to-mouth resuscitation
non-English-speaking patient
non-insulin-dependent diabetes
self-addressed envelope
self-inflicted knife wound
through-and-through sutures
two-pack-a-day smoker
well-known speaker
hard-and-fast rule
tried-and-true method

She is a well-developed, well-nourished, 35-year-old black female.

An end-to-end anastomosis was performed.

The resident consulted the alcoholism counselors on his two MAST-positive patients.

This is a very up-to-date reference for drug names.

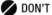 **DON'T** use a hyphen when the phrase follows the verb.

I want these records brought *up to date.*
She appears to be *well nourished.*

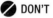 **DON'T** make a compound modifier with an adverb ending in *ly.*

That was a poorly dictated report.
She is a moderately obese waitress.
He is an exceptionally gifted diagnostician.

EXCEPTIONS

a friendly-sounding voice   *a motherly-looking woman*

✓ **DO** make sure that a compound is intended.

We applied a long-leg cast. *(The cast is for a long leg.)*
We applied a long leg cast. *(The cast for the leg is long.)*

There was a soft-tissue lesion on the surface. *(The lesion is composed of soft tissue.)*
There was a soft tissue lesion. *(The lesion is soft.)*

DO   use a hyphen to join two or more words used to describe a noun when clarity is required.

brown-bag lunch   long-awaited diagnosis
in-hospital cardiac arrest   little used-book store
small-town physician

 DO   hyphenate modifiers with a capitalized second element.

pro-American advertising   pre-Elizabethan period
anti-Asian outburst   non-English speaking

DO   hyphenate a compound adjective that consists of a noun and an adjective both before and after the noun.

user-friendly   top-heavy   bone-dry
accident-prone   nerve-racking   habit-forming

The skin covering the graft was paper-thin.

The lull in the storm of patients crowding into the emergency department was short-lived.

8–4 COORDINATE EXPRESSIONS
See also Rule 8-11, Prefix-Compounded Proper Nouns.

DO   use a hyphen to join certain coordinate expressions. The compounds are always hyphenated, regardless of their placement in a sentence.

The waiting room was painted a sort of yellow-orange.
The patient's expression was happy-sad.
That income was tax-exempt.
The old gentleman was stone-deaf.
The tools were stored in a lean-to.

8–5 LATIN COMPOUNDS

DON'T   use hyphens with Latin compounds such as *ad hoc, bona fide, prima facie,* and *per capita.*

Carcinoma was found in situ.
She was part of the in vivo fertility program.

8–6 NAMES, SURNAMES, AND EPONYMS COMPOUNDED

DO   use a hyphen to join compound nouns, compound surnames, and compound eponyms.

Nonne-Milroy disease
Arnold-Chiari type II malformation
Legg-Calvé-Perthes disease
A Davis-Crowe mouth gag was used.
Mary Smyth-Reynolds was in today for her annual Pap smear.
Antonio is the new secretary-treasurer.
He was born right on the Texas-Oklahoma border.
Dr. Asser is Cedar's chief-of-staff.
He is doing research with the Epstein-Barr virus.

EXCEPTIONS: *She was a 35-year-old African American patient.*

American Indian   *native American*   *Mexican American*

🚫 **DON'T**   hyphenate names that are unhyphenated names of a person.

Austin Moore hip prosthesis *not* Austin-Moore

NOTE: *There is no hyphen between the words* Austin *and* Moore *because the prosthesis was invented by Dr. Thomas Austin Moore and not, as one might think, by two persons respectively surnamed Austin and Moore. Check your references when you are not sure.*

8–7   NUMBERS AND FRACTIONS COMPOUNDED WITH WORDS

✅ **DO**   use a hyphen when numbers are compounded with words and they have the force of a single modifier.

✅ **DO**   hyphenate fractions used as an adjective

The auditorium was two-thirds full.
one-third share   35-hour week
four-fifths majority   2-inch incision

Four-vessel angiography showed a narrowing of the left carotid artery.

EXCEPTION: *There is only a 3 percent difference.*

🚫 **DON'T**   use a hyphen when the compound follows the noun.

He is a 56-year-old janitor in no acute distress.
The janitor is 56 years old.

8–8 NUMBERS, COMPOUND AND MULTIPLE

 DO use a hyphen to separate compound written-out numbers from 21 through 99 and written-out simple fractions.

Fifty-five medical transcriptionists attended the meeting last night.

Ninety-nine percent of the time I am confident of the diagnosis.

Paresis was noted in one-half of her left thumb.

✓ DO use the hyphen to attach the number modifier to the noun when the number is preceded by another number.

inserted two 8-inch drains
ordered six 2-gauge needles

8–9 PLURAL FORMATION OF COMPOUNDS

✓ DO add the appropriate plural ending to compound nouns written as one word.

fingerbreadths   teaspoonfuls   spokesmen

✓ DO add the appropriate plural ending to the word that is the essential noun in compound nouns written with hyphens or spaces.

sisters-in-law   surgeons general
chiefs-of-staff   go-betweens
runners-up   know-it-alls

NOTE: *See also Chapter 31, Plural Forms.*

8–10 PREFIX-COMPOUNDED COMMON NOUNS AND ADJECTIVES

✓ DO use a hyphen with compound words beginning with *ex, self,* and *vice;* also use a hyphen to join various other prefixes to avoid an awkward combination of letters, such as two or three identical vowels in a sequence.

self-inflicted wound   ex-patient
vice-president   micro-orchidia

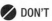 DON'T use a hyphen with the compound words beginning with the prefixes *ante, anti, co, contra, counter, de, inter, intra, multi, non, out, over, post, pre, pro, pseudo, re, semi, trans, un, sub, supra,* and *under* unless the word has identical letters in a sequence.

antemortem	intra-abdominal	pre-evaluation
antenatal	nondrinker	preoperative
antidepressant	outpatient	retype
anti-immune	postmortem	semiprone
anti-inflammatory	postoperative	undernourished
co-op	post-traumatic	

NOTE: *The prefixes* co, pre, *and* re *rarely require a hyphen even if the vowel is doubled.*

No hyphen

coordinate	preempt	reenact
intraarterial	preenzyme	reenlist
preeclampsia	preepiglottic	reenter
preelection	preeruptive	reevaluate
preemergent	preexisting	reexamine
preemployment	reemploy	transsacral

With hyphen

non-Hodgkin *(See 8–11.)*
pre-position *(to position ahead of time)*
re-collect *(collect again)*
re-cover *(cover again)*
re-creation *(to create again)*
re-form *(to form again)*
re-infuse *(to infuse again)*
re-mark *(to mark again)*
re-present *(to present again)*
re-sign *(sign again)*
re-sort *(sort again)*
re-treat *(to treat again)*

 DO use a hyphen with the following words for ease of reading.

re-do   co-op

 DO use a hyphen with compound words beginning with the prefix *extra* when the meaning is *additional* or the word root begins with an *a.*

extra-large   extra-apical

DON'T use a hyphen with compound words beginning with the prefix *extra* when the meaning is *outside.*

extradural   extrathoracic   extracurricular

8–11 PREFIX-COMPOUNDED PROPER NOUNS

✓ **DO** use a hyphen to join a prefix to the proper noun in a compound.

un-American
pseudo-Christian
non-Hodgkin
The estimated date of confinement is sometime in mid-May.

8–12 "STATUS POST"

 DON'T hyphenate the expression *status post.*

status postoperative
status post knee joint prosthesis

 DON'T use a hyphen to join *status post* to the word that follows it.

status post hernia repair
status post vascular shunt
status post myocardial infarction

8–13 SUFFIX COMPOUNDS

✓ **DO** use hyphens to form compounds with the suffixes *plus, elect, designate, odd,* and *in.*

president-elect   shoo-in
thirty-odd minutes   ambassador-designate
She appeared to be fifty-plus years old.

✓ **DO** use a hyphen when a compound consists of an adjective plus a noun plus *ed.* This combination is used both before and after the noun.

She was a good-natured patient.
The patient was good-natured.
The middle-aged man was interviewed.
The man we interviewed was middle-aged.

I removed a medium-sized tumor.
The tumor was medium-sized.
There was a short-lived break in the schedule.
The break was short-lived.

8–14 SUSPENDING HYPHEN

 DO use a suspending hyphen to connect a series of compound modifiers.

There were small- and large-sized cysts scattered throughout the parenchyma.

He has a two- or three-month convalescence ahead of him.

I delivered her baby, but she saw Dr. Thomas for her pre- and postnatal care.

8–15 VERBS

DON'T hyphenate or close up compound verb forms. *(Some verbs form compounds with prepositions or adverbs.)*

Please check up on Jen Mossie in the ICU.
Dr. Jeremy will work up the study protocol for approval.
I will do the surgery but Dr. Buckford will follow up the postoperative results.
Please follow through with this revision.

NOTE: *When used as modifying adjectives, these forms are hyphenated or closed up as a single word.*

follow-up *or* followup
check-up *or* checkup
work-up *or* workup

She was seen today in final follow-up examination. (*also* followup)

NOTE: *As nouns, these forms are closed up as a single term.*

Followup was done in the outpatient clinic.
We informed him that his final checkup would be done just before he was released to return to work.
No workup on preoperative patients was scheduled for any of the interns today.

NOTE: *See Appendix F, Homonyms and Sound-alike Words, for more combinations of solid, hyphenated, and two-word combinations.*

Dash

INTRODUCTION

A dash is less formal than a colon and more direct than parentheses. Its primary use is to create emphasis by switching direction. It is created on the keyboard with two hyphens. It can also be created by pressing the "hyphen" key and the "alt" key at the same time. There is no space before, between, or after the two hyphens.

✓ DO   use the dash *very* sparingly; with overuse, it loses its effect.

⊘ DON'T   use a dash when another punctuation mark will do.

9–1 AMPLIFY OR EXPLAIN

✓ DO   use a single dash to emphasize, amplify, define, explain, or summarize a statement.

As I told you before, she is scheduled for internal mammary artery implantation--not femoral artery implantation.

The diagnosis is grim--I feel helpless.

We may be so busy analyzing physical signs that we miss--or dismiss--clues to frame of mind.

For this patient, a polyp meant a fatal malignancy--and all the awful experiences that attend it.

9–2 APPOSITIVES

 DO   use the dash instead of commas when commas have been used to punctuate the expression itself.

The entire x-ray department–physicians, technicians, therapists, transcriptionists, secretaries, clerks–was completely engrossed in the demonstration of the new equipment.

 DO   consider using parentheses instead of a dash in this situation unless you wish emphasis.

9–3 INTERRUPTION

 DO   use a pair of dashes for a forceful break in thought or an interruption.

I want you to–no, I insist that you–consult a surgeon about the growth in your breast.

9–4 OMISSION

 DO   use a single dash to indicate the omission of letters or words.

His not showing up on time for surgery put us in one h–of a bind.

🚫 **DON'T**   use the dash to indicate an omission when you simply have nothing particular in mind to say.

9–5 SUMMARY

✓ **DO**   use a single dash for summary.

She soon became bored with the nontranscription details of her job–editing, printing, collating–but finally realized it was part of the fabric of the position.
Dr. Praycroft, Dr. Meadows, Dr Lo–all were standing by to assist.

🚫 **DON'T**   begin a new line with a dash. You must carry the last word before the dash to the following line along with the dash.

Drugs and Drug References

10–1 ABBREVIATIONS

 DO　　avoid keying an abbreviation if it can be misread and/or misinterpreted in a chart note. See Table 1-1, p. 20.

DC can be translated as discharge or discontinue; thus a patient could be sent home too early or taken off medication too soon.

The acronym *DPT* stands for two different injectables: (1) a painkiller/tranquilizer combination (Demerol, Phenergan, and Thorazine) and (2) an immunization (diphtheria/pertussis/tetanus).

DW indicates dextrose (sugar) in water, distilled water, or deionized water.

OD for once daily can also be translated to mean right eye *(oculus dexter)*, overdose, on duty, or doctor of optometry.

ON can be misread as the word on, overnight, Ortho-Novum *(birth control pills)*, or every night.

✓ DO use the abbreviated form when metric units are dictated following a number. They are not made plural.

25 mg   0.5 mg   50 gm

✓ DO key dosage instructions in lowercase letters with periods separating the initials.

b.i.d.   p.o.   p.r.n.   q.4 h.   q.i.d.   t.i.d.

NOTE: *Pharmaceutical authorities suggest that the following abbreviations are inappropriate in medical records and that the spelled-out version be used if the abbreviation is dictated.*

Write out the following:
daily   for *o.d.*
orally   for *per os*
every day   for *q.d.*
nightly   for *q.n.*
nightly at bedtime for *q.h.s.*
every other day   for *q.o.d.*
subcutaneous   for *sub q*
subcutaneous   for *SC*
unit   for *U or u.*
bedtime   for *BT* or *h.s.*
each ear   for *a.u.*
three days   for *x3d*

10–2 BRAND NAMES

✓ DO capitalize trade names and brand names of drugs, other trademarked materials, and methods of administration; generic and chemical names are not capitalized.

Brand names	Generic names
Cortisporin	alcohol
Darvon	analgesic
Dermalon	catgut
Gelfoam	cotton
Nitora	ether
pHisoHex	hydrocortisone
Surgicel	potassium iodide
Theokin	silk

✅ **DO** maintain any idiosyncratic capitalization used by the proprietor of the brand name or capitalize only the first letter of brand or trade names.

> Di-Delamine   NegGram   GoLYTELY
> HydroDIURIL *(Hydrodiuril is also correct.)*
> Phisohex *(pHisoHex is also correct.)*
> Eryc (ERYC)

🚫 **DON'T** use lowercase after a hyphen.

> Ser-Ap-Es *(See 10-17.)*

10–3   CHEMICAL NAMES

✅ **DO** begin the chemical name of a drug in lowercase, inserting commas and hyphens as the formula warrants.

> 2-methyl-2-n-propyl-1-1,3-propanediol dicarbamate

10–4   CHEMOTHERAPEUTIC DRUGS

✅ **DO** use acronyms when a patient receives combination chemotherapeutic agents for treatment.

> **Write**
> B-DOPA *(bleomycin, DTIC, Oncovin, prednisone, Adriamycin)*
>
> 5-FU *(5-fluorouracil)*

10–5   DESIGNER DRUGS

✅ **DO** key acronyms or slang names when a physician dictates such in reference to designer drugs in medical reports.

> MDMA *also called* ecstasy *or* Adam
> PCP *or* angel dust
> heroin *or* China White

10–6   DOSAGE

✅ **DO** be careful in transcribing drug dosages. Incorrect numbers could mean a fatal error. Check a reliable drug reference to be sure that you heard the correct dosage if you are unsure. Flag your document so the author can verify the dosage is correct if there is any doubt. *(See also 10-1.)*

For example, you hear "fif . . . mg." A check of the drug reference indicates the drug is given in amounts of 50 mg and 100 mg. Your selection of 50 rather than 15 will be correct.

10–7 EXPERIMENTAL DRUGS

✓ DO use the manufacturer's code number to identify an experimental unapproved drug not yet assigned a USAN name.

PAA-3854 *(clamoxyquin HCl)*

10–8 GENERIC NAMES

✓ DO key or use lowercase letters to spell nonproprietary or generic names. *(One of the examples given is not a drug.)*

Generic name	Brand name
cellophane tape	Scotch tape
meprobamate	Miltown tablets

✓ DO use the generic spelling if the generic and brand names sound alike unless it is certain that the brand name is being referenced.

adrenaline   Adrenalin

10–9 INTERFERONS

✓ DO begin in lowercase and spell out the Greek letter or use the Greek symbol for general classes of compounds or single compounds.

interferon alfa *or* IFN-α

✓ DO use a hyphen and an arabic number with lowercase letter for individual, pure, identifiable compounds.

interferon alfa-2a

✓ DO use a hyphen, a lowercase *n*, and an arabic numeral for names of mixtures of interferons from natural sources.

interferon alfa-n1

10–10 MULTIPLE-DRUG REGIMENS

✔ DO   use the abbreviation for a multiple-drug regimen when it is
         dictated, but make sure it does not have another meaning or
         may be mistaken for another drug.

> CMFPT *(cyclophosphamide, methotrexate, fluorouracil,
> prednisone, tamoxifen)*
> **Incorrect: MOP**
> **Correct:** Mustargen, Oncovin, procarbazine, prednisone
> *(MOPP)*

✔ DO   use generic names with trade names when first mentioned in
         a document.

> In this instance, the drug of choice was Coumadin
> (warfarin).

10–11 NUMBERS

✔ DO   use figures in all expressions pertaining to drugs, including
         strength, dosage, and directions.

> b.i.d. *or* twice a day *or* 2 times a day
> q.4 h. *or* every 4 hours

> He is to take Tofranil, 75 mg/d × 3 days to be increased to
> 100-150 mg/d if there is no response.
> The directions for her Motrin were 400 mg q.4 h. p.r.n.
> for pain.

> One generally gives 6.2 mg/kg to 9.4 mg/kg for those
> children 9 years old or younger.

EXCEPTION: *The number one (1) may be written out or expressed
as a numeral. If it is followed by an abbreviated unit of measure,
the numeral should be used.*

NOTE: *It is helpful to leave a space between the number and the
abbreviation that follows for ease of reading the number.*

> Triaminic 1 tsp. q.8 h.

✔ DO   use metric units of measure in abbreviated form with numerals;
         leave a space between the number and the metric unit.

> 25 mg   0.5 mg *(lowercase with no period)*

DON'T separate the number at the end of the line from the units or symbols that may follow.

Correct . . . . .5 mg
Incorrect . . . . .25 mg

 DON'T use either the lowercase or capital "oh" on the keyboard for zero; use the zero symbol.

Correct:
50 mg
Incorrect:
5O mg, 5o mg

 DO for the sake of clarity, omit commas between drug names, dosages, and instructions.

The patient was given Pen-Vee K 500 mg q.i.d. for ten days.

NOTE: *Because this example shows a nonessential clause, it should have commas and may be seen with commas as a variable.*

The patient was given Pen-Vee K, 500 mg q.i.d., for ten days.

 DO use a comma or semicolon when keyboarding a series that includes drugs, dosages, and instructions.

The patient was sent home on Norpace 150 mg q.6 h.; Procardia 20 mg q.6 h.; and digoxin 0.125 mg q.a.m.
or
The patient was sent home on Surmontil 25 mg t.i.d., nitroglycerin 0.4 mg sublingual p.r.n., and Benadryl 50 mg q.6 h. p.r.n.
or
A complex string can be typed as a list:
MEDICATIONS:
1. Continue his 1800-calorie ADA diet.
2. Estradiol (micronized) 2 mg/d for 25 or 30 days.
3. Flurazepam HCl 30 mg at bedtime.
4. Hydrocodone bitartrate 5 mg b.i.d.
5. Acetaminophen 500 mg b.i.d.
6. Ibuprofen 600 mg q.i.d.
7. Levothyroxine sodium 0.15 mg/d.

8. Metoprolol tartrate 25 mg/d.
9. Prednisone 5 mg/d.
10. Propoxyphene HCl 65 mg q.i.d. (which is an increase from his current t.i.d. regimen).

10–12   RADIOACTIVE DRUGS

✓ DO   begin radioactive pharmaceuticals and associated tests with a capital letter and use hyphens where indicated. It is optional to show super- or subscript.

Iodotope I 131 ^{131}I
Tc-99m   Glofil-125
T3 uptake T_3 uptake
T4 (thyroxine) T_4

NOTE: *When spelling out the isotope name, put the isotope number on the same line in the same font and font size; do not use superscript, subscript, or hyphens.*

gallium 67   indium 111   technetium 99m

✓ DO   capitalize trademarked isotopes.

Glofil-125   Hippuran I 131

10–13   REFERENCES

✓ DO   carefully check any drug names in question for the correct spelling, and if still uncertain about what drug name was dictated, leave a space on the line and write a note to the dictator, describing how the drug name sounded. *(See Chapter 37, Reference Materials and Publications, for a listing of pharmaceutical reference books.)*

✓ DO   check your medical dictionary rather than drug reference book, because a drug class may sound like a drug name.

✓ DO   use your spell-checker feature to help locate the spelling of drugs.

✓ DO   become familiar with complex drug references such as the *Physicians' Desk Reference (PDR)* before you need to use them.

✓ DO   research easy-to-use drug reference books written for medical transcriptionists and have one ready for your research before you need it.

10–14   SOUND-ALIKE, LOOK-ALIKE DRUG NAMES

✓ **DO**   flag a transcript if you are unable to decipher a physician's handwriting from the patient's record or are unable to understand the dictated sound-alike or look-alike drug.

Lamictal	Lamisil
Bicillin	V-Cillin
Cerebyx	Celebrex
Desoxyn	digoxin *(pronounced di-JOX-in)*

NOTE: Saunders Pharmaceutical Word Book *by Drake and Drake provides an extensive list of drug sound-alikes. This list will help you double-check a drug name or dosage when there are any doubts. See also 4-4, Flagging, Carding, Tagging, or Marking, in Chapter 4.*

10–15   STREET DRUG SLANG

🚫 **DON'T**   modify or edit street drug slang when such words are dictated.

Belushi *(cocaine and heroin)*
Charley or Charlie *(cocaine or heroin)*
liquid ecstasy, liquid E, liquid X *(gamma-hydroxybutyric acid)*
Rohypnol *(date rape drug)*

NOTE: Saunders Pharmaceutical Xref Book *by Drake and Drake includes a comprehensive list of street drug slang so you can confirm spelling.*

10–16   SYMBOLS

🚫 **DON'T**   use a slash mark between drug names and dosage because it may be misread as the number one.

Incorrect:
6 units regular insulin/20 units NPH insulin *(May be mistakenly read as 120 units of NPH insulin.)*

10–17   TRADEMARKS

✓ **DO**   capitalize trademark names.

Obenix	ProSom	Levoxyl

✓ **DO**   capitalize the trademarked name for the delivery system of drugs.

Spancaps   Captabs   Wyseal
Inhal-Aid   Gy-Pak

10–18   VITAMINS

✓ **DO**   keyboard *vitamin* in lowercase, capitalize the letter designation, and use arabic numerals.

vitamin B_{12} *or* vitamin B12

⊘ **DON'T**   use a hyphen or space between letters and numerals.

B_{12} vitamin *or* vitamin B12

11

Editing

INTRODUCTION

✓ DO   transcribe *exactly* what is dictated, keeping the following rules or exceptions in mind. Far more editorial latitude is permitted in private medical offices and small hospital departments than in large institutions or transcription services.

✓ DO   use careful proofing. Use diligence to prevent a critical error from appearing in the transcribed report.

⊘ DON'T   tamper with the author's style when editing. In other words, don't rephrase what is dictated to suit your personal preference. Transcribe with accuracy what is meant, which may not be what is actually said.

⊘ DON'T   delete essential information.

✓ DO   rely on hospital policy and the author's preference when editing medical documents.

☑ DO   use the patient's medical record when it is available to you to clarify dictated information.

☑ DO   edit obvious errors when transcribing dictation done by a person who speaks English as a second language. *(See 11-5.)*

☑ DO   transcribe all findings—negative, normal, and positive.

11–1 ABBREVIATIONS

☑ DO   spell out abbreviations in the diagnosis section of medical reports so there is no chance for misinterpretation. The diagnosis section may appear as an impression, preoperative or postoperative diagnosis, discharge diagnosis, or differential diagnosis.

Incorrect:
Final Diagnosis: ASHD
Correct:
Final Diagnosis: Arteriosclerotic heart disease

Incorrect:
Impression: CVA
Correct:
Impression: Chronic villous arthritis

Incorrect:
Preoperative Diagnosis: DVIU
Correct:
Preoperative Diagnosis: Direct vision internal urethrotomy

Incorrect:
Discharge Diagnosis: GVHD
Correct:
Discharge Diagnosis: Graft-versus-host disease

Incorrect:
Differential Diagnosis: VZV
Correct:
Differential Diagnosis: Varicella-zoster virus

11–2 ARTICLES

☑ DO   insert or delete articles *(a, an, the)* to grammatically improve sentences in formal narrative copy when they have been inadvertently added or omitted from the dictation. This situation may occur when the dictator is foreign born or is distracted or speaking hurriedly.

Incorrect:
Patient had colitis in past.
Correct:
The patient had colitis in the past.

11–3 BRIEF FORMS

 DO   spell out most brief forms. However, when a brief form is
dictated, it may be typed as a brief form unless it might be
misread and/or misinterpreted in the report. Likewise, brief
forms may be typed in chart notes unless the brief form
might be misread or misinterpreted.

Incorrect:
Temp 101.
Correct:
Temperature 101.

Incorrect:
The sputum culture grew out H. flu.
Correct:
The sputum culture grew out Haemophilus influenzae.
Correct also:
The sputum culture grew out H. influenzae.

Incorrect:
The patient had a right thoracotomy for removal of cocci
nodules.
Correct:
The patient had a right thoracotomy for removal of
coccidioidomas.

11–4 FLAGGING, CARDING, TAGGING, OR MARKING

 DO   leave a blank and flag, mark, or electronically query any
phrase or word you cannot quite hear or understand. Attach a
note to the transcript with a brief description of where the
blank is located *(See Figure 11–1 at the end of the chapter.)*

Sounds like:
The middlehear was hair contain' . . .
Dictated:
The middle ear was air containing . . .
Note:
Williams, Maribeth #18-74-78. Under PX, Respiratory
(page 2, line 8) "respirations present." Sounds like "chain
smokes." Judy, 5-17-0X
Reply reads:
Cheyne-Stokes respirations present.

Sounds like:
The lab withdrawn on June 1, 200X
Reply:
The lab work drawn . . .

 DO   flag a medical inconsistency you have corrected so the dictator may review it for accuracy.

 DON'T   close up a space where a difficult word, phrase, or sentence belongs.

DON'T   keyboard a line or insert a series of question marks where you encounter a word problem.

11–5   FOREIGN ACCENTS

Dictators who have foreign accents can be difficult to understand, and the grammar occasionally may need correction. *(For further guidelines on grammar correction, see Chapter 17.)*

 DO   tune your ears to the different aspects of your author's voice and develop listening skills to detect patterns.

- *Some languages have no articles, so the author may drop an, a, and the before a noun.*
- *Some words with* ch *and* r *are often very difficult for some speakers learning English as a second language.*
- *Some languages require an article before every noun, so authors may add articles when speaking English.*
- *A* v *may be pronounced as a* b.
- *The word* de *or* ze *may be spoken instead of the word* the.
- *Word endings such as* s, ed, al, *and* ing *may be omitted.*
- *It is very common to omit the past tense of a word.*
  He wait (waited) *over two hours before being seen.*
- *A final* d *may be pronounced as a* t.
  Thus, good *may become* goot.
- *The letters* us *may sound like* oose.
  Thus, venous *becomes* venoose.
- *An extra syllable may be added to a word.*
  Thus, worsen *may become* worsen-ed.
- *The* th *sound may sound like a* t *or an* s.
  Thus, thigh *becomes* tie *or* sigh.
- *An* x *may become an* s.
  Thus, excretion *becomes* escretion; *sounds like* essa-cretion.
- *Additional word endings, such as an* s, *may be added.*
  Thus, abdomen *becomes* abdomens.

- Some speakers of Spanish may add an eh *sound before words that begin with an* s.
  Thus, otolk becomes ehstalk *and stat becomes* ehstat.
- The letter a *may be pronounced* ah.
  Thus, vasodilator *may become* vahsodilator.
- The g *sound may be replaced by a* k *sound.*
  Thus, tingling *becomes* tinkling.
- The l *sound may be replaced with an* r *sound.*
  Thus, cloak *becomes* croak, *and* locked knee *becomes* rocked knee.
- The letter c *is pronounced with a* k *sound.*
  Thus, cephalic *sounds like* kephalic.
- Final consonants may have an added syllable at the end.
  Thus, crest *becomes* cresteh.

NOTE: *Therefore, use your own understanding of medical terminology and the words surrounding the difficult word to assist in determining the meaning of the word. If you hear* iliac cresteh, *you have a distinct clue to the words* iliac crest *intended by the speaker.*

11–6 GRAMMAR

Correction of grammar is often necessary, but material should be edited only to the extent that the editing does not change the meaning of the dictation. Sentence structure may need rearrangement. Remember that medical language may not be changed without permission from the author. *(See also 11–14, Verb-Subject Agreement, and Chapter 17, Grammar.)*

 DO   make sure that the verb and noun match in number.

Incorrect:
The adnexa was negative.
Correct:
The adnexa were negative.

Incorrect:
Then 5 ml of solution were injected into the intravenous fluid.
Correct:
Then 5 ml of solution was injected into the intravenous fluid.

Incorrect:
No evidence of any overlapping sutures are seen.
Correct:
No evidence of any overlapping sutures is seen.

RATIONALE: *The verb must agree in number with the subject of the sentence and not with an intervening prepositional phrase.*

Incorrect:
No adenopathy, lumps, or masses is seen in the chest.
Correct:
No adenopathy, lumps, or masses are seen in the chest.

RATIONALE: *When there is a series, the verb agrees in number with the nearest subject.*

Incorrect:
Sections of the cervical tissue shows mild dysplasia.
Correct:
Sections of the cervical tissue show mild dysplasia.

 DO be careful of collective nouns.

Incorrect:
This group of diagnoses are proposed.
Correct:
This group of diagnoses is proposed.

Incorrect:
Then 2 cc were injected.
Correct:
Then 2 cc was injected.

Incorrect:
Review of systems were negative.
Correct:
Review of systems was negative.

 DO use proper parts of speech. *(See Chapter 17, Grammar, for help with difficult words.)*

Incorrect:
The patient was found laying on the floor.
Correct:
The patient was found lying on the floor.

Incorrect:
Give this to whomever sees the patient.
Correct:
Give this to whoever sees the patient.

Incorrect:
The Tumor Board agreed that they would meet on the first Friday.
Correct:
The Tumor Board agreed that it would meet on the first Friday.

DO   use proper words.

Incorrect:
She neither smokes or drinks.
Correct:
She neither smokes nor drinks.

Incorrect:
There was no reoccurrence of his tumor.
Correct:
There was no recurrence of his tumor.

Incorrect:
He should of been admitted immediately.
Correct:
He should have been admitted immediately.

Incorrect:
It looked like he would begin the procedure unassisted.
Correct:
It looked as if he would begin the procedure unassisted.

Incorrect:
The patient was seen yesterday and is doing well.
Correct:
The patient was seen yesterday and was doing well.

 DO   use nouns and adjectives correctly.

Incorrect:
He was scheduled for replacement of his aorta valve.
Correct:
He was scheduled for replacement of his aortic valve.

DO   use proper singular or plural nouns.

Incorrect:
The conjunctiva were bilaterally inflamed.
Correct:
The conjunctivae were bilaterally inflamed.

 DO   position modifiers correctly.

Incorrect:
The patient had a hysterectomy leaving one tube and ovary in Jacksonville.
Correct:
The patient had a hysterectomy in Jacksonville, leaving one tube and ovary.

DO   use the proper tense.

Past tense is used in the past history part of a report, in discharge summaries, and to discuss patients who have died.

Present tense is used in describing the current illness or disease and in the history and physical.

The patient has had left sciatica for the past two years; this is now exacerbated.

 DO   check unfamiliar words to be sure that you are using them correctly.

Homonyms and sound-alike words may be dictated incorrectly, but often the transcriptionist perceives the word incorrectly or is unaware that another word exists that sounds like or is similar to what was said. *(See Appendix F, Homonyms and Sound-alike Words; and Chapter 17, Grammar.)*

Incorrect:
Mucus membranes were intact.
Correct:
Mucous membranes were intact.

Incorrect:
After delivery of the placenta, the peroneal tear was suture ligated.
Correct:
After delivery of the placenta, the perineal tear was suture ligated.

Incorrect:
A colpocentesis was performed, which revealed pooling of blood. (Colpocentesis *is not a word but sounds logical because* colpo *has to do with the vagina and the dictation concerns a gynecologic problem.*)
Correct:
A culdocentesis was performed, which revealed pooling of blood.

11–7   INCONSISTENCIES AND REDUNDANCIES

 DO   delete redundancies and repair inconsistencies and inaccuracies.

Incorrect:
The patient has no sisters and no siblings.
Correct:
The patient has no siblings.

Incorrect:
The patient fell off of the examining table.
Correct:
The patient fell off the examining table.

Incorrect:
Her appointment is on Friday.
Correct:
Her appointment is Friday.

Incorrect:
WBC was 10,000 with 71 segs, 21% lymphs, and 8% monos.
Correct:
WBC was 10,000 with 71% segs, 21% lymphs, and 8% monos.

NOTE: *A differential white blood count reveals the numbers of different white cell types in a blood sample. The total of the percentage adds up to 100%. Thus it is more accurate, as well as more consistent, to type the % symbol after each number.*

Incorrect:
Babinski negative
Correct:
Babinski present *or* Babinski absent

NOTE: *If you recognize an inconsistency or an inaccuracy but are not technically knowledgeable, ask for help.*

11–8   MISUNDERSTANDINGS

✔ DO   double-check drug names or medical words even if the author has spelled them out if you have any doubt about their accuracy.

✔ DO   determine what a foreign speaker intends to say, and when necessary, edit to preserve the integrity of the meaning of the sentence if the dictator uses grammar rules governing his or her own language.

Incorrect:
The incision was prolonged.
Correct:
The incision was extended.

Incorrect:
The patient's painful feets had disappeared.
Correct:
The patient's foot pain had disappeared.

11–9   NORMAL AND NEGATIVE FINDINGS

 DON'T   delete negative or normal findings.

Allergies: There were no known allergies to food or drugs.

11–10   ORGANIZATION AND WRITING STYLE

✔ **DO**   adjust or rephrase, but preserve the exact meaning of the author or dictator.

Incorrect:
The patient drinks several beers per day, occasional cigars and cigarettes.
Correct:
The patient drinks several beers per day and occasionally smokes cigars and cigarettes.

 DON'T   delete essential information or alter the author's style.

✔ **DO**   expand clipped sentences *(omitting articles, subjects, or verbs)* in formal documents and in documents composed of complete sentences.

Dictated:
Fluid removed but patient still short of breath.
Transcribed:
The fluid was removed, but the patient is still short of breath.

Dictated:
Tubes and ovaries removed.
Transcribed:
The tubes and ovaries were removed.

DON'T   expand most clipped sentences in chart notes, histories, physical exams, operative reports, and so on.

11–11   PROOFREADING
See Chapter 34, Proofreading and Revisions.

✓ **DO**   check for unintended expansions when you are using a text expander.

Don't let *Memphis, Tennessee,* end up as *Memphis, Tenderness,* because your abbreviation *TN* expands to cause this problem.

Rectal exam Morris should have been *Rex Morris.*

11–12   SLANG, VULGAR, AND INFLAMMATORY REMARKS
Brief forms, short forms, and medical slang that are acceptable and are commonly used by physicians are in Chapter 4, Brief Forms, Short Forms, and Medical Slang. Rules presented in this section refer to questionable language.

✓ **DO**   check with your supervisor before transcribing or editing questionable remarks.

The patient was stupid, a crock (hypochondriac), and just plain dumb.

✓ **DO**   have a written policy and procedures manual to describe exact procedures to be carried out with any questionable dictation.

The lousy surgeon used a quack treatment. The nitwit charge nurse should have brought it to my attention.

✓ **DO**   contact the author and diplomatically and tactfully question his or her use of the questionable words before they become a permanent part of the patient's medical record.

✓ **DO**   use appropriate terms for persons. Patients should be described as *infants, boys, girls, men, or women.* Terms to avoid are *male* and *female.*

Term	Age
neonate	birth to one month
newborn	birth to one month
infant	one month to one year
child	1 to 12 years
boy/girl	1 to 12 years
adolescent/youth	13 to 17 years
teenager	13 to 17 years
adult	18 years or older
man *or* woman	18 years or older

✓ DO   correct reference to parents or caregivers as *mom, dad, babysitter,* and so on.

Incorrect:
Mom says the baby has had a temp of 104°.
Correct:
The mother says that the baby has had a temperature of 104°.

✓ DO   spell out slang or short-form expressions.

Incorrect:
After repeated attempts at resuscitation, the patient went flat line and was pronounced. *(Substitute* expired *and finish the sentence with* dead *and the time of day.)*
Incorrect:
After three hours of labor, this primip's contractions fizzled out and she was sent home. *(Change to* primipara's *and consider the use of* stopped *or* diminished.)
Incorrect:
She was sent to the mental health unit for a psych eval. *(Insert* psychiatric evaluation.)

NOTE: *Check the list of short forms or slang expressions in the Appendix and see which of these are acceptable in transcription. Expressions that may be fine in an office chart note or emergency department note are not acceptable in a letter or consultation report.*

11–13   TECHNICAL ERRORS

✓ DO   correct technical errors.

Incorrect:
A *2-mm* incision was closed above the left eyebrow. *(too small)*
Correct:
A *2-cm* incision was closed . . .

Incorrect:
The baby weighed 3½ kg. *(incorrect use of metric)*
Correct:
The baby weighed 3.5 kg.

Incorrect:
There was a $2 \times 3 \times 3$ ovarian tumor.
Correct:
There was a $2 \times 3 \times 3$-cm ovarian tumor. *(This information is confirmed by the pathology report, operative report, or dictating physician.)*

Incorrect:
We removed *1800 mg* of serosanguineous fluid. *(wrong unit of measurement)*
Correct:
We removed *1800 mL* of serosanguineous fluid.

Incorrect:
The *suture* was closed with #6-0 silk sutures.
Correct:
The *wound* was closed with #6-0 silk sutures.

NOTE: *When you are working and errors such as this one occur, you will have to ask your supervisor or the author for the correct word unless you are positive you know what word was intended but not dictated.*

11–14   VERB-SUBJECT AGREEMENT
See 11–6 and Chapter 17, Grammar.

To_____ Date_____

Document#_____

Patient_____

Date of dictation_____

Type of report_____

   Please see blank   page_____

                          paragraph_____

                          line_____

         sounds like_____

☐ need spelling for drug_____

☐ need clarification of drug dosage_____

☐ need spelling for test/procedure_____

☐ need spelling for patient's name_____

☐ need patient's age_____

☐ need patient's hospital number_____

☐ need title for document_____

☐ need final diagnosis_____

☐ need clarification of surgical instrument_____

☐ year/date missing_____

☐ courtesy copy to?_____

☐ need address_____

☐ missing_____

☐ did not understand abbreviation_____   please spell out

_____

☐ please see the area of this report indicated by the penciled check-
    mark for accuracy.

☐ my edit correct?_____

Comments_____

_____

Thank you. Please return this flag with your dictation to:

Transcriptionist_____

Figure 11–1   An example of a flagging or tagging note to be appended to a medical transcript for solving problem dictation. This form may be printed on colored paper.

12

Electronic Mail

INTRODUCTION

Electronic mail (email or e-mail) is the process of sending, receiving, storing, and forwarding medical records, messages, and other forms of electronic communication (e.g., newsletters, photos, attachments, and reports) over computer networks and the Internet. Time and money are saved by using this system of sending and receiving communications. You may set the importance level of your documents by marking them if you desire to do so. When sending email, it is important to follow ethical standards and etiquette guidelines, which are listed in the following material.

12–1   ATTACHMENTS

✓ DO   add a cover note when sending an attached file, so the receiver will know to look for it.

✓ DO   avoid attachment problems by copying the text and pasting it into the body of your message.

⊘ DON'T   forward large files without compressing them.

12–2   CONFIDENTIALITY

✓ DO   observe confidentiality issues with regard to sending and receiving email messages.

DON'T   send a message that you do not want made public. Some courts have ruled that a company's email is company property, and employers are allowed access to their employees' email files.

DO   use password protection, encryption, and authentication in transmission of patients' records. Data security must be ensured.

DON'T   use or disclose protected health information without a signed consent form. *(Patients must acknowledge they understand the risks of emailing information.)*

DON'T   use patient identifiers in the subject field.

12–3   CONTENT

DO   write your message with the same tone and style as that of a business letter or memo.

DO   use an informal greeting comparable to that used for a postcard.

DO   insert a meaningful subject line for an email message.

DO   choose words carefully when expressing emotion or describing feelings in an email message. These comments can be misinterpreted because the receiver cannot see the body language or hear the tone of voice.

DO   number requests when you have more than one.

DO   use bullets to emphasize action items.

DON'T   incorporate fancy fonts; they may be received as confusing characters.

DON'T   capitalize full words in email messages; doing so implies that you are shouting at the recipient. Instead, put asterisks around sentences or phrases that you want to emphasize.

DO   use acronyms or email shorthand to convey your message if the recipient understands them. Some examples of email shorthand are *FYI (for your information)* and *ASAP (as soon as possible)*.

✓ **DO** retain portions of an original email message so the recipient can see what is referred to.

✓ **DO** snip *(delete)* text by inserting *<snip>* or *<SNIP>* where you have eliminated extraneous portions of the original message, retaining only relevant text.

✓ **DO** update the subject line when you send a reply.

✓ **DO** be careful to address the email correctly so it reaches the correct destination. There are no spaces in email addresses, and the exact configuration, with uppercase and lowercase letters, numbers, the @ symbol, and domain name tag, must be given.

> griffis@aol.com   http://www.agedwards.com

✓ **DO** end each email message with a signature file of about four lines. This file should contain your name, email address, and telephone and fax numbers. It may be optional to include your address, depending on the relationship with the recipient.

✓ **DO** use only essential punctuation.

🚫 **DON'T** use tabs or make columns, because these elements can change during electronic transmission. The recipient generally receives the message restructured, and these odd arrangements make the message difficult to read.

✓ **DO** check spelling, grammar, and accuracy.

12–4 COPIES

✓ **DO** retain copies of your messages for a specific period so you can refer to them if necessary. Some systems allow you to organize messages into files. However, if you let messages pile up in your mailbox, they can slow down the system, and it may be difficult to locate them when needed.

✓ **DO** print and file messages when there is a need for a paper record.

12–5 DISTRIBUTION LISTS

✓ **DO** include all individuals who have a legitimate need to receive the information when you distribute an email message.

✅ **DO**   suppress and blind copy *(bcc)* distribution lists when you send a document to a large group of recipients, both to cut down on the length of the document and to guard the name and address privacy of the recipients.

12–6   ETIQUETTE

🚫 **DON'T**   write anything racially or sexually offensive or sarcastic or use language that could be considered off-color.

🚫 **DON'T**   gossip or send remarks about other individuals or discuss proprietary information.

🚫 **DON'T**   write about bad news or delicate issues that would be better dealt with in person.

🚫 **DON'T**   send chain letters.

🚫 **DON'T**   respond immediately to any message that upsets you.

✅ **DO**   follow policies instituted by the employer on use of electronic mail for employees' personal correspondence.

✅ **DO**   inquire about the company's policy for subscribing to news groups or lists.

✅ **DO**   follow company guidelines for retaining and deleting email messages.

✅ **DO**   respond promptly to email messages you have received. If you are unable to give a complete response, at least acknowledge receipt and let the sender know when you will respond in full.

✅ **DO**   check your mailbox frequently—at least twice a day.

✅ **DO**   respect the sensitivity level that the sender has applied to the communication.

🚫 **DON'T**   forward personal mail unless you have the original sender's permission to do so.

✅ **DO**   credit the individual if you are quoting someone in the email message.

🚫 **DON'T**   send messages to those in your employ pointing out errors or shortcomings.

✓ DO   use "automatic reply" when you are unable to respond to your email on a regular basis, notifying the sender of your targotod roturn date.

✓ DO   keep messages short.

13

Envelope Preparation

13–1 FOLDING AND INSERTING
See Chapter 22, Letter Format.

13–2 MAILING ADDRESS

✓ DO   use the envelope feature of your computer to print the mailing address and delivery point bar code *(see 13-5)*.

✓ DO   use the nine-digit ZIP code to expedite and reduce mailing costs when using bulk mail processing.

San Diego, CA 92109-3602

✓ DO   use single spacing, and block each line at the left, giving the name of the person to whom you are writing, the street address (post office box number or rural route number), and city *(written in full)*, state, and ZIP code.

Marvin O'Connor, MD
2458 West Main Street
Dayton, OH 45439-2017

✓ DO   put the apartment or suite number after the street address or on the line above.

Mrs. Arthur Gildea
1826 Lucretia Road, Apt. 3D
Oxnard, CA 93030-8213

or

Mrs. Arthur Gildea
Apartment 3D
1826 Lucretia Road
Oxnard, CA 93030-8213

🚫 **DON'T**   place the apartment number or suite number on the line below the street address.

✅ **DO**   capitalize the first letter of each word except prepositions, conjunctions, and articles used in a name or title. The United States Postal Service optical character readers (OCRs) now read both uppercase and lowercase letters. Punctuation *(periods with abbreviations and commas)* can be read when used. Optical character readers can read both the traditional style of address and the all-cap style.

Traditional
James B. Peter, MD
4500 Oregon Street
Portland, OR 97204-2628

All-cap style
JAMES B PETER MD
4500 OREGON STREET
PORTLAND OR 97204 2628

✅ **DO**   give a two-letter abbreviation for the state name. *(See Chapter 2, Address Formats for Letters and Forms of Address; Chapter 49, ZIP Codes; and Table 1–2.)*

✅ **DO**   leave one or two spaces between the state name and the ZIP code.

✅ **DO**   list the ZIP code on the last line immediately below the city and state if space will not permit the traditional format.

✅ **DO**   type an attention line *(when one is necessary)* on the second line below the inside address starting at the left margin or as the second line of the address.

National Paper Company
Attention Frank Honeywell
1492 Columbus Avenue, North
New York, NY 10005-4101

Mail to Canada
Ms. Adrianna Marie Praycroft
Manager, Abbott Realty
1804 31st Avenue SW
Calgary, AB T2T 1S7
CANADA

International mail
Mr Tom Walters
566 Kenton Lane
Harrow Weald
Middlesex HA3 7lJ
ENGLAND
or
PROF WOLFGANG HINZ
ART DIRECTOR RHINELAND INST
SCHULSTRASSE 21
SIEGELBACH
PFALZ 6751
GERMANY

Mail to military
JONATHAN R PEZINOSKI WO
COMPANY R
5th INFANTRY REGT
APO NEW YORK NY 09801

 DO use the name of the foreign country on the last line in all capital letters.

 DO insert the private mailbox number *(rented from private company)* above the delivery address.

Mr. Steven R. Madruga
PMB 9982
115 South Olive Street
Philadelphia, PA 10101

13–3 OPTICAL CHARACTER READER

An example of address placement on an envelope for OCR processing is shown in Figure 13–1 at the end of the chapter.

 DO use the name of the institution or company name as the first line if no person's name is available.

 DO type the address block for OCR processing no higher than 2¾ inches from the bottom edge of the envelope, no lower than ⅝ inch from the bottom edge, and no closer than 1 inch from either the left or the right edges of the envelope.

137

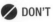

✅ **DON'T** use both post office box number and street address when both are known.

✅ **DO** use the post office box number.

✅ **DON'T** allow any notations to fall alongside or below the area established for the mailing address; material not in the proper area will interfere with OCR processing.

✅ **DON'T** use a script or italic typeface.

13–4 PERSONAL NOTATIONS

✅ **DO** list personal notations *(confidential, personal, please hold, forwarding or address service requested)* below the return name and address beginning on line 9 or on the third line below the return address. Begin each main word with a capital and align at the left with the return name and address.

13–5 POSTAL (MAILING) NOTATIONS

✅ **DO** list mailing notations *(special delivery, registered, certified, hand cancel)* in all-capital letters in the upper right corner of the envelope beginning on line 9 or on the third line below the bottom edge of the stamp. The notation should end about ½ inch from the right margin. Be sure to leave room for the postage.

✅ **DO** insert the USPS POSTNET or FIM-A *(Facing Identification Mark)* code above or below the address when mailing to US addresses. These codes are read by the USPS automated mail-handling equipment and speed mailing service. *(See Figure 13–1 at the end of the chapter.)*

13–6 RETURN ADDRESS

✅ **DO** list a return name and address in the upper left corner of the envelope beginning on line 3 about ½ inch in from the left edge.

13–7 ZIP CODE
See Chapter 49, ZIP Codes.

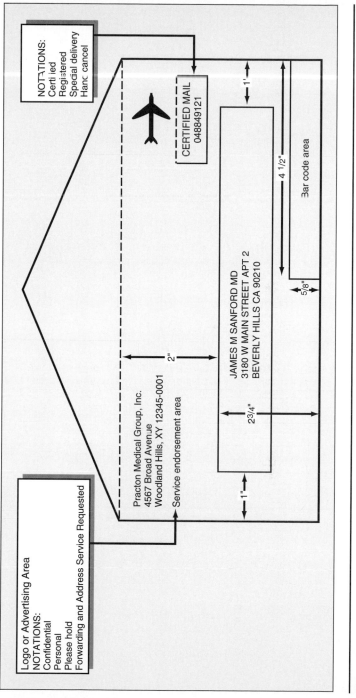

Figure 13–1 Suggested address placement on a number 10 envelope showing locations for notations and special services label.

14

Eponyms

INTRODUCTION

Medical eponyms are proper names used as adjectives to describe specific treatments, operations, surgical instruments, diseases, parts of the anatomy, laboratory procedures, and pharmacological and microbiological terms. Each of these words uses the surname of an individual who is prominently connected with the development or discovery of the disease, instrument, surgical procedure, and so forth.

This chapter is not a reference list of eponyms, but it is important that you have one. Always carefully check the spelling of these difficult terms by consulting a dictionary or other reference book. Look for the eponym by checking under the noun that accompanies it; for example, to find the correct spelling for *Abbe anemia* look under the listing *anemia*. In looking for *Pott paralysis,* look under *paralysis,* and if you cannot find it there, look under *disease*. *Syndrome* is another key word that may be used instead of *disease*. Other terms that accompany eponyms include *sign, test,* and *phenomenon*. If the eponym has a prefix, look first under that prefix and then with the prefix dropped. For example, the tumor, disease, and canals named for *von Recklinghausen* may be listed under *Recklinghausen*. If it is the stylistic preference of the author of your document who dictates the possessive form, then follow the rules for forming the possessive.

DO   capitalize all eponyms but not the nouns that accompany them.

14–1 ANATOMY

There are literally thousands of eponyms that refer to various parts of the human body. If generic terms are available to describe a body part or organ, they should be used in preference to the eponym.

 DO   capitalize an eponym that refers to a part of the anatomy and show the possessive *(s'* or *'s)* when appropriate to do so and the author dictates it.

With possessive

Stensen's duct   Bartholin's gland

Without possessive

Deiters nucleus	Flack node
Beale ganglion	Golgi complex
Broca area	Hensen body
bundle of His	Houston value
Chopart joint	islands (or islets) of Langerhans
circle of Willis	Mauthner membrane
Couvelaire uterus	Purkinje fibers

🚫 DON'T   capitalize most words derived from eponymic names.

eustachian tube   fallopian tube   malpighian bodies

14–2 DISEASES AND SYNDROMES

This list is constantly growing as new diseases are identified and named or combinations of symptoms are grouped into a new syndrome. Some diseases have a common name, an eponymic description, and an abbreviation.

HW syndrome
or
Hayem-Widal syndrome
or
acquired hemolytic jaundice

 DO   capitalize an eponym that refers to a disease, condition, reflex, crisis, ulcer, palsy, phenomenon, or syndrome and show the possessive *('s)* when appropriate to do so if the author dictates it. *(Both are illustrated.)*

Bell's palsy	Laennec cirrhosis
Biermer anemia	MacCallum patch
Shiga bacillus	Escherich's reflex
Graves' disease	tetralogy of Fallot
Hirschsprung disease	Tietze syndrome

DON'T capitalize most words *derived* from eponymic names.

Addison disease *but* addisonian
Cushing syndrome *but* cushingoid facies
Parkinson disease *but* parkinsonism

cesarean	kocherize
coxsackievirus	marfanoid
graafian	pagetic
gram-positive	skenitis

 DON'T use the possessive with an eponym if the eponym is preceded by an article.

Dupuytren's contracture
but
the Horner syndrome
the Babinski sign
a Pfannenstiel incision

☑ **DO** when writing for publication, it is preferred that the author substitute the specific descriptive term for a disease for the equivalent eponymic term. Further, if the author prefers the eponym, avoid using the possessive form. Different rules apply when writing for publication.

Preferred:
alopecia parvimaculata syndrome
Second choice:
Dreuw syndrome
Not:
Dreuw's syndrome

Preferred:
pancreatic exocrine insufficiency syndrome
Second choice:
Clarke-Hadfield syndrome

NOTE: *It is important to note that more and more writers are making exceptions to the possessive rule by not showing the possessive with an eponym. In fact, some dictionaries and other reference books may show conflicting spellings, one showing the eponym with the possessive and another showing it without.*

14–3 INCISIONS, PROCEDURES, AND OPERATIONS

 DO capitalize an eponym that refers to a particular surgical incision or operative procedure and show the possessive *('s)* when appropriate to do so and when dictated by the author.

Billroth II gastric resection
Buck operation *or* Buck's operation
Eloesser flap
Esser graft
Girdlestone-Taylor procedure
Maisonneuve amputation
Pfannenstiel incision
Roux anastomosis

14–4 MICROBIOLOGY

 DO capitalize an eponym that refers to a particular microorganism and show the possessive *('s)* when appropriate to do so and when dictated by the author.

Dutton spirochete
Epstein-Barr virus
Escherich bacillus *or* Escherich's bacillus
Whitmore bacillus
Zimmermann virus

14–5 PHARMACOLOGY

 DO capitalize an eponym that refers to a particular pharmaceutical, drug, or substance and show the possessive *('s)* when dictated by the author. *(See Chapter 10 concerning drugs and drug references.)*

Bamberger fluid
Fothergill pills
Pover powder *or* Pover's powder
Ringer's lactate *(always shows the possessive)*

14–6 PLURALS
See 31–6 in Chapter 31, Plural Forms.

14-7 POSITIONS

 DO capitalize an eponym that refers to a particular patient position for a surgical or diagnostic procedure and use the possessive *('s)* when appropriate to do so and when dictated by the author

Caldwell position
Fowler's position *or* Fowler position
Gaynor-Hart position
Rose position
Sims' position *or* Sims position
Trendelenburg position

14-8 POSSESSIVE

 DO form the possessive of eponyms that refer to parts of the anatomy, diseases, signs, or syndromes when use of the possessive is preferred by the author of the document.

Signs and tests
Ayer test *or* Ayer's test
Babinski sign
Hoffmann reflex
Anatomy
Bartholin glands *or* Bartholin's glands
Beale ganglion
Mauthner membrane
Diseases and syndromes
Fallot tetralogy *or* Fallot's tetralogy
Hirschsprung disease
Sjögren syndrome
Tietze syndrome

 DO use the possessive when the eponym closes the sentence.

The infant shows early signs of Reye's. *(syndrome is understood)*

DON'T show possession for eponyms that describe surgical instruments, are compounds, or represent the names of places or patients.

Surgical instruments
Foley catheter
Liston-Stille forceps
Mayo scissors
Richard retractors

Names of places or patients
Chicago disease
Christmas factor
Lyme disease
Compound names
Adams-Stokes disease
Bass-Watkins test
Gruber-Widal reaction
Leser-Trélat sign
Stein-Leventhal syndrome
But the following is not a compound:
Blackberg and Wanger test

NOTE: *Be careful to check the correct spelling of the name. Is it* Water's view *or* Waters' view? *(The second choice is correct.)* *Other names that cause problems are* Coombs, Deiters, Desjardines, Graves, Homans, Krebs, Langerhans, Sims, Treves, Wilkins, *and* Wilms.

14–9 SIGNS, TESTS, AND OTHER THEORETICAL KNOWLEDGE

✓ DO   capitalize an eponym that refers to a particular sign, rule, postulate, classification, test, law, theory, formula, constant, reaction, and so forth and show the possessive *('s)* when appropriate to do so and when dictated by the author.

Maurer dots *or* Maurer's dots
Babinski sign *(or reaction)*
Hoffmann reflex *(or reaction)*

Apgar score	Pfeiffer phenomenon
Bowie stain	Pignet formula
Buergi theory	Planck constant
Coombs test	Tyndall effect
Dubois method	Wassermann test

14–10 SURGICAL AND OTHER INSTRUMENTS

✓ DO   capitalize an eponym but *do not show the possessive ('s)* when the eponym describes surgical and diagnostic instruments, materials, solutions, and so forth.

Castroviejo knife	Glassman clamp
Crozat appliance	Liston-Stille forceps
DeBakey prosthesis	Mayo scissors
Foley catheter	Richard retractors
Gigli saw	Starr-Edwards valve

14–11   TREATMENT

✔️ DO   capitalize an eponym that describes a particular treatment or test and show the possessive *('s)* when the author dictates it.

Dubois method *or* Dubois' method
Balfour treatment
Ebstein diet
Fliess' therapy *or* Fliess therapy
Rollier radiation

15

Exclamation Mark

15–1 DASHES

✓ **DO** use dashes to set off an exclamation within a sentence. The exclamation mark should be placed before the closing dash.

The new staff physician–I couldn't understand him!–dictated as though he were chewing peanuts.

✓ **DO** use an exclamation point at the end of an exclamatory sentence that uses a closing dash.

STAT Transcription Service delivers the reports–on time!

15–2 PARENTHESES

⊘ **DON'T** use an exclamation point inside the closing parenthesis unless it refers to the parenthetical item and the sentence ends with a different mark of punctuation.

Be sure to send the medical report to the state hospital in Washburn, Maine (not Washburn, Wisconsin!).

✓ **DO** use an exclamation point outside the closing parenthesis if the phrase in parentheses is to be incorporated at the end of a sentence.

What a terrific outcome (a once in a lifetime opportunity)!

15–3 PUNCTUATION

✓ DO   use an exclamation point following a word, phrase, clause, or sentence to indicate a forceful statement or great surprise.

Physicians have had enough of governmental interference in medical practice!

No!

Congratulations! Your baby is completely healthy.

✓ DO   use a comma or period if the exclamation is mild.

Yes, tell Ms. Seitz to come to the office tomorrow.

Well, I think you had better deliver this good news in person.

15–4 QUOTATION MARKS

✓ DO   use an exclamation mark inside the closing quotation mark when the exclamation mark applies to the quoted material.

She keeps telling me, "I'm leaving this job!"

✓ DO   place the exclamation mark outside the closing quotation mark when the exclamation mark applies to the entire sentence.

I can't believe the sign read, "Smoking allowed"!

✓ DO   use quotation marks outside the closing exclamation mark when a quoted sentence stands alone or is at the beginning or end of a sentence.

"I won't accept that as payment in full!" I told him.

15–5 SPACING

✓ DO   use one or two spaces after an exclamation mark at the end of a sentence.

NOTE: *There is no space after an exclamation mark when another mark of punctuation* (closing quotation mark, parenthesis, or dash) *immediately follows.*

16

Faxing Documents

16–1   CONFIDENTIALITY

✓ **DO**   fax only to machines located in the secure areas of a business or office that is inaccessible by any individual not bound to a HIPAA compliance contract. The area should be locked when the fax is unattended. *(See Chapter 18 for further HIPAA information.)*

⊘ **DON'T**   fax to machines in mail rooms, office lobbies, or other open areas unless the machines are secured with passwords.

✓ **DO**   have the patient sign a properly completed authorization form for release of confidential medical information if such data must be faxed.

✓ **DO**   use a transmittal sheet with each fax transmission that includes a statement about the receiving of confidential information and that includes language clearly outlining the confidential nature of the data being transmitted. *(See Figure 16–1 at the end of the chapter.)*

✓ **DO**   monitor incoming faxes frequently to be certain confidential messages are not left *lying around* for others to view.

✓ **DO**   verify the telephone number and make arrangements with the recipient for a scheduled time of transmission or send the fax to a coded mailbox to maintain confidentiality.

✓ **DO**   notify the authorized recipient immediately upon receipt of a faxed record.

✓ **DO**   check with local hospitals and clinics about their fax policies before releasing any patient information.

✓ **DO**   monitor incoming faxes frequently to maintain confidentiality.

16–2   RECORD KEEPING (LOGGING)

✓ **DO**   keep a log of all fax transmissions indicating the date, time, and destination.

16–3   TRANSMISSIONS

✓ **DO**   use a transmittal sheet with each fax transmission indicating to whom the fax is directed, date, time, fax number, number of pages including the transmittal sheet, who the fax is from and that person's telephone number, and a confidentiality statement.

✓ **DO**   fax health information only when it is absolutely necessary to save time critical to the patient's welfare rather than using a fax for convenience.

✓ **DO**   consult an attorney to make sure documents *(contracts, proposals, outlines, charts, graphs, plans, artwork comps, or photographs)* requiring signatures are legal if faxed.

✓ **DO**   spell numbers to avoid misinterpretation when preparing a document to be faxed *(five hundred* rather than *500).*

✓ **DO**   keep fax transmissions short *(not more than 10 pages).* When you have a lengthy fax to send, telephone the recipient and ask when it is a good time to transmit.

⊘ **DON'T**   fax a patient's financial data.

✓ **DO**   program frequently used numbers into the fax machine to avoid misdirecting faxed communications.

KARL ROBRECHT, MD
Internal Medicine

ADRIANNA SACHS, MD
Cardiology

Gulf Medical Group, Inc.

800 Gulf Shore Drive
Naples, FL 33940

Telephone 813 649-1111   FAX 813 987-5121

FAX COMMUNICATION TRANSMITTAL COVER SHEET

To:_____Date:_____

Fax #_____Time:_____

Telephone #_____

Number of pages (including this one):_____

From: **Gulf Medical Group, Inc.; Karl Robrecht, MD; Adrianna Sachs, MD**

If you cannot read this fax or if pages are missing, please contact
Gulf Medical Group at 813-649-1111.

Remarks:_____

_____

Note: This transmittal is intended only for the use of the individual or
entity to which it is addressed and may contain information that is
privileged, confidential, and exempt from disclosure under applicable law.
If you are not the intended recipient, any dissemination, distribution, or
photocopy of this communication is strictly prohibited. If you have received
this communication in error, please notify this office immediately by
telephone and mail the original fax to us at the address above. Thank you.

Instructions to the authorized receiver
Please complete this statement of receipt and return to sender via this fax
number: 813-987-5121

I, _____, verify that I have received_____
        (name)   (no. of pages including cover sheet)
from **Gulf Medical Group, Inc.**

Figure 16–1   Example of a fax cover sheet for medical document transmission
illustrating a message for retaining confidentiality and a statement of receipt.

Grammar

INTRODUCTION

Although the medical transcriptionist should key exactly what is dictated, it is important to keep the rules of proper grammar in mind. Frequently, correction of grammar is necessary, but the text should be edited only to the extent that the editing does not change the intended meaning. When a statement is ambiguous, the astute medical transcriptionist will recognize the discrepancy and query the author. When the intended meaning is clear, but the text is grammatically faulty, it is vital that corrections be made to enhance clarity and readability.

✔ **DO**   go over the following when you need help with grammar.

17–1 ADJECTIVE MODIFIERS

✔ **DO**   be sure that you use an adjective to modify a noun.

aortic aneurysm *not* aorta aneurysm
mucous membrane *not* mucus membrane
urethral meatus *not* urethra meatus
hemorrhagic episode *not* hemorrhage episode

17–2 ANTECEDENTS, USE OF PRONOUNS

 DO   be sure that each pronoun has a clear antecedent; if it does not, substitute a noun for it.

Dr. Johnson observed the operation on Mr. Spokes after which he was taken to the recovery room. *(You would assume that Mr. Spokes was taken to the recovery room, but the sentence is unclear.)*
Recast
Dr. Johnson observed the operation on Mr. Spokes after which the patient was taken to the recovery room.

Pull the patient's record and notify the doctor of the emergency; then give him the record. *(You would guess that the physician is to receive the record, but this is unclear.)*
Recast
Pull the patient's record; notify the doctor of the emergency; give the doctor the record.
or
Pull the patient's record. Notify the doctor of the emergency and give him the record.

17–3 COLLECTIVE NOUNS

Collective nouns include words such as team, class, committee, group, family, jury, number, set, variety, and staff and units of measure and sums of money. These nouns take a singular verb when thought of together as a set.

 DO   use a singular verb for a collective noun that represents a single entity or set.

Then 450 mg of clindamycin was prescribed by the clinic physician.
This group of diagnoses is proposed.
The Review of Systems was negative.
He felt $500 was a lot of money.
Only twenty percent of the fluid was examined.

✓ **DO**   use a plural verb for a collective noun when the individuals making up the group are being considered.

The family were crowded into the small room.
The jury were overcome by the fumes in the hallway.
The parents, as well as the child, were reassured.

17–4 DANGLING CONSTRUCTION AND MISPLACED MODIFIERS

Words, phrases, or clauses may all be modifiers. A misplaced modifier occurs when the writer does not make clear what is being modified. In some instances, the "word" being modified may be missing altogether and so the modifier "dangles." Misplaced modifying words or phrases often produce humorous results. Therefore, you must reconstruct or recast the sentence so that all the parts are in agreement. Ambiguous or illogical placement of a modifier can usually be avoided by placing the modifier close to the word it modifies.

Sentences can become confusing when phrases are misplaced.

 DO   recast awkward sentences so that it is clear what each phrase refers to.

After recovering from a coma, the physician reassured him.
Recast:
After the patient recovered from the coma, the physician reassured him.

He was referred to a urologist with advanced pyleonephritis.
Recast:
He had advanced pyelonephritis and was referred to a urologist.

She has protruding eyes, which have been present all her life.
Recast:
All her life she has had protruding eyes.

Walking down the road, the ambulance passed me.
Recast:
The ambulance passed me as I was walking down the road.

Wishing to get to the accident, the ambulance sped through the light.
Recast:
The ambulance sped through the light on the way to the accident. *(Note also that the ambulance cannot "wish." The ambulance driver may "wish" of course.)*

Before the patients are placed on gurneys, they are thoroughly scrubbed.
Recast:
Scrub the gurneys thoroughly before patients are placed on them.

17–5 *INDEFINITE PRONOUNS*

Indefinite pronouns such as *everybody, anybody, anyone, each, everyone, nobody, no one, somebody,* and *someone* are usually singular.

 DO   use a singular verb with an indefinite pronoun.

Nobody *is* on the roster to work the p.m. shift.
Everyone *is* invited to attend the Utilization Review Meeting.

No one is going to take responsibility for leaving the file unlocked.

I hope that everybody is happy.

17–6   PARALLEL STRUCTURE

Parallel ideas must be expressed in parallel form in a sentence. This rule applies to lists as well. Each part of speech *(adjective, noun, verb, and so on)* must be matched in parallel structure.

 DO   use the same parts of speech as subjects or objects in a sentence.

Incorrect:
Learning to write is a challenge and interesting.

NOTE: *In this sentence, writing is described with an adjective (interesting) and with a noun (challenge). It would be better to use two adjectives and change the sentence.*

Recast:
Learning to write is challenging and interesting.

Incorrect:
To be accurate and meet your production level are important here.
Recast:
To be accurate and to meet your production level are important here.
Better:
It is important to be accurate and to meet your production level here

Incorrect:
Pull the patient's record, notifying the doctor of the emergency, then give the record to him and be sure to relate any information you have received.
Recast:
Pull the patient's record; notify the doctor of the emergency; give the record to the doctor; relate any information you have received.

NOTE: *Notice also that the antecedent for the pronoun* him *was unclear and so a noun was substituted.*

Because lists are often used in reports, remember to match nouns with nouns, verb with verbs, and so on.

Incorrect:
Considerations for your work station include the following:
* *Get a comfortable, adjustable chair.*
* *You should have a glare-protected screen.*
* *Ergonomic keyboards help prevent injury.*
* *It is important to have adequate room lighting.*
* *Be sure that your reference placement is convenient.*
* *If you need it, an adjustable foot rest is helpful.*
* *Adequate storage for your personal things.*
* *Keep the environment quiet or use white noise.*

Recast:
Considerations for your work station include the following:
* *a comfortable, adjustable chair*
* *a glare-protected screen*
* *an ergonomic keyboard*
* *adequate room lighting*
* *convenient reference placement*
* *an adjustable footrest*
* *adequate storage*
* *a quiet environment (or white noise)*

✔ DO   use the pairs *either/or* and *neither/nor* properly. *(These are called correlative conjunctions, and elements on both sides must match.)*

Either I get this correct or I resign myself to going over the entire document again.

Neither the consultant nor the family physician was prepared for the outcome.

Not only the emergency department but also the urgent care center was overwhelmed by the crisis.

Both the full-time staff and the per diem staff were pleased with the raise.

Incorrect:
She will be discharged to her home or go to the nursing center.
Correct:
She will be discharged either to her home or to the nursing center.

Incorrect:
She does not agree to have radiation nor chemotherapy.
Recast:
She will agree to neither radiation nor chemotherapy

17–7 PERSONAL PRONOUNS

 DO   select the appropriate pronoun on the basis of its position in the sentence.

Pronouns used as the subject of the sentence: *I, you, he, she, we, they*
Dr. Johnson and I prepared the rotation schedule together.

NOTE: *Mention yourself second if you are included.*

The residents and we could not agree on it, however.

Pronouns used as the objects of verbs and prepositions: *me, you, him, her, us, them*

She asked him to deliver the report to her and me. *(The word* him *is the object of the verb;* her *and* me *are objects of the preposition* to.*)*

She gave the reports to them and us.

Just between you and me, these often cause me to pause.

Dr. Johnson and I prepared the rotation schedule together.

However, the PM staff and we disagreed on the holiday schedule.

DON'T   use the objective form with the verb *to be (am, is, are, were, was, will be, been).* Always use the subjective.

It is *I.*
That could not have been *she* who called.
Dr. Jones said it was *he* whom we saw.
Aurora was sure it was *they* who attended the concert.
I know Robert said it was *we* who made all the noise, but I know it was *they.*

HELP: *How do you check this? Ask who made the noise. We* did *or* they *did.*

NOTE: *Sentences that contain a linking verb in the form of to be (am, is, are, were, was, will be, been, become) do not take a direct object. The object of such a verb is called a predicate complement. These linking verbs may join a plural subject with a singular complement or a singular subject with a plural complement. We must be sure that the verb agrees with the subject.*

 DO   be sure to make the correct choice when using a contraction. Spell out your contraction and you will be sure.

their *or* they're *(they are)*
its *or* it's *(it is)*
whose *or* who's *(who is or who has)*

 DO   use reflexive pronouns *(myself, herself, ourselves, yourself, himself, itself, yourselves, themselves)* to emphasize or to refer to the subject of the sentence.

She herself did not realize what was going on until too late.

You call yourself an artist?

The physician herself called that in.

Incorrect:
Give that to him and myself.
Correct:
Give that to him and me.

17–8 PLURAL PRONOUNS WITH SINGULAR ANTECEDENTS

In order to avoid sexist language, use of plural pronouns with singular antecedents is becoming acceptable, thereby avoiding the tedious repetition of *his or her* and so on.

 DO   attempt to recast the sentence, if you can, to avoid this construction.

May be acceptable:
Each medical transcriptionist must have their own books and research materials.
Correct:
All medical transcriptionists must have their own books and research materials.

May be acceptable:
Every one of the participants enjoyed learning a new method to proofread their own on-screen documents.

Correct:
The participants enjoyed learning a new method to proofread their own on-screen documents.

17–9   PLURALS AND SINGULARS

 DO   use a plural verb with compound subjects.

The patient and his parents *were* accommodated quickly by the night supervisor.

 DO   use a plural verb with plural subjects. *(Find the subject of the sentence, not just the word close to the verb.)*

The conjunctivae *were* bilaterally inflamed.
Fifteen members of the board *were* present.
Sections of the cervical tissue *show* mild dysplasia.
The urinalysis was negative, as *were* the chest x-ray and drug screen.

 DO   use a singular verb with singular subjects. *(Find the subject of the sentence, not just the word close to the verb.)*

The cost of the diagnostic procedures *is* increasing.

The scalene node biopsy *is* scheduled for tomorrow morning.

The Language of Medicine, along with three other texts, *is* recommended for study.

Bronchoscopy of the right upper lobe bronchus, right lower lobe bronchus, and left lower lobe bronchus *revealed* bronchiectasis.

 DO   be sure to match the verb to the subject and not to explanatory material that may follow the subject.

The family, both child and parents, *was* reassured. *(compound subject thought of as singular)*

The admission workup (CBC, urinalysis, and chest-ray) *was* carried out the previous day. *(singular subject)*

 DO   use a singular verb with most collective nouns *(team, group, committee, units of measurement).*

Then 450 mg of clindamycin *was* prescribed by the clinic physician.

This group of diagnoses *is* proposed.

The Review of Systems *was* negative.

Only twenty percent of the fluid *was* examined.

✓ **DO** watch for verb-subject agreement in *either/or* and *neither/nor* constructions. *(Parts of a compound subject joined by or or nor take a singular verb when the subjects are singular.)*

Neither the primary care physician nor the consultant *was* available to confirm a "do not resuscitate" order.

Either a nursing home or a skilled nursing facility *is* her destination.

NOTE: *Parts of a compound subject joined by or or nor take a plural verb when the subjects are plural or the subject closest to the verb is plural.*

Neither the Dorland's nor the specialty reference books *were* available.

Neither the specialty reference books nor the Dorland's *was* available.

Either the residents or the doctor on call *was* responsible for the change in the rotation.

Either the pathology reports or the operative report *is* left to be transcribed.

✓ **DO** watch for verb-subject agreement in not only/but also construction. *(A compound subject joined by not only/but also takes a singular verb when the subject closest to the verb is singular; use a plural verb when the subject closest to the verb is plural.)*

We found that not only the oviducts but also the uterus *was* involved.

We found that not only the uterus but also the oviducts *were* involved.

✓ **DO** use either a singular or a plural verb with *none,* depending on its use in the sentence. When *none* means *not a single one* or *no one person,* use a singular verb.

None of our staff *was* available to serve on the safety committee. *(not one)*

When none means not any or no part of, use a plural verb.

None of the members *were* available to serve on the safety committee. *(not any)*

17-10   SENTENCE STRUCTURE

 DO   use complete sentences when transcribing most reports.

> NOTE: *Clipped sentences are correct, however, when dictated in chart notes/progress reports or in the history and physical examination. Generally, the missing words are suggested and you can insert them easily.*

Clipped:
Chest clear to percussion and auscultation.
Expanded clipped (for physical exam note)
Chest: Clear to percussion and auscultation.
Complete (for a formal document):
The chest is clear to percussion and auscultation.
Clipped:
Closed with 3-0 silk sutures.
Complete:
The incision was closed with 3-0 silk sutures.

Be sure the sentence says what you know the speaker intended.

He went to the emergency department in Douglas where they told him that he had chest discomfort.
Intended:
He went to the emergency department in Douglas with chest discomfort.

She has well-documented diabetic retinopathy with hemorrhages throughout both lung fields.
Intended:
She has well-documented diabetic retinopathy with hemorrhages throughout both eye fields.

He has some transient ischemic event, resulting in the loss of his eye for a short period of time.
Intended:
He had a transient ischemic event, resulting in the loss of his vision for a short period of time.

Mrs. Johnson was diagnosed with diabetes mellitus.
Intended:
Mrs. Johnson's diagnosis was diabetes mellitus.
or
Mrs. Johnson's problem was diagnosed as diabetes.
(A disease is diagnosed, not a patient.)

There is sublingular or submandibular swelling.
Intended:
There is no sublingular or submandibular swelling. *(Left out the word no.)*

He was late because he had to see the bullet wound in the ED.
Intended:
He was late because he had to see the patient with the bullet wound in the ED. *(Patients are not referred to as their problem.)*

17–11   TENSE OF VERBS

 DO   use the past tense in the following situations:

- *in the "past history" part of a report,*
- *in discharge summaries, and*
- *in discussing patients who have died.*

The patient *has had* sciatica on the left side for the past two years.

The patient *complained* of pain in the epigastrium that radiated to the right lower quadrant. There *was* no rebound tenderness when I examined her.
Incorrect:
The patient *was seen* yesterday and *is* doing well.

 DO   use the present tense to describe the physical examination.

Abdomen: There is no rebound tenderness.

The patient has had sciatica on the left side for the past two years; this condition is now exacerbated.

Heart: There is normal sinus rhythm.
Abdomen: It is flat. There is no rebound tenderness.

Because the physical is generally typed in clipped sentences, this example generally appears as follows:

Heart: Normal sinus rhythm.
Abdomen: Flat. No rebound tenderness.

Do not use clipped sentences in formal documents such as letters and medicolegal documents.

17–12   WORD CHOICES

✓ DO   use the proper terms for persons.

In descriptions for persons, patients are described as infants, boys, girls, men, or women. Terms to avoid are *male* and *female.*

Term	Age
neonate	birth to one month
newborn	birth to one month
infant	one month to one year
child	1 to 12 years
boy/girl	1 to 12 years
adolescent/youth	13 to 17 years
teenager	13 to 17 years
adult	18 years or older
man/woman	18 years or older

It is dehumanizing to refer to a patient as a diabetic. Use *diabetic patient* or *patient with diabetes.*
Incorrect:
She is a 32-year-old female diabetic.
Correct:
She is a 32-year-old woman with diabetes.

✓ DO   be aware of the many homonyms that exist in English and medical terminology and be careful to make the proper selection

Homonyms are the most difficult of the "word demons" in both English and medical words, and a good deal of experience may be required to choose the correct term. Homonyms, as you recall, are words that are similar in pronunciation but different in meaning and spelling. A few English examples are *hair/hare, weak/week, too/two/to.* When you hear these words dictated, you know which one to choose because you know its meaning. But what happens when you do not even know that a homonym exists and you choose a correctly spelled word that is the homonym of the correct word? That possibility is what this next set of words is about: To make you aware of these words and to be on the alert for the many more that exist. Mastery of some of the more challenging homonyms can save you time and possibly embarrassment. *(The spell checker cannot make the proper choice.)*

A • An
a: used with a word that begins with a consonant or that sounds like a consonant
- a transcript
- a mistake
- a one-day turnover

an: used with a word that begins with a vowel sound and with an unsounded *h*
- an hour
- an eight-hour work day
- an outcome
- an abbreviation
- an MD degree
- an EKG

Abrasion • Aberration
abrasion: a scraping away of the surface
- She came in with multiple abrasions and contusions.

aberration: deviation from the normal course
- The patient's illness showed an aberration in his condition.

Absorption • Adsorption • Abruption
absorption: soaking up, assimilation
- There was rapid absorption of the drug into the system.

adsorption: attachment of one substance to the surface of another substance
- The charcoal was responsible for the adsorption of the poison.

abruption: a tearing away or detachment
- She experienced a placental abruption during her seventh month.

Accept • Except
accept: to receive or to take
- His family could not accept his diagnosis.

except: to leave out
- His family understood everything except the diagnosis.

Adapt • Adopt
adapt: to modify
He was able to adapt the instrument for this procedure.

adopt: to take as one's own
- plan to adopt the positive attitude held by the quality assurance manager.

Adherence • Adherents

adherence: the following of an idea; a faithful attachment; sticking to something
- The adherence of the bandage caused the patient to break out in a skin rash.

adherents: followers or believers of an advocate
- Many at the hospital are adherents to his line of thinking.

Advise • Advice

advise: to counsel, to notify *(verb)*
- Dr. Blake will advise her to have surgery.

advice: a recommendation *(noun)*
- The quality assurance manager gave her good advice.

Affect • Effect

The first step in having power over these two words is to determine how they are being used in the sentence: as a noun or verb.

Noun form: effect (result):
- Estrogen effect appears adequate for her age.

Verb form: affect (to influence): *Affect* means to produce a change but implies a lack of intent.
- The surgeon doubted that this finding would affect the final diagnosis.

This is how these words are used most of the time. But the big problem arises when we encounter the exceptions for each of these words.

EXCEPTION: effect *used as a noun. When used as a verb, the word* effect *means to bring about a change or cause a change to happen. It implies power, creation, and administration.*

- He single-handedly effected the changes in our department.

EXCEPTION: affect *used as a noun. The word* affect *is seldom used as a noun in everyday speech. In psychiatry, the noun affect (af-fect) refers to the emotional reactions associated with an experience and is generally qualified by an adjective.*

- The patient had a blunted affect.

We can now begin to exercise our power over this set. The first step when we encounter one of them is to firmly determine if it is a noun or a verb. In doing so, the correct word choice will be produced, and things will work pretty well. Because the exception for *affect* is so narrow, once you memorize the exception, this usage is no longer a problem. Now just the final hurdle is left. When do you use *effect* as a *verb*. In fact, this last "question" is usually the one to cause the problem. You can answer it by doing the following:

1. You decide you need a verb choice.
2. Now you examine just how this verb is going to be used. Remember that generally you will select *affect*; now you have to see if the exception is coming into play.
3. Does the use of *affect* denote power and so on? If not, that is the end of the thinking process. If it does, then your choice changes to *effect*.

Aid • Aide
aid: a form of help *(noun)*; to help or assist *(verb)*
• We need to readjust her hearing aid.

aide: a person who helps or assists *(noun)*
• They are going to find a home health aide for her to help with the housework.

Allusion • Illusion
allusion: an indirect reference
• I got the point when she made an allusion to the fact that we were late again this morning.

illusion: deception or misleading impression
• Combing his hair over the bald spot fails to give the illusion that he has a full head of hair!

Already • All ready
already: previously
• The transcription had already been done by the night shift.

all ready: each individual is prepared
• They were all ready for the surgery to begin.

Alternately • Alternatively
alternately: by turns *(alternating)*
• He was alternately discouraged and hopeful.

alternatively: a possible choice *(an alternative)*
• Alternatively, there is the option of doing nothing at all.

Altogether • All together
altogether: wholly, entirely, completely *(adverb)*
• The two medical cases are altogether different.

169

all together: collectively, in a group
- We must leave for the clinic tour all together.

Alumna • Alumnus
Alumna: one woman graduate
Alumnae: women graduates
Alumnus: one man graduate
Alumni: men graduates, men and women graduates collectively

Apposition • Opposition
apposition: placement of things in proximity
- The drug was in apposition to the cellular structure of the target site.

opposition: a contrary action or condition
- The neurologist was in opposition to the plan to discharge the patient today.

Appraise • Apprise
appraise: evaluate or size up
- The consultant was asked to appraise more than her current problem.

apprise: inform
- He asked Dr. Wilson to apprise the residents of the new surgical team rotation.

Assure • Ensure • Insure
assure: provide positive information; implies removal of doubt
- We will do all that we can to assure your family of the favorable prognosis.

ensure: make certain
- He is unable to ensure the results of this procedure.

insure: take precautions beforehand
- She plans to insure her travel arrangements this time.

Awhile • A while
awhile: briefly *(adverb)*
- We must wait awhile before we will be able to see the patient.

a while: a space of time *(noun)*
- It took a while for him to telephone the diagnosis to the charge nurse.

Bad • Badly

bad: acceptable when discussing illness *(adjective)*
- The patient has felt bad for several days. *(Substitute sick for bad to catch this usage.)*

badly: describes how something is done *(adverb)*
- She performed badly and was eventually fired.

Beside • Besides

beside: by the side
- He sat beside the patient.

besides: in addition to, moreover
- Besides, he was not on call.

Bolus • Bullous

bolus: a concentrated mass of a pharmaceutical preparation given all at once
- We prepared a chemotherapy bolus of several drugs to be injected intravenously.

bullous: referring to bullae, which are large vesicles containing fluid
- There were many bullous sacs scattered throughout the pleura.

Breech • Breach

breech: buttocks; a part of a gun
- The infant was delivered from a frank breech position.

breach: a gap or break
- We continued the discussion in order to avoid a breach in communication.

Bridle • Bridal

bridle: a loop; referring to part of the tack for a horse
- A single bridle suture was placed.

bridal: belonging to a bride or a wedding
- We finished our work early so we could attend the bridal shower together.

Callous • Callus

callous: hard, insensitive, uncaring *(adjective)*
- A painful, callous area appeared on the palm of her hand after a long day of gardening.

callus: hardened skin *(noun)*
- The patient complained of a solitary callus on the outside of his left heel.

Chord • Cord

chord: series of musical notes *(A chord with an* h *is the one you* hear.*)*
- He refused to leave until the final chord was played.

cord: strands twisted together *(spinal cord, umbilical cord, vocal cord)*; a cable; a unit of measurement of wood
- The vocal cords were viewed with indirect mirror laryngoscopy.

Cite • Sight • Site, see *Sight.*

Compare to • Compare with

compare to: with dissimilar things
- The pace in the emergency department was frantic compared to the placid movements of the triage clerk.

compare with: with similar things
- Compared with the rotation in the abdominal surgery unit, the rotation in orthopedic surgery was a breeze.

Complement • Compliment

complement: that which completes
- Massage therapy was a complement to the physical therapy.

compliment: admiration or praise
- He gave a compliment to each member of the committee.

Continual • Continuous

continual: repetitive, recurring
- She made continual visits to the emergency department.

continuous: unbroken, without interruption
- Her stay with the child was continuous, lasting throughout the visiting hours.

Dilate • Dilation • Dilatation

dilate: to expand or open *(verb)*
- The pupils were able to fully dilate.

dilation: the act of dilating
- She was scheduled for dilation of her esophagus.

dilatation: the condition of being stretched or dilated
- He discovered that the dilatation was not as uncomfortable as he imagined.

Discrete • Discreet
discrete: separate
- There was total involvement of the right fallopian tube and a discrete mass on the right ovary.

discreet: wise, showing good judgment
- He was being very discreet in keeping the confidential files locked.

Disinterested • Uninterested
disinterested: impartial
- We are going to need a disinterested party here to make the final decision.

uninterested: unconcerned, indifferent
- We could not understand why the parents seemed so uninterested.

Dysphagia • Dysphasia • Dysplasia
dysphagia: difficulty swallowing
- She had dysphagia following her esophageal dilatation.

dysphasia: impairment of speech faculty
- After suffering a stroke, Mr. James had dysphasia for six months.

dysplasia: poorly formed
- The child continues to have problems due to his spinal dysplasia.

Elicit • Illicit
elicit: to draw forth *(verb)*
- He attempted to elicit the appropriate response.

illicit: unlawful *(adjective)*
- It is illicit to give out information about a child without written permission from the parents or guardian.

e.g. • i.e.
e.g.: for example

- We asked for clarification of the work hours (e.g., who can plan on overtime, who will work on holidays, who is available for per diem). *(Note use of the comma.)*

i.e.: that is
- I noticed only one difference (i.e., the increased strength in her right biceps).

NOTE: *The same function can often be accomplished with a colon.*

- I noticed only one difference: the increased strength in her right biceps.

Emigrate • Immigrate (Emigrant • Immigrant)
emigrate: to leave one's country to reside elsewhere *(emigrant: one who emigrates)*
- He has yet to decide if he wishes to emigrate from Scotland.

immigrate: to reside permanently where one is not a native *(immigrant: one who immigrates)*
- The entire family recently immigrated to Russia.

NOTE: *To help you remember:* emigrant *begins with* e, *as does* exit; immigrant *begins with* i, *as does* in.

Eminent • Imminent • Immanent
eminent: famous, superior
- The speaker was the eminent surgeon, Dr. Adrianna Battencourt.

imminent: impending, about to happen
- He continues to be very fearful of his imminent demise.

immanent: present, dwelling within
- She was very serene, relating to me that perfect peace was always immanent.

Enervated • Innervated
enervated: to be weakened, debilitated
- He was enervated by just a few steps to the bathroom.

innervated: to be supplied with nerves
- That part of the arm is innervated by the ulnar nerve.

Ensure, see *Assure.*

Etiology • Ideology

etiology: all the possible causes of a disease or problem
• The etiology of the syndrome is still undetermined.

ideology: a systematic body of concepts; theories of a program
• We were unable to get a clear picture of the primary ideology of his group.

Every day • Everyday

every day: each day
• I will see the patient every day.

everyday: ordinary
• She is unable to do her everyday chores.

Every one • Everyone

every one: each one
• Every one of the diagnoses was ruled out.

everyone: all persons
• Everyone was present at the board meeting.

Farther • Further

farther: to or at a more distant or remote point in space *(distance)* or time
• He cannot think farther than his next meal.

further: additional
• I do not believe that further tests need to be carried out at this time.

Followup • Follow Up • Follow-Up

followup: the care given to a patient subsequent to a procedure (e.g., surgical or diagnostic procedure, office call, or treatment for an accident or illness *(noun)*; pertaining to care given to a patient after a specific medical service was performed *(adjective)*
• She was seen for daily followup in the hospital.

follow up: to provide patient care such as reexamination or brief history subsequent to the patient's illness, accident, or procedure *(verb)*
• I will want to follow up this problem daily for the next week at least.

follow-up: *adjective*
- Her follow-up examination was scheduled as early as possible. (*also* followup)

Formerly • Formally
formerly: earlier *(states when)*
- He was formerly a patient in the Green Valley Sanitarium.

formally: officially *(states how)*
- He was formally greeted by the president of the association.

Illusion, see *Allusion.*

Imply • Infer
imply: hint at, insinuate; what the speaker suggests
- We were afraid that he would imply that the tumor was cancerous.

infer: presume from what another said or wrote, to draw a conclusion
- From your response, I infer that you are angry.

NOTE: Infer *is what the listener takes in or perceives the speaker to be saying.*

In Toto • Total
in toto: totally; referring to a specimen sample in which an entire piece of tissue is submitted
- The specimen was removed and sent to pathology in toto.

total: entire, the whole
- The patient had total involvement of the right fallopian tube within the mass.

Incidence • Incidents
incidence: frequency
- The incidence of accidents on the ward has greatly decreased.

incidents: subordinate to something else; consequences or events
- That is likely to be one of the unfortunate incidents to expect when alcohol is mixed with driving an automobile.

Its • It's
its: belonging to it; a personal pronoun

- She noticed its smell before she noticed its appearance.

it's: it is or it has; a contraction *(one of the most commonly misused words in English)*
- It's going to take a long time for me to get used to it. (*Written out:* it is)

Last • Latest
last: final
- It was his last request.

latest: most recent
- The latest diagnosis is pelvic inflammatory disease.

Lie • Lay
lie: a falsehood *(noun and verb) (not a problem, grammar-wise, that is)*

lie: to recline *(verb) (the most incorrectly used verb in English)*
- I asked the patient to lie on the examining table. (*recline, present tense, now*)

NOTE: *The past tense of lie is lay, which we will consider next. The verb lie never takes an object.*

lay: to place *(This verb always takes an object; we have to have something to place.)*
- I asked her to lay the dictionary on the table. *(place)*

NOTE: *The present tense word lay is also the past tense of lie.*

Look at all the principal parts of *lie: lie, lay, lain, lying.* The patient was asked to lie on the table; luckily, he lay there a short time; he has lain there too long in the past and knows he will be lying here again in the future.

Look at the principal parts of *lay: lay, laid, laid, laying (place)*
I asked her to lay the dictionary on the table. Yesterday she laid it on the printer where it has been laid often in the past. The students are fond of laying it there because it is closer to the monitor and the keyboard.

Here is a hint to help you choose the correct version of the word: substitute the word *place* for your word. If it works, then *lay* or one of its principal parts fits. If it

does not fit, then *lie* or one of its principal parts fits.
(*lay:* place and *lie:* recline)
- I need to (lie/lay) this heavy box down. *(Place the box? Yes. So it is* lay *the box.)*
- The nurse said he (lay/laid) awake most of the night. *(Placed awake? No. So it is* lay *awake.)*
- I (lay/laid) the medical records on the top of the filing cabinet. *(Placed the records? Yes. So it is* laid*.)*
- He had been (lying/laying) tile for the past several years. *(Placing tile? Yes. So it is* laying*.)*
- She has never been accused of (lying/laying) down on the job. *(Placing down? No. So it is* lying*.)*

Lose • Loose
lose: sacrifice; to suffer a loss
- He was afraid he would lose his concentration with the music playing.

loose: relaxed; not dense
- She complained of nausea and loose stools.

Maybe • May be
maybe: possibly *(adverb)*
- Maybe you could ask him about it before we get our hopes up.

may be: perhaps *(verb)*
- He may be ready to start surgical rounds

Most • Majority
most: nearly all
- Most of us wanted to begin work earlier; John was a holdout.

majority: the number greater than half a total *(used with things you can count)*
- The majority of the voters said no to the proposal. Most of the eligible voters sent in ballots.

Mucus • Mucous • Mucosa
mucus: a fluid secreted by mucous membranes and glands *(noun)*
- There was thick mucus occluding both nares.
- She complained of coughing up a mucuslike substance in the morning.

mucous: resembling mucus *(adjective)*
- The mucous membranes were inflamed and reddened.

mucosa: the mucous membrane *(noun)*
- There was some tearing of the vaginal mucosa.

Nauseated • Nauseous
nauseated: to be sick
- He has been nauseated since he woke up this morning.

nauseous: to cause to be sick
- The fumes were nauseous.

Navel • Naval
navel: the umbilicus
- There was an exquisitely tender spot just to the right of the navel.

naval: having to do with the navy, ships, or sailing
- A huge naval deployment was planned for the end of the year.

Only One Of • The Only One Of • One Of
the only one of (used with a singular verb)
- He is the only one of the surgeons who was available.

only one of and one of (used with a plural verb)
- He is only one of the surgeons who were available.
- She is one of those who were always eager to respond.

Opposition • Apposition, see *Apposition*.

Palette • Palate • Pallet
palette: an artist's paint board
- Her work is said to be the results of her wide and wonderful palette.

palate: the roof of the mouth; taste
- He was able to close the cleft lip and palate with ease.

pallet: a bed; a platform for moving materials
- The pallet slipped and fell, and a splinter flew into her hand.

Past • Passed
past: recent or preceding *(adjective)*
- There was nothing in his past history to indicate he was at risk.

passed: approved or to go beyond *(verb)*
- The ambulance passed us as we hurried to the hospital.

Persons • People
persons: emphasizes the individual
- He recommended that two persons should be appointed to the committee.

people: an undifferentiated group
- She is one of those people who never speaks bad about anyone else.

Proceed • Precede
proceed: advance, go on
- She must proceed with her initial assessment.

precede: introduce, to go before
- History taking precedes the physical examination except in an emergency.

Principle • Principal
principle: rule, regulation
- We have a new class in the principles of medical ethics.

principal: main, head
- We need to turn our attention to the principal diagnosis.

Recur • Reoccur
recur: repeat, return
- He was frightened that his symptoms would recur during his holiday

reoccur: *not a word in the English language; do not use*

Regardless • Irregardless
regardless: despite
- Regardless of our advice, he checked himself out of the hospital.

irregardless: *not a word in the English language; do not use*

Regime • Regimen • Regiment
regime: a period of rule or form of government
- Nothing much can be planned during this regime.

regimen: a systematic schedule set up to improve or maintain the health of a patient
- The patient has a strict regimen to follow as soon as he is discharged.

regiment: a military unit

Repeat • Repeated
repeat: to say or perform again
- We need to repeat the sonograms as soon as possible.

repeated: occurring again and again
- She had repeated bouts of doubling-up pain.

Root • Route
root: underlying support, origin or source
- The cannula was placed near the aortic valve root.

route: a line of travel
- The route between surgery and recovery is nearly blocked with ladders and paint cans.

Sit • Sat • Set
sit: to assume a particular position; does not take an object *(sit, sat, sat)*
- You go get the car while I sit here.

sat: the past tense of *sit*
- He sat in the emergency department for three hours before being seen.

set: to place; takes an object *(The past tense is* set.*)*
- Please set the Mayo stand closer to the work area.

EXCEPTIONS: *The sun sets, and milk and pudding set.*

Sight • Site • Cite
sight: vision
- Her sight was greatly improved after the cataract surgery.

site: location
- The site of the injury was extensive.

cite: quote
- He can cite you that regulation in the hospital bylaws.

Sometime • Some Time • Sometimes
sometime: at some unspecified time

- We need to consider doing a complete physical exam sometime.

some time: a period of time
- I do think we have some time to indulge in "watchful waiting."

sometimes: now and then
- He takes a walk sometimes after his evening meal.

Super • Supra
super: (as a prefix) means over, above, more than normal, excessive; used mainly with everyday word roots
- A superabundance of medical records is waiting to be reviewed.

supra: (as a prefix) means over, above; used mainly with medical word roots *(generally refers to location)*
- There is tenderness in the suprapubic area.

Then • Than
then: at that time *(adverb)*
- We then closed the incision with #3-0 Dacron.

than: used in comparing or contrasting *(conjunction)*
- Don has always proofread on screen faster than I have.

Tortuous • Torturous
tortuous: winding, full of turns, tricky
- His right ankle was fractured on a tortuous ski trail.

torturous: painful, very unpleasant
- He spent a torturous time waiting to be rescued.

Which • That
which: a relative pronoun that introduces a nonrestrictive clause, enclosed in commas
- The instruments, which you sterilized, were not returned to the drawer.

that: a relative pronoun that introduces a restrictive clause, not enclosed in commas (Do not use in reference to persons.)
- The instruments that you sterilized were not returned to the drawer.

Use *which* and *that* for things and *who, whose, whom* for persons

- She is the patient who needed to be seen immediately.
- This is the pacemaker that I am using on Mrs. Silvanis.
- This pacemaker, which we found was not defective, was used on Mrs. Silvanis.

Who · Whom

The words *who* and *whoever* are used as subjects; the words *whom* and *whomever* are used as objects.

- To determine the correct form, first separate the clause containing the target word and disregard the rest of the sentence.

If *he, she,* or *they* would be correct, use *who* or *whoever*. If *him, her,* or *them* would be correct, use *whom* or *whomever*.
- Who/whom did you say was on call?
1. Separate the clause: *who/whom* was on call?
2. Substitute the helper pronouns: *he/she* was on call.
3. Select *who*.

- The internist, the only one whom/who we had a pager number for, arrived immediately.
1. Separate the clause: we had a pager number for *whom/who*?
2. Substitute the helper pronouns: we had a pager number for *him*.
3. Select *whom*.

Who · Whom and Verb forms with Only One Of · The Only One Of · One Of

the only one of: used with a singular verb
- He is the only one of the surgeons who *was* available.

only one of and **one of:** used with a plural verb
- He is only one of the surgeons who *were* available.
- She is one of those who *were* always eager to respond.

Workup · Work Up

workup: the diagnostic study *(noun)*
- He has to do the workup on about six more patients before he begins rounds.

work up: to perform the history and/or physical examination *(verb)*
- She will work up each of the patients for the attending physician.

Worse · Worst

worse: bad or ill to a great degree
- By morning, the patient was feeling much worse.

worst: bad or ill to the greatest degree
- I am sorry, but it is the worst possible diagnosis

18

HIPAA Guidelines

INTRODUCTION

The Health Insurance Portability and Accountability Act of 1996, usually referred to by the acronym "HIPAA," requires health care providers to safeguard an individual's protected health information (PHI). PHI refers to any part of an individual's identifiable health information that is collected by the health care provider and is maintained or transmitted by electronic media. The provider must address both privacy and security issues in maintaining and transmitting patient information. Since many medical transcriptionists are independent contractors or business owners, they are acting on behalf of the health care provider and must implement clear policies and procedures that ensure appropriate safeguards are in place to protect PHI. The independent transcriptionist that is not an employee of the provider is a "Business Associate" under HIPAA.

18–1   AMENDING PATIENT RECORDS

✓ DO   understand your office's policy on the patient's right under HIPAA to request an amendment to his or her health records.

✓ DO   know that request for amendment under HIPAA may be denied by the health care provider—be sure to get permission BEFORE you change anything!

⊘ DON'T   assume that you know the provider will automatically agree with the patient's request.

DO keep requests from patients for amendment and the health care provider's determinations for amendment in their health records, clearly documented.

DON'T amend anything in a patient's record if you are a Business Associate and directly contacted by the patient to do so.

DO direct patients to the Covered Entity's compliance officer to assist them with their amendment requests.

18–2 ELECTRONIC MAIL

DON'T email protected documents without written permission to do so by the provider.

DO observe confidentiality issues with regard to sending and receiving email messages.

DO use password protection, encryption, and authentication in transmission of patients' records. Data security must be ensured.

DON'T use or disclose protected health information without a signed consent form. *(Patients must acknowledge they understand the risks of emailing information.)*

DON'T use patient identifiers in the subject field.

18–3 FAXING DOCUMENTS

DO save and log all fax transmission and receipt confirmation reports.

DO fax only to machines located in a secure area of a business or office that is inaccessible by any individual not bound to a HIPAA compliance contract. The area should be locked when the fax is unattended.

DON'T fax to machines in mail rooms, office lobbies, or other open areas unless the machines are secured with passwords.

DO have the patient sign a properly completed authorization form for release of confidential medical information if such data must be faxed.

DON'T fax protected documents without written permission to do so by the provider.

✓ DO   use a transmittal sheet with each fax transmission that includes a statement about the receiving of confidential information and that includes language clearly outlining the confidential nature of the data being transmitted. *(See Figure 16–1.)*

✓ DO   verify the telephone number and make arrangements with the recipient for a scheduled time of transmission or send the fax to a coded mailbox to maintain confidentiality.

✓ DO   notify the authorized recipient immediately upon receipt of a faxed record.

✓ DO   check with local hospitals and clinics about their fax policies before releasing any patient information.

18–4 PRIVACY AND SECURITY

✓ DO   understand that medical transcriptionists are affected by the new HIPAA regulations, regardless of whether they are employees or independent contractors. *(See Figure 18-1 at the end of the chapter.)*

✓ DO   adhere to the federal HIPAA regulations that affect your responsibility to patient confidentiality.

✓ DO   understand that disclosure of PHI is prohibited only except as required to fulfill your contractual obligations.

✓ DO   understand and abide by individual state laws that may further provide legal protection of medical documents. Some state laws will take precedence over HIPAA regulations.

✓ DO   have a written policy and procedures manual concerning HIPAA required responsibilities. It's your duty to the health care provider since you act on their behalf!

✓ DO   know that you must have strict measures in place to guard the privacy and confidentiality of patient information.

✓ DO   use HIPAA-compliant security and privacy safeguards to manage the entire transcription process from voice capture to electronic reports.

✓ DO   maintain security with networking partners to ensure they meet HIPAA regulations.

DO   be aware that all paper records and media records must be stored, transmitted, secured, and labeled according to HIPAA regulations at all times.

DO   see that an obvious measure such as shredding protected health information when it is no longer needed is documented as policy.

DO   be aware that it is inappropriate to include a patient's name in another patient's document.

DON'T   discuss medical information with others unless there is written authorization to do so.

DON'T   carry your compliance to the extreme: a covered entity is permitted to disclose protected information for treatment, payment, or health care operations.

DO   guard the privacy and confidentiality of **all** patient information.

DO   know that you may disclose protected health information only with the patient's written consent to do so.

DO   know that you may provide access to those who do quality assurance or record review of your medical transcripts as long as there is a contract in place with the reviewer of the records outlining permission to access.

DO   know that you may give patients access to records concerning protected health information about themselves, unless you are a Business Associate.

DO   know that MTs who are employees of hospitals, private physicians offices, government agencies, and clinics must follow the policies and procedures as outlined by those organizations.

DO   seek out training regarding updates on policies and procedures by attending lectures and seminars on HIPAA.

DO   place prominent notices in your public areas regarding privacy practices mandated by HIPAA.

DO   make yourself knowledgeable about HIPAA issues so you can make appropriate modifications to your business.

DO   have a signed contract or a written agreement with all business associates and subcontractors who receive protected health information from you outlining their limits to disclose protected health information. (These are the same conditions and restrictions that protect all medical records.)

✓ DO   shred all documents when they are no longer needed.

✓ DO   keep all papers, tapes, discs and removable drives in a locked fireproof container or file cabinet.

⊘ DON'T   retain voice or text records longer than necessary and appropriate to carry out your functions.

⊘ DON'T   reuse tapes or disks unless the data are thoroughly erased.

⊘ DON'T   work at home in an area that is accessible to unauthorized individuals such as family, neighbors, delivery persons, and so on.

✓ DO   immediately report to the health care provider any instance when PHI is endangered. This includes cases of unauthorized access or theft of software, hardware, or patient data.

✓ DO   use a bonded courier when transporting medical records. The records should be sent in a sealed and tamper-proof container with no patient data information visible to the courier or any third party. Use a service that provides tracking of delivery and require recipient signature upon receipt.

✓ DO   remember that being compliant with HIPAA regulations is an ongoing process.

18–5   ROLE OF THE BUSINESS ASSOCIATE

✓ DO   determine if you are a Business Associate under HIPAA.

✓ DO   have appropriate Business Associate Agreements in place.

✓ DO   understand that even after termination of contract or Business Associate Agreement, disclosure of PHI is prohibited indefinitely.

⊘ DON'T   give patients access to records concerning protected health information about themselves. Instead, direct the patient to contact the provider's office for access.

18–6   USE OF THE COMPUTER

✓ DO   remove all PHI, if feasible, when hardware needs repair.

DO   keep a record of who accessed your software programs to resolve technical problems and/or, repaired hardware.

DO   be certain that you have completely erased your reusable media before the media are used for new dictation.

DO   make sure your computer screen is protected from unauthorized viewing by those passing your work station.

DO   carefully purge electronic files from computer hard drives.

DO   have data back-up plans for disaster and emergency recovery of data.

DO   use password protection for access to your computer and to transcription databases.

DO   monitor all user activity on your computer and document any unauthorized access.

DO   have an automatic screen saver or timed log-out of computer when left unattended.

DON'T   share passwords, not even with your family members, when you are working from home.

DO   utilize firewall protection software on your computer when working from home.

DON'T   use the same computer for Internet use and your transcription work. (There are too many viruses and, remember, your documents can become attachments in your emails without your knowledge!)

DO   acknowledge to the health care provider that you will only use the computer for transcription.

NOTE: *For further information, order* HIPAA for MTs: Considerations for the Medical Transcriptionist as a Business Associate with Sample HIPAA Business Associate Agreement *from AAMT (800-982-2182) or research online at www.hipaa.org.*

Medical Record Confidentiality Agreement

As a condition of my employment with _____,
I agree to the following provisions:

- All information received that relates to patients of this facility will be considered private, confidential and privileged.

- Patient information will not be accessed unless needed in order to perform my job.

- No patient information will be removed from the premises in any form without permission.

- Email and fax transmission of patient data will be restricted to that permitted by the facility.

- Computer passwords will be safeguarded and not posted in any public place or where they could be misplaced.

- Computer passwords will not be shared with any other employee for any reason.

- Computer passwords of other employees will not be used to log on for any reason.

- Patient information obtained while an employee of this facility will continue to remain private, privileged, and confidential even upon cessation of employment with the facility.

- HIPAA policies and regulations will be complied with at all times.

I understand that violation of any part of this agreement could result in termination of employment.

Signed_____ Date_____

Printed name_____ Witness_____

Figure 18–1   Confidentiality agreement

19

History and Physical Format

INTRODUCTION

✓ **DO** use the formats and standard outlines preferred in your locality or hospital facility. Remember that appearance and ease of readability are important considerations; however, most transcription services have a preset format for every document so you will not have to be concerned about which format to select. The formats shown in the figures here are just to give you an idea of some different types of formats and to point out that you want to be consistent with capitalization, indents, underlining, spacing, and so on, no matter what format you use.

✓ **DO** make templates, macros, and boilerplates to speed up transcription of reports. The main topics and subtopics are entered and those needed are used; the others are discarded for that document.

BIG FOUR

Medical reports referred to as the "Big Four" consist of four types of reports:

- *History and physical examination (in this chapter)*
- *Operative report (see Chapter 24)*
- *Consultation report (see Chapter 24)*
- *Discharge summary (see Chapter 24)*

19–1 CONTINUATION SHEETS

✅ **DO** key headings for page 2 and subsequent pages; use the format preferred by your employer, client, or facility. These headings would include the patient's name, medical record number, page number, and other optional statistical information *(type and date of report or name of attending physician).*

✅ **DO** key flush with the left margin or use a horizontal format.

Robert J. Newton
#45700
Page 2
or
Robert J. Newton #45700 Page 2

✅ **DO** key *continued* on the bottom of each incomplete sheet beginning with the first page when there is more than one sheet.

🚫 **DON'T** carry a single line of a medical report to a continuation page.

🚫 **DON'T** include only the signature block and closing data on a continuation page.

19–2 DATES

✅ **DO** use the date the author dictated for the heading, *not* the day it was transcribed.

✅ **DO** spell out the date in full in either the traditional or the military style.

December 22, 200X *(traditional)*
22 December 200X *(British and military)*

✅ **DO** key the dates of dictation and transcription at the end of each report on two lines below the reference initials.

DO   key in the time after the date when it is the custom to do so.

lrd *(transcriptionist's initials)*
D: 10-12-0X *(D indicates the date dictated)*
T: 10-13-0X *(T indicates the date transcribed)*

or (using the year date in full)
lrd
D: 10-12-200X
T: 10-12-200X

or (using slashes)
lrd
D: 10/12/200X
T: 10/12/200X

or (with 24-hour clock time)
lrd
D: 10/21/200X 1430
T: 10/22/200X 1020

19–3   FORMAT STYLES

Full Block Format *(See Figure 19–1, p. 206.)*

Statistical Data: As determined by the medical facility. *(In some medical transcription services, the entire statistical heading is printed for the medical transcriptionist including the patient's name, ID number, and so on.)*

Robert Sudeerlund, NO. 7659-98-45
REF: Kai Hay Fong, MD

 DO   begin all lines including headings and subheadings at the left margin.

 DO   show the history of the patient as one report with a signature line and the physical examination as a second complete report if this is the custom of the author of the document. Most are typed as a single document.

Title:	*History* or *Physical Examination* centered on the page introducing that section of the report. All capital letters.
Main Topics:	All capitals and may be underlined. On a line by itself. Begun on edge of left border.
Example:	CHIEF COMPLAINT

Subtopics:	Capitalized or all capital letters followed by a colon if the data is on the same line.
Example:	Habits: The patient is a light social drinker.
Data:	Begun on the *same* line as subtopic. Single spaced. All lines return to the left margin. Double space between the last line of one topic and the next heading.
Margins:	Narrow (½ inch to ¾ inch is appropriate).
Close:	Keyed line for signature. Author's typed name. Transcriptionist's initials. Date of dictation (D). Date of transcription (T). Time of day after the date, when requested to do so. **Example:** See Figure 19–1.
Variations:	1. Double space below main topic. 2. Subtopics grouped after heading in paragraph format.

Indented Format (See Figure 19–2, p. 208.)

This style is somewhat fussy and takes time to format but may be chosen for ease of readability.

Statistical Data:	As determined by the medical facility.
Title:	*History* or *Physical Examination* centered on the page introducing that section of the report. All capital letters, may be underlined.
Main Topics:	All capitals, underlined, followed by a colon. Begun flush with the left margin.
Subtopics:	All capitals, followed by a colon. Indented one tab stop (or five spaces) under main topics.
Data:	Begun on the *same* line as the topic or subtopic. First *and* second lines tabulated to an indentation of 25 characters or spaces, which is the 2.5 tab stop. To prepare the tab stops for this format,

clear all tabs and set the first tab stop at 0.5, the second at 2.5, and the third at 4.0. These will clear the outline when you are ready to tabulate. *Third* and *subsequent* lines brought back to the left margin *(as long as they clear the outline—if too brief, block under first two lines)*.

Example

SOCIAL: She does not smoke or drink. She lives with her husband who is an invalid and for whom she cares. She is a retired former municipal court judge.
Single spaced.
Double space between topics.

Margins: Narrow (½ inch to ¾ inch).

Close: Keyed line for signature at the tab stop of 4.0.
Dictator's typed name.
Transcriptionist's initials.
Date of dictation (D).
Date of transcription (T).

Variations: 1. No underlining.
2. Subtopics not indented. *(Not indenting subtopics makes this format quicker and easier to do.)*

✓ **DO** **begin all data single spaced on the same line as the topic or subtopic.**

SOCIAL: She does not smoke or drink. She lives with her husband, who is an invalid and for whom she provides care. She is a retired municipal court judge.
or
SOCIAL: She does not smoke or drink. She lives with her husband, who is an invalid and for whom she provides care. She is a retired municipal court judge.

Modified Block Format *(See Figure 19–3, p. 210.)*

Statistical Data: As determined by the medical facility.
Title: *History* or *Physical Examination* centered on the page introducing that section of the report.
All capital letters.

Main Topics:	All capitals, followed by a colon. May be underlined. Begun on edge of left border.
Subtopics:	Indented one tab stop (five spaces) under main topics. All capitals, followed by a colon.
Data:	Begun on the same line as the topic or subtopic. Data input begun at the 2.5 tab stop after the heading. *(All other data are tabbed and blocked to this same point under the previous line. The initial tab at this place is adequate so that all data are evenly blocked.)* Single spaced. Double space between the last line of a topic and the next heading.
Margins:	Narrow (½ inch to ¾ inch).
Close:	Keyed line for signature. Dictator's typed name. Transcriptionist's initials. Date of dictation (D). Date of transcription (T).
Variations:	1. No underlining. 2. Single space between subtopics. 3. No indent on subtopics

Example

CHIEF COMPLAINT:	Prolapse and bleeding after each bowel movement for the past 3-4 months.
PRESENT ILLNESS:	This 68-year-old white female says she usually has three bowel movements a day in small amounts, and there has been a recent change in frequency, size, and type of bowel movement she has been having. She is also having some pain and irritation in this area. She has had no previous anorectal surgery or rectal infection. She denies any blood in the stool itself.

Run-on Format (See Figures 19–4 and 19–5, pp. 211 and 212.)

The run-on format is the easiest to do and that may be why it is the most popular. Often we have no choice but just need to know how to follow the proper pattern for whatever format we do carry out.

Statistical Data:	As determined by the medical facility.
Title:	*History* or *Physical Examination* may be centered on the page or flush left. All capital letters.
Main Topics:	All capitals, followed by a colon. Begun flush with the left margin.
Subtopics:	Uppercase and lowercase, followed by a colon. Data continued within the paragraph.
Data:	Begun on the same line as the outline, a double space after the colon. Single spaced. Double space between topics.
Margins:	Narrow (½ inch to ¾ inch).
Close:	Keyed line for signature. Dictator's typed name. Transcriptionist's initials. Date of dictation (D). Date of transcription (T).
Variations:	1. Single space between topics. 2. Topics on a separate line not closed with a colon. 3. Subtopics begun on a separate line and typed in caps, not closed with a colon.

Allergies

 DO   key in all capitals, underline, and/or use bold font when the patient has allergies to food or drugs.

PAST HISTORY
Illnesses: The patient had polio at age 8, from which she has made a remarkable recovery. She was paralyzed in the right lower extremity and now has use of it.

Allergies: **ALLERGIC TO PENICILLIN.** She denies any
other drug or food allergies.
or
PAST HISTORY:ILLNESSES: The patient had polio at age
8, from which she has made a remarkable recovery. She
was paralyzed in the right lower extremity and now has
use of it.
ALLERGIES: **ALLERGIC TO PENICILLIN.** She denies any
other drug or food allergies.

Diagnosis

 DO   spell out any abbreviations in the diagnosis part of a history
and physical.

Incorrect:
DIAGNOSIS: ASHD
Correct:
DIAGNOSIS: Arteriosclerotic heart disease

 DO   use numbering if dictated; it is optional if not dictated.

DIAGNOSES: Gastritis.
               Pancreatitis.
or
DIAGNOSES
1. Gastritis.
2. Pancreatitis.

DON'T   use a number if there is only one diagnosis.

19–4 HEADINGS

 DO   key in all capital letters for major headings followed by a
colon; do not use a colon if the heading is on a line by itself.
Format determines if you underline or put the main topic on
a line by itself.

HEENT
There is marked hypertrophy of the nasal turbinates with
obstruction of the airways. The conjunctivae were not
injected. The tonsils were hypertrophic but did not appear
actively infected.

19–5 INTERVAL HISTORY OR NOTE
A complete history and physical does not have to be done to follow
up a patient who is being admitted within a month after discharge
from the hospital and who is being readmitted. An interval history
or note *(see Figure 19–6, p. 213)* may be dictated. The present com-

plaint and interval history are emphasized in the report. The physical examination would include any new findings since the last examination and may also include a brief check on vital body systems. A more extensive examination would be done if the patient were readmitted to the hospital for a completely new problem or extended stay.

19–6 MARGINS

✓ DO   use ½-inch to ¾-inch margins both right and left and top and bottom. Ragged right margins are preferred over justified margins.

⊘ DON'T   justify the right margin in medical reports.

⊘ DON'T   hyphenate at the end of a line *(except for words with hyphens)* for enhanced readability.

19–7 NUMBERING

✓ DO   number all or none of the entries when typing if the dictator numbers some but not all items in a series. Be consistent.

> MEDICATIONS: 1. Mylanta 1 tsp a.c.
>   2. Mellaril 25 mg q.i.d. in liquid form.

19–8 OUTLINES

⊘ DON'T   use abbreviations unless they are approved by the author of the document or your employer.

✓ DO   key in main headings whether dictated or not and insert those subheadings as dictated. The following are standard headings. Main headings are typed in all capital letters. Subtopics are capitalized.

> HISTORY
> CHIEF COMPLAINT
> HISTORY OF PRESENT ILLNESS
> PAST HISTORY
> ALLERGIES
> Medications
> Immunizations
> Habits
> Social
> Family
> Medical

Surgical
Psychiatric
Alcohol and Substance Abuse
REVIEW OF SYSTEMS
General
Skin
Head
Eyes
Ears
Nose
Mouth and Throat
Neck
Breasts
Respiratory
Cardiac
Gastrointestinal
Genitourinary
Gynecologic
Musculoskeletal
Neurologic
Hematologic
Endocrine
Psychiatric
PHYSICAL EXAMINATION
GENERAL
VITAL SIGNS
SKIN
HEAD, FACE, NECK
HEAD, EYES, EARS, NOSE, AND THROAT (*or abbreviated*
HEENT.)
MOUTH, THROAT, TEETH
NECK
LYMPH NODES
THORAX AND LUNGS
BREASTS
HEART
ABDOMEN
PELVIS
PERIPHERAL VASCULAR
MUSCULOSKELETAL
EXTREMITIES
NEUROLOGIC
PSYCHIATRIC
FINDINGS
DIAGNOSIS
PLAN

19–9 PARAGRAPHS

✅ DO   Insert a new subtopic title to separate narrative blocks within sections when emphasis shifts; all paragraphs have a heading.

19–10 PAST AND PRESENT TENSE

✅ DO   use the past tense in the past history part of a report, in the discharge summary, or to discuss a patient who has died.

PAST HISTORY: His only previous illnesses were tonsillitis, measles, and chickenpox with no complications or sequelae.

✅ DO   use present tense when describing the current illness or disease in the history and physical.

PRESENT ILLNESS: The pain is mainly in his right lower quadrant. He has never had an attack like this before. He is urinating without discomfort. There is no splitting or deviation of the stream.

19–11 REFERENCE INITIALS

✅ DO   use a double space below the typed signature line and type initials flush with the left margin.

✅ DO   key the author's, the signer's, and the typist's initials when the author differs from the person who signs the history and physical.

mjp/lrc/wpd *or* mjp:lrc:wpd
(Here, mjp *stands for the dictator,* lrc *stands for the signer, and* wpd *stands for the typist.)*

✅ DO   use either all capital letters or all lowercase letters for both sets of initials, with a colon or virgule between the initials

🚫 DON'T   use humorous or confusing combinations of reference initials.

crc *(rather than* cc*)*
db *(rather than* dmb*)*
dg *(rather than* dog*)*

19–12 SHORT-STAY RECORD
When a patient is admitted for 48 hours or less *(diagnostic or minor operative procedure)*, a shorter form of the history and physical examination record is acceptable in most hospitals *(see Figure 19–7, p. 214).*

19–13 SIGNATURE LINE

✓ DO   leave three blank lines below the last line of the report and key the signature line; placement should be consistent with the format of the report.

✓ DO   key the author's full name. It is optional to insert a line for the signature. If a title is required, put it directly below the dictator's name.

19–14 SPACING OF HEADINGS

✓ DO   use double spacing between the last line of one section and the next heading. It is optional to use no space below the main topic. When data are dictated without a heading, insert the heading for clarity.

19–15 STATISTICAL DATA

✓ DO   include the required information and use the format preferred by your employer and/or hospital facility. The following is statistical data that may or may not be listed.

Patient's name
Age and date of birth
Date of admission
Date of dictation
Medical record number
Hospital room number
Insurance plan or coverage
Name of attending physician
Name of referring physician
Name(s) of anyone who is to receive a courtesy copy of the report

19–16 SUBHEADINGS

✓ DO   key subheadings in all capital letters or uppercase and lowercase followed by a colon. It is optional to begin each subtopic on a separate line. Subheadings not dictated may be inserted, but this too is optional.

HEENT
EYES: Pupils are equal and react to light and accommodation.
EARS: Tympanic membranes are intact.
NOSE AND THROAT: Essentially unremarkable.

or

HEENT: Eyes: Pupils are equal and react to light and accommodation. Ears: Tympanic membranes are intact. Nose and throat. Essentially unremarkable

 DO   be consistent in numbering. Either number all items or none of them.

 DO   double-space between major sections of medical reports.

DON'T   space between subheadings that are listed vertically.

REVIEW OF SYSTEMS
Eyes: No double vision.
Ears: No ringing of the ears.
Gastrointestinal: No weight change. No change in bowel habits or any blood in bowel movements.
Genitourinary: No difficulty urinating. No blood in the urine.
Cardiac: Denies any chest pain or radiation of any pain into left arm.

DON'T   use a hyphen or dash instead of a colon following a heading or subheading.

Incorrect:
CHIEF COMPLAINT–Acute onset, severe abdominal pain and indigestion.
Correct:
CHIEF COMPLAINT: Acute onset, severe abdominal pain and indigestion.
Also correct:
CHIEF COMPLAINT
Acute onset, severe abdominal pain and indigestion.

DO   use a colon after a heading or subheading when the data continue on the same line as the heading.

FAMILY: There is no family history of breast cancer.

19–17 *TITLES*

DO   center all titles on the page and key in all capital letters. Underlining the title is optional.

Interval History

ADMIT NO: 7802870
MR NO: 787307
PATIENT: REZNEK, MARYLOU

DATE: 07/18/OX
DOB: 08/03/XX SEX: F AGE: 68
PCP: JENNI APONTE, MD

HISTORY

CHIEF COMPLAINT
This 68-year-old lady was brought to the emergency room by the parmedics this evening.

HISTORY OF PRESENT ILLNESS
She apparently came out of a swimming pool complaining of chest pain, difficulty breathing and collapsed. The paramedics were called. The patient was described as gurgling. The patient had collapsed to the floor and was described as having vomited and aspirated. The patient could not be intubated due to a clenched jaw. Blood pressure was recorded 280/140. The patient was transported to the ER where she was noted to be in pulmonary edema with hypertension, hyperglycemia and respiratory distress. The patient's symptoms have been relieved with nitroglycerin and BiPAP. Initial enzymes are normal. Blood sugar is 260.

PAST HISTORY
The patient apparently has been a life-long cigarette smoker. She has been treated for hypertension with unknown medications. Her only listed medication is Glyburide for diabetes for three years. The family brings in medicine bottles that are up to 15 years old. The patient does not appear to take most of these medications on a regular basis. There is outdated tetracycline, as well as Darvocet N, which is 15 years old, and penicillin, which is also out of date.

SURGICAL: The patient apparently has had multiple surgeries, but the nature of these is uncertain. She indicates she has had nine surgeries.

ALLERGIES: She has no known drug allergies or sensitivities.

HABITS: She currently smokes ten cigarettes a day.

FAMILY HISTORY: Not available.

REVIEW OF SYSTEMS: A review of systems is not possible.

PHYSICAL EXAMINATION

GENERAL
The patient is a well-developed, heavyset elderly lady. She is presently resting comfortably on BiPAP 15/5, FiO2 of 1.0. She arouses and seems to be oriented to person and place. She is afebrile to touch.

VITAL SIGNS
Pulse is 110 per minute and regular, blood pressure 140/80, respirations 25, pulse ox 97%.

HEENT
Normocephalic. The sclerae are without evident icterus. Conjunctivae are well perfused. The mucous membranes are moist. BiPAP mask is in place and is fairly well tolerated.

Figure 19–1 Example of a full block format

ADMIT NO: 7802870
MR NO: 787307
PATIENT: REZNEK, MARYLOU

DATE: 07/18/OX
DOB: 08/03/XX SEX: F AGE: 68
PCP: JENNI APONTE, MD

Page 2 H&P

NECK
Without jugular venous distension. The trachea is in the midline.

THORAX AND LUNGS
Symmetrical on auscultation. There are bilateral rales and some rhonchi. Wheezes are not heard. Cardiac tones are distant. The rhythm is rapid and regular. Possible third heart sound is present along the left sternal border.

ABDOMEN
Soft, slightly distended and tympanitic to percussion. Organomegaly is not evident. Multiple surgical incisions are well healed from remote procedures.

EXTREMITIES
Absence of edema. There are some stasis changes about the ankles. Dorsalis pedis and posterior tibial pulses are present bilaterally. Toes are downgoing on plantar stimulation bilaterally.

LABORATORY
Troponin-I less than 0.6. CPK 111. Urinalysis clear except for 100 mg% protein. Blood gases pH 7.22, pCO2 60, and pO2 66. Subsequently on BiPAP, pH 7.24, pCO2 58, pO2 146.

Electrocardiogram shows a sinus tachycardia, left atrial enlargement and nonspecific ST-T wave abnormalities.

Blood sugar 263, BUN 13, creatinine 1.0, sodium 139, potassium 3.9. White count 14,600, hemoglobin 16.5, hematocrit 50.

IMPRESSION
1. Pulmonary edema, probably precipitated by hypertension with resultant respiratory failure.
2. Hypertension.
3. Diabetes.
4. Probable aspiration.
5. Probable chronic obstructive pulmonary disease.

DISCUSSION
The patient will be admitted to the Intensive Care Unit. She will be continued on her nitroglycerin drip, given morphine if necessary, in addition to Pepcid, nifedipine, Lovenox. Clindamycin will be started after obtaining a sputum specimen for culture and sensitivity. Followup laboratory work will be obtained in the morning.

Ralph P. Huber, MD

RPH:rlo
D: 07/18/200X 23:13:00 #687
T: 07/19/200X 10:27:58 #17116

CC: MILLER, KENNETH MD
    APONTE, JENNI MD

Figure 19–1   Cont'd

RE: Coselli, Ralph   DOB: 9-27-XX

June 5, 200X

HISTORY

CHIEF COMPLAINT: This 26-year-old male was a passenger in
                                    a vehicle on 02/29/0X when the car was
broadsided and spun around again by a semi-trailer truck. The vehicle was thrown
into the center divide. He was wearing a seat belt, but struck his head against the
window. He had the sudden onset of neck pain and some low back pain over
the next 24-48 hours.

HISTORY OF PRESENT ILLNESS: He has noted increasing pain in his neck and
                                    has difficulty moving. The pain is located at
the base of the skull, radiating infrascapularly. It is an aching pain which is moderate
in the morning and more severe at night. It is aggravated by coughing, sneezing,
prolonged sitting. The headaches are not associated with any nausea or vomiting.
There is no history of syncope. The back pain is in the lumbar region, radiating to
the buttocks, a constant aching pain which is moderate in the morning and more
severe at night, aggravated by sitting. The patient has been fatigued, irritable, has
nightmares. He has been taking Tylenol, with little relief.

PAST HISTORY
        Medical: Noncontributory.
        Surgical: None.
        Accidents: None reported.
        Allergies: None.
        Medications: Tylenol.
        Social: The patient is a flight attendant. He is
                            married without children. He does not
                            smoke and rarely drinks alcohol.
        Family: Noncontributory.

PHYSICAL EXAMINATION

GENERAL: The patient is a well-developed, well-nourished
                            young man in no acute distress at this time.

VITAL SIGNS: BP 130/60. Height 72 inches. Weight 198 lb.

SKIN: Symmetrical and normal with respect to color
                            and temperature without atrophy; normal
                            hair growth.

HEENT: Eyes: Pupils are equal and reactive to light
                            and accommodation. Conjunctivae clear.
Funduscopic examination reveals no hemorrhage or exudate. Extraocular movements
are intact. Mouth: Oral mucosa is clear. Trachea is midline. Neck: Supraclavicular
fossae empty and thyroid not palpable. No lymphadenopathy noted.

LUNGS: Clear to auscultation and percussion. No rales,
                            rhonchi or extra sounds. Quiet precordium.

Figure 19–2   Example of indented format.

RE: Coselli, Ralph
page 2, H&P

CARDIAC: The PMI is within the midclavicular line.
                            No rubs, gallops or murmurs. Normal sinus
                            rhythm. Heart sounds appear normal.

ABDOMEN: Soft, without organomegaly. Liver, kidney
                            and spleen not palpable. Abdomen is
tympanic to percussion, without rebound. Bowel sounds normoactive. No
lymphadenopathy or inguinal hernia noted.

RECTAL/GENITALIA: Deferred.

EXTREMITIES: No cyanosis, clubbing, spooning, or
                            peripheral edema. Good peripheral pulses.

MUSCULOSKELETAL:
        Cervical spine: There is pain on palpation of the occipital
                            prominences bilaterally and the paraspinal
muscles at the C4 through C6 level and the trapezius muscles, primarily on the left,
are painful to palpation (the patient winces and pulls away). There is markedly
diminished range of motion with lateral rotation of 30° bilaterally. Anterior flexion,
chin-to-chest, is limited at four fingerbreadths. Cervical compression positive with
pain at the C5-6 level. There is weakness on anterior flexion of the neck musculature.
The deltoids, biceps and triceps are normal.

        Lumbar spine: There is pain on palpation at the L4-5 level
                            with full anterior flexion to 80°. Straight leg
                            raising negative; toe/heel walking normal.

NEUROLOGIC: Symmetrical deep tendon reflexes, vibratory
                            sense, position sense and pinprick; cranial
                            nerves and cerebellar examination grossly
                            intact.

DIAGNOSES: 1. Cervical spraining injury, moderately severe.
                            2. Lumbar spraining injury, moderate.
                            3. Blunt trauma to the skull; no evidence
                               of concussion.

DISCUSSION AND PLAN: This patient appears to have suffered mostly
                            a cervical spraining injury and will be treated
with physical therapy. X-rays of the spine will be reviewed and Parafon Forte
provided for pain relief. The patient will be reevaluated in one to two weeks.

Evans T. Orr, M.D., Inc.

rgk
D: 6/20/0X
T: 6/21/0X

Figure 19–2   Cont'd

PATIENT: Stephen Shess   RECORD#: 17-65-00
DOB: 2-17-0X
REF: William A. Berry, MD

HISTORY

DATE OF ADMISSION: June 1, 200X

CHIEF COMPLAINT: Tongue-tied.

HISTORY OF PRESENT ILLNESS: This is a 3-year-old Caucasian male being admitted to Children's Hospital for an elective frenuloplasty. The patient has been known to have limited tongue motion since birth. When examined, the patient was noted to have a mobile anterior tongue, which extended to the lips. The parents were told that frenuloplasty was elective and not mandatory, and that speech articulation could still meet the requirements with the assistance of a speech therapist. Despite this, the parents desire to have this procedure performed.

PAST MEDICAL HISTORY

     SURGICAL: Negative.

     ALLERGIES: Negative

REVIEW OF SYSTEMS: Negative.

PHYSICAL EXAMINATION

HEENT: Negative otoscopic and rhinoscopic examination. Oral examination reveals the presence of a tied frenulum with mobility of the anterior tip of the tongue to the lips. Presently, speech articulation appears to be acceptable.

NECK: Supple, without adenopathy.

LUNGS: Clear to auscultation and percussion.

HEART: Normal sinus rhythm without murmur.

ABDOMEN: Soft, nontender, without masses or organomegaly; bowel sounds within normal limits.

EXTREMITY: Grossly within normal limits.

DIAGNOSIS: Tongue tied.

PLAN: 1. Admit to Children's Hospital.
     2. Elective surgery

ret   _____
     Kyle Singh, MD

D: 6/1/0X
T : 6/1/0X

Figure 19–3   Example of modified block format.

TITLE OF NOTE: H&P
SOCIAL SECURITY NUMBER: 532-07-1199
VISIT DATE/TIME: 09/21/0X@1623
AUTHOR: Moira Jordan, MD
CLINIC NAME: UROLOGY/ONCOLOGY
DATE OF NOTE: 09/21/0X @1623

PATIENT NAME: CARUFEL, DAVID

HISTORY: The patient is a new patient to our clinic having sought to transfer his care to the VA. He was diagnosed with prostate cancer by Dr. Harold Hamlyn by biopsy in 200X or so. He was placed on watchful waiting. His PSA has varied between 9 and 25 since the time of diagnosis. The last PSA that he can recall was 9.6 in May 1999. He has had no PSA and no laboratories drawn here. He denies voiding complaints, specifically he reports a good force of stream and no obstructive symptoms; however, he does have nocturia x2 to x3. He denies hematuria.

PAST MEDICAL HISTORY
1.   Hypercholesterolemia.
2.   Coronary artery disease status post angioplasty in 2003 and status post coronary artery bypass grafting x2 in 2001.
3.   Glaucoma.
4.   Cataracts, bilaterally, status post vitrectomy.

MEDICATIONS
1.   Zocor.
2.   Baby aspirin.
3.   Glaucoma eye drops.

ALLERGIES: **PENICILLIN.**

SOCIAL HISTORY: The patient denies tobacco and alcohol use.

PHYSICAL EXAMINATION: Reveals a viable pleasant man in no apparent distress. There is no costovertebral angle tenderness. The abdomen is benign. The penis is circumcised and normal. The testes are normal bilaterally; however, there are bilateral varicoceles, right greater than left in size. Digital rectal examination reveals a firm prostate bilaterally consistent with stage 3 prostate cancer.

ASSESSMENT: Prostate cancer. Watchful waiting is a good option as is expectant therapy. We will check a PSA and a chem 7 today. I will also check an ultrasound given the physical finding of the right varicocele to rule out any renal abnormality. We may consider a bone scan in the future though I think it is very unlikely that he has bony metastasis at this time. Now that we have him in our clinic, we can follow serial PSAs. We will see him in six weeks after the ultrasound.

Moira Jordan, MD

D: 09/21/0X 1623
T: 09/22/0X 1142
EL/TR73/PP/61407

Figure 19–4   Example of run-on format.

JOHN MICHAEL ZELLER, JR.   RECORD Z-842-98-12

HISTORY

CHIEF COMPLAINT
This is a 26-year-old man who complains of an approximately eight-month history of
recurrent nasal congestion with frequent sneezing and eye tearing.

HISTORY OF PRESENT ILLNESS
Patient notices most while at work and also in the mornings on the weekdays but not on
the weekends. He will have a large amount of clear nasal discharge with sneezing. This is
unaccompanied by fever, sinus tenderness, ear fullness, cough or shortness of breath. He
does have occasional frontal headache. He has used Sudafed for this with some relief.
He does not notice any specific precipitants, specifically, change in temperature, humidity,
alcohol. He states he keeps his house clean with frequent vacuuming, dusting and washes
the bed sheets frequently.

PAST HISTORY
He has no history of asthma. Patient also complains of a number of warts on his right
forearm and fingers for the past couple of years. No operations. He does have chronic
low back pain for which he has been treated in the past with physical therapy.

Allergies: None.

Medications: None.

Family History: His mother is 60 years old with coronary artery disease and hypertension.

Social History: Patient works as a CEO in a local electronics firm. He is married without
children. He does not smoke and rarely drinks alcohol.

REVIEW OF SYSTEMS
Unremarkable.

PHYSICAL EXAMINATION

VITALS
Vital signs normal. This is a well-appearing man.

SKIN
Exam reveals several verrucae vulgaris. Two, half-centimeter lesions on the right anterior
wrist and a few smaller ones on the index and second fingers.

HEAD AND NECK
Exam revealed no sinus tenderness, The ears were clear. The nasal mucosa was normal
appearing; there were no swollen turbinates or polyps. Throat was clear. Neck was supple.

DIAGNOSIS
Patient's symptoms are that of most likely vasomotor rhinitis, although I cannot rule out
allergic rhinitis at this time.

PLAN: I have suggested that the patient use Seldane twice a day and Ocean Spray nasal
spray twice a day for the next three weeks on a trial basis. If this does not result in
improvement, we will consider a steroid nasal inhaler. I have applied liquid nitrogen to
the warts on his arm and referred him to Dermatology for followup of the warts. I will
see him back in one month. He will get a cholesterol screening today.

jbtr
D: 05/14/0X
T: 05/15/0X   Jorge R. Gonzales, MD

Figure 19–5   Example of medical clinic run-on format.

Children's Hospital and Health Center
1234 Children's Way • Blue Flower, XX 09090

Patient: Robert R. Kern

Date of Admission: 06/08/200X

H19413571

DOB: 01/13/200X

ADMITTING PHYSICIAN: Judith B. Thornberg, M.D.

INTERVAL HISTORY

HISTORY OF PRESENT ILLNESS

Robert is a 3-year-old with rhabdomyosarcoma involving the left inferotemporal fossa. He underwent an initial incisional biopsy on May 17, 200X, and received his first course of chemotherapy shortly thereafter. He developed drainage from the incisional area proximal to the left ear which showed Pseudomonas, and he was admitted for antibiotic therapy. He is currently receiving radiation therapy to his lesion. He is due at this time to be admitted for his second course of chemotherapy with vincristine and Cytoxan. His mother reports no additional concerns at this time.

PHYSICAL EXAMINATION

VITAL SIGNS AND STATISTICS: Physical examination revealed a weight of 16.3 kg, a height of 97 cm, temperature 97.7, pulse 115, respirations 26, blood pressure 110/46.

GENERAL: He is a somewhat small-appearing Caucasian male.

SKIN: Skin examination reveals no rashes.

HEENT: Examination reveals swelling over the left side of the face, which is still prominent. The suture line is well-healed. His left eyelid continues to droop, although he does open it more than he was previously opening it. The TMs are clear. Mouth and throat are clear.

CHEST: Clear to auscultation. There is an indwelling right atrial catheter.

LUNGS: Clear.

HEART: Regular rate and rhythm.

ABDOMEN: Soft without tenderness to palpation or hepatosplenomegaly.

EXTREMITIES: Normal.

NEUROLOGIC: Neurologic examination reveals a left seventh nerve paresis.

IMPRESSION: Rhabdomyosarcoma of the inferotemporal region, status post incisional biopsy and one course of chemotherapy with continuing radiation therapy and today is being admitted with vincristine and Cytoxan.

_____

Judith B. Thornberg, M.D.

nr15-32987

D: 06/08/200X 11:00

T: 06/08/200X 12:17

Figure 19–6   Example of an interval history.

Children's Hospital and Health Center
1234 Children's Way • Blue Flower, XX 09090

Patient: Robert R. Kern
Date of Admission: 06/08/200X

H19413571
DOB: 01/13/200X

ADMITTING PHYSICIAN: Judith B. Thornberg, M.D.

SHORT STAY RECORD

HISTORY

Robert is a 3-year-old with rhabdomyosarcoma involving the left inferotemporal fossa. He underwent an initial incisional biopsy on May 17, 200X, and received his first course of chemotherapy shortly thereafter. He developed drainage from the incisional area proximal to the left ear which showed Pseudomonas, and he was admitted for antibiotic therapy. He is currently receiving radiation therapy to his lesion.

PHYSICAL EXAMINATION

VITAL SIGNS AND STATISTICS: Physical examination revealed a weight of 16.3 kg, a height of 97 cm, temperature 97.7, pulse 115, respirations 26, blood pressure 110/46.

GENERAL: He is a somewhat small-appearing Caucasian male.

SKIN: Skin examination reveals no rashes.

HEENT: Swelling over the left side of the face, which is still prominent. The suture line is well-healed. His left eyelid continues to droop, although he does open it more than he was previously opening it. The TMs are clear. Mouth and throat are clear.

CHEST AND LUNGS: Clear to auscultation.

HEART: Regular rate and rhythm. There is an indwelling right atrial catheter.

ABDOMEN: Soft without tenderness to palpation or hepatosplenomegaly.

EXTREMITIES: Normal.

NEUROLOGIC: Neurologic examination reveals a left seventh nerve paresis.

IMPRESSION: Rhabdomyosarcoma of the inferotemporal region.

PLAN: Course of chemotherapy with continuing radiation therapy with vincristine and Cytoxan.

_____
Judith B. Thornberg, M.D.

JY/NR15 32987
D: 06/08/200X 11:00
T: 06/08/200X 12:17

Figure 19–7 Example of a short-stay record.

20

Hyphen Use and Word Division

See topics in Chapter 8 (listed in italics) for additional information on hyphens and compounds.

INTRODUCTION

Hyphens are used primarily to aid the reader and avoid ambiguity. Whenever possible, avoid the use of hyphens when corresponding online via electronic mail. Please refer to Chapter 8 for additional help with hyphens.

20–1 AMINO ACID SEQUENCES

 DO   use a hyphen to separate the abbreviations for known amino acid sequences.

Lys-Asp-Gly

NOTE: *Unknown sequences are enclosed in parentheses and separated by commas.*

20–2 CHEMICAL ELEMENTS AND RADIONUCLIDES

✓ **DO**   use a hyphen to join the isotope number to the radiopharmaceutical brand names.

Glofil-125

⊘ **DON'T**   use a hyphen in the generic form.

sodium iodide I 131   iothalamate sodium I 125

NOTE: *Elements are written with superscripts:* ^{131}I.

✓ **DO**   use a hyphen with words and numbers describing chemical elements.

HDL-cholesterol   P-glycoprotein
aquaporin-1   5-FU
M-protein   5-azacytidine
17-hydroxycorticosteroids

✓ **DO**   use a hyphen with words and numbers describing immunostimulants and interleukins.

interferon alfa-n3   interferon gamma-1b
IL-16   IL-1RA

20–3 CLARITY

✓ **DO**   use a hyphen to join two or more words used to describe *(modify)* a noun when clarity is required.

brown-bag lunch
small-town physician
long-awaited diagnosis
There was a soft-tissue lesion on the surface. *(The lesion is composed of soft tissue.)*
little used-book store

new car salesman *(new at the job)*
new-car salesman *(sells new cars)*

NOTE. It is necessary to join certain modifiers to convey a single concept. *Except in instances of combined color terms, the compound modifier before the noun is hyphenated, but generally is not when it comes after the noun.*

The large blue-green bruise on her right cheek had begun to fade.
The large bruise on her right cheek is blue-green.
The well-used reference is well used.
The 2-cm incision is 2 cm long.
The O-positive patient is O positive.
The 28-year-old patient is 28 years old.
The well-nourished infant is well nourished.

However, look at this example:
The poorly nourished infant is poorly nourished.

20–4   DISEASE NAMES

🚫 **DON'T**   hyphenate most compound disease names when the term is used as a unit.

atrial septal defect
chronic obstructive pulmonary disease
congestive heart failure
pelvic inflammatory disease
sickle cell anemia

✓ **DO**   use a hyphen between two or more individuals' names used to describe a disease. *(See 14–2, Diseases and Syndromes, in Chapter 14.)*

Guillain-Barré syndrome
Laurence-Moon-Bardet-Biedl syndrome
Nonne-Milroy disease

20–5   NUMBERS

✓ **DO**   hyphenate numbers 21 through 99 when they are written out.

Fifty-five medical transcriptionists attended the meeting last night.

Ninety-nine percent of the time I am confident of the diagnosis.

DO   hyphenate spelled-out fractions.

She has spent one-third of her life concerned about the appearance of this scar.

☑ DO   hyphenate the modifier attached to a CPT code in narrative copy.

99255-32   69502-99

☑ DO   hyphenate compound modifiers composed of numbers and words.

4-cm long incision
3-month-old infant
5 × 5 × 1-mm glass fragment
35-hour week
4- to 5-year history
.45 caliber weapon
figure-of-8 sutures

20–6   *RANGE INDICATOR*

☑ DO   use the hyphen to take the place of the word *to* or *through* in numeric and alphabetic ranges. *(See 27-10 for further help with numeric ranges.)*

Take 100 mg Tylenol, 1-2 at bedtime
the L2-3 disk
C7-T1 disk
30-35 mEq
Rounds were made in Wards 1-4.
practicing there from 1990-1999
cranial nerves II-XII
Check V2-V6 again.
We eliminated every diagnosis from A-Z.
Note the P-R interval.

 DON'T   use a hyphen to express a range when one or both of the numbers contain a minus or plus sign.

at a −2 to a −3 station

NOTE: *Use* through *to describe ranges of vertebra and spinal nerves.*

The L2 through L5 vertebra were involved.
There was C1 through C6 nerve damage.

20–7 WORD DIVISION

A hyphen is used to divide a word at the end of a line. This situation does not come up very often because of the word-wrap feature of word processing software. It might be a problem if you have to use right-side line justification, of course. However, avoid dividing words at the end of the line whenever you can. Doing so takes time and breaks your rhythm and often confuses the reader. It is also easier to read and understand unhyphenated words. We divide some words to avoid a very ragged right margin. When you must divide a word, follow the rules provided here.

It is preferable to divide at certain points in order to obtain a more intelligible grouping of syllables. When in doubt about proper word division, check your dictionary or word-division manual. A word divided in error is just as incorrect as a word misspelled.

Dividing Words at the End of A Line

✓ DO divide English words only between syllables and in keeping with proper American pronunciation.

knowl/edge (*not* know/ledge)
liga/ture (*not* lig/ature)
sepa/rate (*not* sep/arate)

✓ DO divide medical words either before a suffix, after a prefix, or between compounds.

dys/menorrhea acro/phobia ile/ostomy

✓ DO divide after a one-vowel syllable in the middle of a word.

organi/zation regu/late busi/ness

✓ DO divide between two vowels that appear together within the word.

cre/ative retro/active valu/able

✓ DO divide a word between doubled consonants, *but* divide a word root that *ends* with a double consonant between the root and the suffix.

swim/ming occur/ring control/ling
admit/ting sug/gested misspell/ing

✓ DO divide a solid compound word between the elements of the compound.

over/riding	fiber/scope	off/spring
lack/luster	child/birth	gall/bladder

 DO   divide a hyphenated compound word after the hyphen.

self-/esteem   middle-/aged

 DO   divide a word with a prefix between the prefix and the root.

ante/natal   non/reactive   dys/phagia

Dividing Word Sets

 DO   divide names between the given name and the surname. Include a middle initial with the given name; divide names preceded by long titles between the title and the name.

Annie P./Younger
Claude/Richey
Rear Admiral/John Wentworth
Mary Margaret/Smith

 DO   avoid dividing dates. The only acceptable division of a date is between the comma *(after the day)* and the year.

Correct:
September 1,/200X
Incorrect:
September/1, 200X
Incorrect:
Sep/tember 1, 200X

Hyphenation Errors

 DON'T   divide words of only one syllable or with fewer than six letters.

thought   tumor   edema   weight

NOTE: *Even when* ed *is added to some words, they still remain one syllable and cannot be divided.*

passed   trimmed   weighed

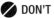 **DON'T**   divide words in a way that will leave a confusing syllable on either line.

ambi/tious *(confusing)*
am/bitious *(better)*

coin/cide *(confusing)*
co/incide *(better)*
inter/pret *(confusing)*
in/terpret *(better)*

🚫 **DON'T** leave a one-letter syllable at the beginning or the end of a divided word. Leave at least two characters *(plus the hyphen)* on the upper line and at least two characters *(plus a punctuation mark)* on the next line.

Incorrect:
i/deal
pian/o
a/mount
bacteri/a
Correct:
ad/ducent
de/capsulation
bi/lateral

🚫 **DON'T** divide names, other proper nouns, abbreviations, numbers, or contractions.

PhD   ASCVHD   f.o.b.   can't   CMA-A   wouldn't
Incorrect:
Wiliam/son

✅ **DO** write out a contraction to divide it.

can/not   would/not

NOTE: *Avoid writing contractions in any case.*

🚫 **DON'T** divide identifying information from accompanying numbers.

2 cm   6 lb 4 oz
December 20XX   1400 hours
page 84
Incorrect:
Diagnoses: 1. / Respiratory tract infection
Correct:
Diagnoses: / 1. Respiratory tract infection

🚫 **DON'T** divide word sets.

5 feet 6 inches   6 lb 4 oz   x-ray
6 cm   co-op

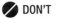 **DON'T** divide a street address between the number and the street name. You may divide an address after the name of the street and before the word *street, avenue, circle,* and so forth.

Incorrect:
3821/Ocean Street
Correct:
3821 Ocean/Street

Correct:
821 East Hazard/Road
Incorrect:
821 East/Hazard Road

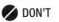 **DON'T** hyphenate a Latin compound

in vitro testing   ad hoc committee

 DON'T divide the last word on a page.

DON'T divide a word that would change its meaning when hyphenated. If unsure of the meaning of a word that has been dictated, look up the word in the English dictionary so you do not make a mistake.

Dr. Cho re-treated the inflamed area.
She retreated to Hawaii for a vacation.

I will re-collect the patient daily slips.
He had to recollect the operative procedure.

Meg re-marked the x-ray cassette.
Mrs. Avery remarked to me about the case.

Please re-sort the ledger cards.
She had to resort to turning the patient's account over to a collection agency.

21

Laboratory Terminology and Normal Values

See Appendix G, p. 577, for a list of laboratory tests and normal values.

21–1   ABBREVIATIONS
See also Chapter 1, Abbreviations and Symbols.

✓ **DO**   key a laboratory abbreviation if it is dictated.

RBC	WBC	BUN
SMAC	AT-III	pH

🚫 **DON'T**   key an abbreviation if the dictator has used the full word without a number in the expression or sentence.

There was a high sodium level noted. (*not* a high Na level)

EXCEPTION: *Always abbreviate* pH.

✅ **DO**   use an abbreviation to refer to a test in a report or paper *after* the abbreviation has been used once in its completely spelled-out form.

All newborns are routinely tested for phenylketonuria (PKU). As a result, the incidence of PKU as a cause of infant . . .

🚫 **DON'T**   punctuate those scientific abbreviations written in a combination of uppercase and lowercase letters.

| IgG | mEq | pH |
| mOsm | Hb | Hct |

21–2   BRIEF FORMS

✅ **DO**   key a brief form as dictated but spell it out in headings and subheadings.

| lab | macro | micro | pro time |
| norm | prep | sed rate | |

EXCEPTIONS: *Some laboratory slang expressions or brief forms must always be spelled out.*

Bilirubin	for *bili*
beta-hemolytic streptococcus	for *B strep*
coagulation studies	for *coags*
hematocrit	for *crit*
differential	for *diff*
H. influenzae *or* Haemophilus influenzae	for *H. flu*
Electrolytes	for *lytes*
hematocrit and hemoglobin	for *H&H*

✅ **DO**   add an *s* to a plural laboratory brief or short form.

| bands | basos | blasts | eos | lymphs |
| monos | polys | segs | stabs | |

21-3 CAPITALIZATION

✓ **DO**   use lowercase letters for metric symbols or abbreviations.

kg (for *kilogram*) *not* Kg *and not* kilos
cm (for *centimeters*) *not* CM *and not* Cm *and not* cms

EXCEPTIONS: *L (*for *liter), C (*for *Celsius), mEq (*for *milliequivalent)* not *meq*

21-4 COMPOUNDS

✓ **DO**   use a hyphen to join a number to a word to form a coined compound phrase.

SMA-1	alpha-1	profile-1
ribose-5-phosphate	3-oxobutyric	ytterbium-169

✓ **DO**   use a hyphen when a compound term is used as an adjective.

gram-positive organism   gram-negative stain

✓ **DO**   use a hyphen to join a single letter to a word to form a coined compound.

T-cell leukemia

21-5 DECIMAL FRACTIONS

✓ **DO**   use a period to separate a whole number from a decimal fraction.

PTT 23.9
globulins 2.8
hematocrit 38.6 and hemoglobin 12.9

✓ **DO**   key a whole number followed by a decimal point and the dictated digits.

The arterial gases showed a pH of 7.45.

Urinalysis: straw-colored, cloudy, pH 4.5, glucose 1+, acetone negative.

⊘ **DON'T**   key a whole number with a decimal point and zero, because it may be misread as a larger quantity.

Incorrect:
Potassium 3.0 mEq/L
Correct:
Potassium 3 mEq/L

✓ DO key specific gravity with four digits and a decimal point. Place the decimal point between the first and second digits even though the value may be dictated as "one zero," "one oh," or "ten." The normal range for specific gravity in urine is 1.015-1.025.

Dictated:
Specific gravity ten twenty.
Transcribed:
Specific gravity 1.020. (*not* 10.20)

Dictated:
Specific gravity one point zero three zero.
Transcribed:
Specific gravity 1.030.

✓ DO key pH with at least one digit following the decimal point; if there is none, add a zero.

Dictated:
The "pee h" was seven.
Transcribed:
The pH was 7.0.

✓ DO place a zero before a decimal point so it is not misread as a whole number

Correct:
0.1
Incorrect:
.1

Dictated:
point seventy-five percent basos
Transcribed:
0.75% basos

✓ DO use a decimal fraction instead of a common fraction.

Dictated:
Urinalysis revealed one quarter percent urine sugar.
Transcribed:
Urinalysis revealed 0.25% urine sugar.

Dictated:
Monocytes one and one-half per cent.
Transcribed:
Monocytes 1.5%

21–6 EPONYMS

See also Chapter 14, Eponyms.

☑ DO   capitalize an eponym that refers to a particular test and show the possessive *('s)* when appropriate to do so and the author dictates it.

Gram stain
Eagle medium
Eijkman lactose
Pasteur culture
Pfeiffer's phenomenon *(or reaction)*
Salmonella-Shigella agar
Wassermann test *(or reaction)* *or* Wassermann's test *(or reaction)*

21–7 GENUS

☑ DO   abbreviate the genus name *(but not the species name)* after the genus name has been used once in the text.

The report was negative for Escherichia coli. We had expected to find E. coli . . .

☑ DO   abbreviate the genus name *(but not the species name)* with a period.

E. coli *(Escherichia coli)*
H. influenzae *(Haemophilus influenzae)*

⊘ DON'T   abbreviate the genus name when used alone without the species name.

His serologic test for Mycoplasma will not be repeated.

21–8 HYPHEN

☑ DO   join a number to a word to form a coined compound phrase.

SMA-1   alpha-1   profile-1   ribose-5-phosphate
ytterbium-169   3-oxobutyric   HPA-1

EXCEPTIONS: *T3* or T_3, *T4* or T_4

DO   use the hyphen to take the place of the dictated word *to* when identifying numeric and alphabetic ranges.

30-35 mEq

 DON'T   divide identifying information from accompanying numbers

Hgb 14.8   pH 7.42   CPK 716

NOTE: *Do not separate the abbreviation from the figure that follows it. If the abbreviation occurs at the end of a line, carry the abbreviation to the next line so it will appear with the figure.*

Correct:
Admission WBC 7400, Hgb 14.8, Hct 47%.
Correct:
Admission WBC 7400, Hgb 14.8,
Hct 47%.

Incorrect
Admission WBC 7400, Hgb 14.8, Hct
47%.

NOTE: *Some individuals prefer to do a forced return in front of the set to be carried to the next line.*

21–9   LOWERCASE AND UPPERCASE LETTERS

 DON'T   use periods with scientific abbreviations that include uppercase and lowercase letters.

The arterial gases showed a pH of 7.45.

21–10   METRIC SYSTEM
See Chapter 26, Metric System.

21–11   NUMBERS

 DO   use Arabic numerals to express laboratory values, but avoid beginning a sentence with a number.

PTT 23.9
Globulins 2.8
Hematocrit 38.6 and hemoglobin 12.9
wbc 3.8 thousand *or* WBC 3800

 DO   use commas to group numbers in units of three.

platelets 250,000   wbc 15,000

EXCEPTION: *Four digits are written without a comma.*

wbc 3800

🚫 **DON'T**   use commas with the metric system or with decimals.

Correct:
1000 ml
Incorrect:
1,000 ml

✓ **DO**   write large numbers with a combination of numbers and words.

3,000,000 *or* 3 million

✓ **DO**   use figures when numbers are used directly with symbols or abbreviations.

pH 6.5   pO2 pO_2 pCO2 pCO_2

✓ **DO**   leave a space between the number and the abbreviation.

IgA 60

EXCEPTION: *The Western Blot HIV AIDS test shows no space between the number and alpha character.*

Bands present at p24 and p55.
Bands present at p24, gp160.

✓ **DO**   use figures with metric abbreviations

7 ml   20 kg   1 L

✓ **DO**   use figures and symbols when writing plus or minus with a number.

1+ protein
0 Rh blood

21–12   PLURAL FORMS WITH LABORATORY ABBREVIATIONS
See also 21–2, Brief Forms.

✓ **DO**   use an apostrophe to form the plurals of lowercase abbreviations and abbreviations that include periods.

There were elevated wbc's.

🚫 **DON'T**   use an apostrophe with plural short forms.

The patient's white blood cell count was 4.8 thousand with 58% segs, 7% bands, 24% lymphs, 8% monos, 1% eos, and 2% basos.

🚫 **DON'T**   add *s* to the abbreviation of a unit of measurement.

The length of the incision was 4 cm (*not* 4 cms).

21–13 PUNCTUATION WITH LABORATORY ABBREVIATIONS

✅ **DO**   write most abbreviations in full capital letters without punctuation.

PKU   BUN   CBC   WBC   RBC

🚫 **DON'T**   punctuate those scientific abbreviations written in a combination of uppercase and lowercase letters.

pH   Hb   Hgb   mEq   mOsm

✅ **DO**   use commas when multiple related laboratory test results are reported.

Phosphorus 5.2, BUN 30, creatinine 1.4.
WBC 12.4 with 69 segs, 5 stabs.

NOTE: *It is optional to use commas or colons to separate a laboratory value from the test it describes.*

Creatinine 1.4
Creatinine, 1.4
or
Creatinine: 1.4

NOTE: *For the sake of clarity in some instances it is wise to insert punctuation. The numbers tend to run together when a colon or semicolon is omitted.*

CO_2, 24; pCO_2, 35; 120/80 mmHg
pO_2: 26; 120/80 mmHg

✅ **DO**   use periods to separate unrelated laboratory test results.

White blood cell count 8100. Potassium 3.3. SGOT 20. Albumin 4.4.

🚫 **DON'T**   insert a period after the abbreviation of a unit.

> **Correct:**
> cm (for *centimeter*)
> **Incorrect:**
> cm.

🚫 **DON'T**   separate sets of words incorrectly.

> **Incorrect:**
> Serum electrolytes alkaline, phosphatase BUN, creatinine, glucose and calcium will be checked.
> **Correct:**
> Serum electrolytes, alkaline phosphatase, BUN, creatinine, glucose, and calcium will be checked.

✅ **DO**   use semicolons when a series with internal commas is present.

> Differential showed 60 segs, 3 bands, 30 lymphs, 5 monos, and 2 basos; hemoglobin 16.0; and hematocrit 46.1.

21–14 RATIOS

✅ **DO**   use a colon to express ratios in which the colon takes the place of the word *to*.

> The solution was diluted 1:100.
> We had a 2:1 mix.

21–15 ROMAN NUMERALS

🚫 **DON'T**   use a type font that is sans serif *(a style of printing type with no serifs)*, because the capital letter *I* needed for Roman numerals looks like the number one.

✅ **DO**   use Roman numerals with typical noncounting or nonmathematical listings.

> Factor: Missing factor VII *(blood factor)*
>
> Papanicolaou smears can be reported as class I through class V or by Cervical Intraepithelial Neoplasia (CIN) classes I through III.

21–16 SHORT FORMS
See also 21–2, Brief Forms.

✓ DO   use the short form, or brief form, when dictated, if it does not
         violate any of the rules listed in 21–1.

> Pap smear *(Papanicolaou)*
> sed rate *(sedimentation rate)*
> lymphs *(lymphocytes)*
> monos *(monocytes)*
> eos *(eosinophils)*
> basos *(basophils)*
> chem profile *(chemistry profile)*

21–17 SLASH

✓ DO   use a slash in writing certain technical terms. The slash
         sometimes substitutes for the word *per* in laboratory terms.

Dictated:
The lumbar puncture showed one white blood cell per
cubic millimeter.
Transcribed:
The lumbar puncture showed 1 wbc/cu mm.

⊘ DON'T use a slash to express a ratio.

Incorrect:
1/20,000
Correct:
1:20,000

21–18 SPECIFIC GRAVITY

✓ DO   key specific gravity with four digits and a decimal point
         placed between the first and second digits even though the
         value may be dictated as "one zero," "one oh," or "ten."

Dictated:
Specific gravity ten twenty.
Transcribed:
Specific gravity 1.020.

Dictated:
Specific gravity one point zero three zero.
Transcribed:
Specific gravity 1.030.

21-19 STAINS

✓ DO key the word *Gram* with a capital *G* when indicating Gram stain, method, or solution, because it is an eponym. However, when *Gram* is used as a compound word, it begins with a lowercase *g*.

Gram stain
gram-negative *(means the specimen loses the stain)*
gram-positive *(means the specimen retains the stain)*

21-20 SUBSCRIPT AND SUPERSCRIPT

✓ DO use numeric subscripts with capital letters when typing human blood groups or referring to thyroid tests.

Mrs. James's blood group test showed she is A_2B Rh+.
The patient's T_4 was in the mid range of 7.1.

NOTE: *These expressions can be put on the same line if your equipment is not capable of printing small numbers above or below the line.*

EXCEPTION: *Mathematical exponents must be typed as superscripts (e.g., 10^5).*

21-21 SYMBOLS

✓ DO use symbols only when they occur in immediate association with a number or another abbreviation.

4-5 *(four to five)*
2+ *(two plus)*
diluted 1:10 *(diluted one to ten)*
−2 *(minus two)*
nocturia × 2 *(nocturia times two)*
25 mg/h *(twenty-five milligrams per hour)*
35 mg% *(thirty-five milligram percent)*

✓ DO leave a space between the number and the abbreviation.

50 ml *(not 50ml)*
35 mg *(not 35mg)*

DON'T leave a space between the number or abbreviation and a symbol.

50% (*not* 50 %)
46 mg% (*not* 46 mg %)

✓ **DO** be consistent when keying the percent sign even if the dictator dictates the first percent but does not dictate the rest of the percent symbols in a series of related tests.

The triglycerides were high at 646 mg% and cholesterol 283 mg%.

Blood sugar was 46 mg%.

The patient had a white blood cell count of 4.8 thousand with 58% segs, 7% bands, 24% lymphs, 8% monos, 1% eos, and 2% basos.

✓ **DO** use figures and symbols when writing plus or minus with a number.

1+ protein

 DON'T pluralize symbols or abbreviations.

kg (for *kilograms*) *not* kgs *and not* kilos
m (for *meters*) *not* ms

21–22 *VALUES*

Normal values vary from one laboratory to another, depending on types of equipment. Refer to Appendix G, Laboratory Terminology and Values, p. 577.

Letter Format

22–1 ADDRESS

See Chapter 2, Address Formats for Letters and Forms of Address, for complete information on forms of address.

 DO   use proper forms of address for military ranks and ratings in written correspondence. List full name followed by a comma and branch of service *(abbreviated)* with no punctuation.

NOTE: *Titles of officers are the same in the Army* (USA), *the Air Force* (USAF), *the Marine Corps* (USMC), *the Navy* (USN), *and the Coast Guard* (USCG).

EXCEPTION: *The top rank in the Marine Corps is Commandant of the Marine Corps.*

Captain William Molony, USAF
Capt Alexander Kolin, USMC
Capt Robert LaMacchia, USN
CPT Jerome Stein, USA

22–2 ATTENTION LINE

 DO   key the attention line two spaces below the last line of the address, starting at the left margin. *Attention* may be spelled out in full caps or have only the first letter capitalized.

John R. Parsons, MD
321 Fifth Avenue, Suite B
Altamont Springs, FL 32716

Attention Josephine Simmons, Administrator

 DO   use *Gentlemen* or *Dear Sir or Madam* as the salutation when using an attention line in a letter.

NOTE: *Writers often find it awkward to use* Dear Sir or Madam *after they have used a name in the attention line. To eliminate the problem, eliminate the attention line, and send the letter directly.*

Josephine Simmons, Administrator
c/o John R. Parsons, MD
321 Fifth Avenue, Suite B
Altamont Springs, FL 32716

Now you may say *Dear Ms. Simmons* or *Dear Josephine*, which would have been incorrect with the attention line as first illustrated.

✔ DO	insert the attention line in the inside address between the name of the addressee and the street address or box number if using word processing equipment. This format allows easy generation of the envelope address.

Practon Medical Group, Inc.
Attention Jane Dye, CMA
4567 Broad Avenue
Woodland Hills, CA 91607-4102

⊘ DON'T	abbreviate the attention line or use any punctuation. It is optional to underline the word *Attention*.

22–3 BODY

✔ DO	begin the body of the letter a double space from the salutation or reference line; use single spacing. The first and subsequent lines are flush with the left margin unless indented paragraphs are used, in which case the first line of each paragraph is indented one tab stop *(five spaces)*.
✔ DO	double-space between paragraphs.
✔ DO	leave at least two lines of the paragraph at the foot of one page and carry over at least two lines to the top of the next page.
⊘ DON'T	divide a paragraph of only two or three lines between the bottom of one page and the top of the next.

22–4 COMPLIMENTARY CLOSE

See Figure 22–1 at the end of the chapter, p. 252.

✔ DO	line up the complimentary close with the date and type it a double space below the last typed line. In a full block style letter, begin the closing at the left margin. The closing may be omitted in a simplified letter.

NOTE: *When using word processing software, create a macro that represents the closing of a letter to include the complimentary close.*

✔ DO	capitalize only the first word in the complimentary close.
✔ DO	use a comma after the complimentary close when using *mixed* punctuation; no punctuation mark is used with *open* punctuation.

Sincerely, *(mixed)*   Sincerely yours *(open)*
Yours very truly,   Very truly yours

✔ DO   key the complimentary closing in its regular position, and insert an informal phrase at the end of the last paragraph or as a separate paragraph with appropriate punctuation if using both a complimentary close and an informal closing phrase.

Regards to Janet and the children.

Sincerely,

Robert T. Braun, MD

22–5 CONFIDENTIAL NOTATION
See Figure 22–1 at the end of the chapter, p. 252.

✔ DO   key a personal notation on the second line below the date at the left margin. The notation may be keyed in all capital letters or in uppercase and lowercase letters that are underscored.

PERSONAL *or* <u>Personal</u>
CONFIDENTIAL *or* <u>Confidential</u>

22–6 CONTINUATION PAGES

✔ DO   continue to the second page at the end of a paragraph whenever possible.

✔ DO   leave at least two lines of the paragraph at the foot of one page and carry over at least two lines to the top of the next page.

NOTE: *Some word processing programs have a feature that prevents the creation of orphans* (printing the first line of a new paragraph as the last line on a page) *and widows* (printing the last line of a paragraph as the first line of a new page).

✔ DO   place headings 1 inch from the top of the page. *(See 22–17, Margins.)*

🚫 DON'T   key closer than 1 inch from the bottom of a page.

🚫 DON'T   divide a paragraph of only two or three lines between the bottom of one page and the top of the next.

🚫 DON'T   divide the last word on the page.

✓ DO   leave two blank lines between the last line of the heading and the first line of the continuation of the letter. To do this, press the return or enter key three times at the end of the keyed data in the heading.

Horizontal format

RE: Leah Hamlyn	2	October 3, 200X
(patient's name)	*(page number)*	*(date)*

Vertical format

RE: Leah Hamlyn
Page 2
October 3, 200X

NOTE: *The page number is centered in the horizontal format. In a nonmedical letter, the name of the correspondent is listed in place of the patient's name.*

✓ DO   always check your printout to be sure that the page 2 markings appear where they were intended.

NOTE: *If using a template, the software program may automatically insert a continuation page heading and correctly number each subsequent page.*

22–7 COPY NOTATION

Copy notation is used when a copy is sent to someone else.

✓ DO   type a copy notation flush with the left margin a double space below the reference initials, mailing notation, or enclosure notation, whichever comes last. The abbreviation *cc* remains correct and popular. It used to mean *carbon copy* and now means *courtesy copy*. Since most copies mailed out today are photocopies, some offices prefer to use the abbreviation *pc* or simply *c*. A colon may or may not be used after *cc*. Use the recipient's full name and title if known.

cc: Frank L. Naruse, MD
c: Ruth Chriswell, Business Manager
CC: Hodge W. Lloyd
Copy: Carla P. Ralph, Buyer

Copies: Kristen A. Temple
         Anthony R. McClintock

pc: John B. Smith, MD
If you have a very lengthy list of copy notations, consider making a two- or three-column list rather than a long string that could affect another page.

CC: Claire Duennes, MD   Norman Szold, MD
     Sharon Kirkwood, MD   James Tanaka, MD
     Amrum Lambert, MD   Robert Wozniak, MD
     Clifford Storey, MD   Vell Yaldua, MD

 DON'T   type a copy notation without a name following it.

✓ **DO**   use a blind copy *(bcc)* notation if the addressee is not intended to know that one or more persons are being sent a copy of the letter. This notation is included on the file copy and on the copy to the recipient of the blind copy on the second line below the last item in the letter *(below the reference initials, enclosure notation, mailing notation, cc notation, or postscript)*.

> **HANDY HINT:** *Add the* bcc *notation and print out your file copy and the bcc copy for the recipient. Delete the entire bcc and print the original.*

bcc Ms. Penelope R. Taylor *(This line appears only on the file copy and the bcc copy.)*

✓ **DO**   note on the file copy if enclosures are sent to other recipients of the correspondence. Usually, it is assumed that the enclosures accompany only the original letter.

cc/enc: John L. Blake *(received the letter and the enclosures)*

 DON'T   make a copy notation on the original correspondence if the sender wishes a copy of the correspondence sent to a third party and does not wish the recipient of the original copy to know that this was done. *(See preceding instructions for blind copy notation.)*

✓ **DO**   use a check mark next to the name of the person for whom the copy is intended if copies are to be sent to several people.

cc: Ms. Joan Cannon
Ms. Harriet Newman ✓
(This letter was sent to Ms. Newman. The letter to be sent to Ms. Cannon would have a check mark by Ms. Cannon's name.)

✓ **DO**   give each document a unique file name. This way transcribed documents may be retrieved easily and quickly when needed. You may be able to use your own file name; however, the dictator or organization may prefer that you use their unique codes. If you are able to use your own codes, here are some hints to make it simple.

- Use minimum data: ID # for the dictator, patient name, date.
- Use letters and numbers: for dates, use just the last digit of the year then 1-9 for the first nine months and o, n, d for the last three.
- Use a period for a separation mark.
- Place the code as the last entry on the page.
- Decrease the font size to 8 or 9 points.
- Use the identical code as your "save."
- Use on your file copy and computer copy only.

Example
(using Figure 22–2 at the end of the chapter, p. 251)
(Your ID # for Dr. Berry is B1)
B1.Hall.73X, and in reduced size as you may want to show it: B1.Hall.73X.
Uncoded: Dr. Berry dictated a letter on patient Hall on July 3, 200X.

22–8   DATE LINE

✓ DO   key the date in keeping with the format of the letter and in line with the complimentary close and keyed signature line. The date is keyed three lines below the letterhead *(no closer, but you may drop it farther down for a brief letter)*. The date used is the day the material was dictated, *not* the day it was transcribed.

✓ DO   spell out the date in full in either the traditional or the military style.

December 22, 200X *(traditional style)*
22 December 200X *(British and military style)*

22–9   ENCLOSURE NOTATION

✓ DO   key an enclosure notation flush with the left margin if enclosing one or more items in a letter. The number of enclosures should be noted if there is more than one.

Enc.   Enclosure   Check enclosed
Enc. 2   2 Enc.   2 enclosures
Enclosures: 2
Enclosed: 1. History and physical
          2. Operative report
          3. Pathology report

NOTE: *A one-page enclosure is not clipped or stapled to a letter but is folded the same way as the letter and inserted into the last fold of the letter. An enclosure smaller than the letter is stapled to the top of the letter in the upper left corner.*

22–10 FOLDING AND INSERTING
No. 6-3/4 Envelope (6-½ × 3-⅝ Inches)

✓ DO   bring the bottom edge of the sheet up to within ½ inch of the top edge and fold. From the right edge, fold over one third of the sheet, and crease. From the left edge, fold the sheet so the left edge is ½ inch from the right fold, and crease. Insert the last creased edge into the envelope first.

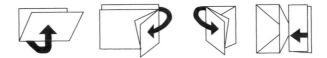

No. 10 Envelope (9-½ × 4-⅛ Inches)

✓ DO   bring up the bottom third of the sheet and crease. Fold down the upper third of the sheet so the top edge is 1 inch from the first fold, and crease. Insert the last creased edge into the envelope first.

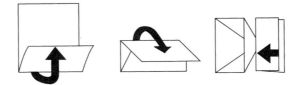

Window Envelope

✓ DO   bring up the bottom third of the sheet and fold. Fold the top of the sheet *back* to the first fold so that the inside address is on the outside, and crease. Insert the sheet so the address appears in the window.

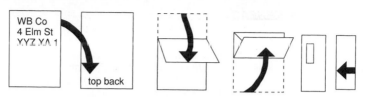

22–11 FORMAT

✓ DO key all lines of the letter flush with the left margin in full block letter format. The lines include date line, address, salutation, all lines of the body of the letter, complimentary close, signature line, and reference line. *(See Figure 22–3 at the end of the chapter, p. 254)*

✓ DO key the date line, complimentary close, and signature line just to the right of the middle of the page in modified block letter format. *(See Figure 22–4, at the end of the chapter, p. 255.)*

✓ DO indent paragraphs one tab stop (five spaces) for modified block indented letter format.

✓ DO replace the salutation with a subject line in all capitals and omit the complimentary close when using simplified style. Begin all lines at the left margin. Key the signature line in all capital letters on one line.

22–12 IN CARE OF

✓ DO use an "in care of" notation if a letter cannot be sent to the addressee's home or place of business and must be directed to a third person. Use the in-care-of notation *(c/o)* to eliminate an attention line. *(See 22-1, Address.)*

Ms. Margaret Shay
In care of Robert D. Hensley, MD
or
Ms. Margaret Shay
c/o Robert D. Hensley, MD

22–13 INSIDE ADDRESS
See Chapter 2, Address Formats for Letters and Forms of Address.

22–14   LETTERHEAD

✓ DO   obtain approval from your employer before changing the letterhead, the type of printing, or the quality of the paper. The letterhead should contain the author's name (or corporate name) and address, telephone and fax numbers, medical specialty, and/or board membership.

22–15   LISTS

See discussion under 22–31, Tabulated Copy, p. 251.

22–16   MAILING OR DELIVERY NOTATIONS

✓ DO   key a mailing notation on the line below the reference initials or enclosure notation, whichever is last, if a letter is to be delivered in a special way.

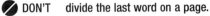

mtf	md	brt
Enc. 2	By Federal Express	Enclosures 3
Certified	cc Ms. Mary Evans	By messenger

22–17   MARGINS

See 22–28, Spacing, on how to lengthen a letter.

✓ DO   use the default *(preset)* feature of the word processing program to keep side margins of letters consistent in dimension.

✓ DO   leave a bottom margin of at least 6 lines *(1 inch)*. However, if there is a second page to the letter, the bottom margin of the first page can be increased up to 12 lines *(2 inches)*.

22–18   PAGE-ENDING CONSIDERATIONS

✓ DO   leave a uniform margin of 6 to 12 lines at the bottom of each page of a letter *(except the last page, which can be short)*.

🚫 DON'T   divide the last word on a page.

🚫 DON'T   divide a paragraph that has only two or three lines. If a paragraph has four or more lines, leave at least two lines of the paragraph at the bottom of the previous page and carry over at least two lines to the continuation page.

🚫 DON'T   use a continuation page to key only the complimentary close of a letter. The closing should be preceded by at least two lines of the body of the letter.

22–19 PARTS OF THE LETTER

See Figure 22–1 at the end of the chapter for the parts of the letter.

22–20 PERSONAL NOTATION

✓ DO   use the words *personal* or *confidential* on the second line below the date, at the left margin, in uppercase letters or in underscored uppercase and lowercase letters to indicate a personal notation. *(See Figure 22–1 at the end of the chapter.)*

PERSONAL *or* Personal
CONFIDENTIAL *or* Confidential

22–21 POSTSCRIPTS

✓ DO   key a postscript *(P.S., PS:, PS)* one double space below the last reference notation, flush with the left margin. If the paragraphs are indented, indent the first line of the postscript and bring the second and subsequent lines flush to the left margin. The P.S. can be an afterthought or a statement deliberately withheld from the body of the letter for emphasis or a restatement of an important thought (e.g., a phone number in a letter of application). If the afterthought reads in such a way that the letter looks poorly organized, insert the statement in the appropriate section of the letter. *(Notice the spacing in the examples.)* It may be handwritten or keyed, with or without the *PS* notation at the end of the letter.

P.S. By the way, I saw Flo Douglas in the elevator in St. Michaels Hospital the other day. She said she enjoyed seeing you at the golf outing last weekend. *(afterthought)*

PS: Please do not hesitate to call on me if I can help you in any way. *(emphasis)*

✓ DO   leave two spaces between the colon or period and the first word.

✓ DO   key *(P.P.S., PPS:, or PPS)* for an additional postscript, and double-space down from the first postscript typed.

PS: Please do not hesitate to call on me if I can help you in any way.

PPS: Will you be attending the board meeting at Cottage Hospital this Friday? I hope to see you there.

245

22–22   *QUOTATIONS*
See also Chapter 36, Quotation Marks.

✅ **DO**   use single spacing and indent one tab stop *(five spaces)* from each side margin for keying a quotation that is four or more lines. Double-space above and below the quotation. If the quotation is the beginning of an indented paragraph, indent the first word an additional tab stop or five spaces.

🚫 **DON'T**   enclose the quotation in quotation marks; the indention replaces the marks.

22–23   *REFERENCE INITIALS*

✅ **DO**   place the initials of the person who keyed and formatted the letter, in lowercase letters, at the left margin, a double space below the last line in the signature block and flush with the left margin. The author's initials are generally omitted but *may* be included and will precede the initials of the preparer of the letter.

> **Preparer's initials alone:** mlo
> **With author's initials:** ARC:mlo *or* ARC/mlo

✅ **DO**   key the dictator's, the signer's, and the typist's initials when the dictator differs from the document signer.

> MJP/arc/wpd *or* MJP:arc:wpd
> Here, *mjp* stands for the dictator, *arc* stands for the signer, and *wpd* stands for the transcriptionist.

🚫 **DON'T**   use humorous or confusing combinations of reference initials.

> crc *(rather than* cc*)*
> db *(rather than* dmb*)*
> dg *(rather than* dog*)*

🚫 **DON'T**   key your reference initials when you prepare a letter for your own signature.

22–24   *REFERENCE OR SUBJECT LINE*

✅ **DO**   key the patient's name a double space *after* the salutation in full block style. *(See Figure 22–3 at the end of the chapter, p. 254.)*

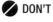 **DO** key the patient's name in the blank space between the last line of the address and the salutation in modified block style. Align the patient's name with the date. *(See Figure 22–4 at the end of the chapter, p. 255.)*

DON'T use a period after a subject line.

DON'T place the reference or subject line in the wrong location, since dictators commonly dictate it out of place.

Incorrect *(placement error)***:**
Matthew R. Bates, MD
7832 Johnson Avenue
Denver, CO 80241

RE: Leah Hamlyn

Dear Dr. Bates:

Incorrect *(spacing error)***:**
Matthew R. Bates, MD
7832 Johnson Avenue
Denver, CO 80241

                                        RE: Leah Hamlyn

Dear Dr. Bates:

Correct:
Matthew R. Bates, MD
7832 Johnson Avenue
Denver, CO 80241

Dear Dr. Bates:

RE: Leah Hamlyn

Correct:
Matthew R. Bates, MD
7832 Johnson Avenue
Denver, CO 80241

                                        RE: Leah Hamlyn

Dear Dr. Bates:
(Note the spacing between the address and the salutation.)

Correct:
Matthew R. Bates, MD
7832 Johnson Avenue
Denver, CO 80241

Dear Dr. Bates:

RE: Leah Hamlyn, Accident report E 14-78-9865

Correct:
Matthew R. Bates, MD
7832 Johnson Avenue
Denver, CO 80241

Dear Dr. Bates:

RE: Leah Hamlyn
      Horizons Insurance Company
      Accident report E 14-78-9865

✓ **DO**   use a subject line in place of the salutation in the simplified letter style. Begin the subject line on the third line below the inside address at the left margin, and type it in all capital letters.

🚫 **DON'T**   use a term such as *Subject* to introduce the subject line in the simplified letter style.

✓ **DO**   key a control reference notation two lines below the date or on the second line below any notation that follows the date.

When replying, refer to VMT-501

✓ **DO**   key the reference notation *Refer to:* or *RE:*. Leave one or two spaces after the colon.

In reply to: Z940 280 100 *(file number)*
Refer to: Policy 90245 *(insurance policy number)*
RE: Jennifer K. Hotta *(name of patient)*

✓ **DO**   key your own reference notation before the addressee's reference notation when there are two reference notations. Key the addressee's reference notation on the second line below your reference notation. Double-space between each notation.

When replying, refer to G-8043

Your reference: BOX-Z-9

NOTE: *When replying to a letter that has a refer-to notation, the notation may be typed in the subject line or below the date line.*

October 2, 200X
Refer to: Policy 90245

22–25 RETURN ADDRESS

✓ **DO**   key a return address when using *plain paper,* listing the street address, city, state, ZIP code, and the date. The telephone number is optional. Allow a top margin of 1½ to 2 inches. For modified block letter style, center the return address. For full block letter style, begin each line at the left margin.

479 East 53 Street, Apt. 45   *or*   Apartment 2B
New York, NY 10011-2706   479 East 53 Street
October 4, 200X   New York, NY
                                          10011-2706
                                          (212) 458-0998
                                          October 4, 200X

22–26 SALUTATION

See Chapter 2 for a comprehensive list of address formats for letters and forms of address.

✓ **DO**   key the salutation a double space after the last line of the address when using mixed punctuation *(a colon)* or open punctuation *(no colon).*

Dear Dr. Hon:
or
Dear Dr. Hon

22–27 SIGNATURE LINE

✓ **DO**   key the dictator's or writer's name exactly as it appears in the letterhead, three blank lines after the complimentary close and aligned with it. Press the return/enter key four times after you key the complimentary close.

✓ **DO**   key the dictator's or writer's official title when preferred. If the title appears on the same line as the name, it should be preceded by a comma. If the title is keyed on the line directly below the name, no comma is needed. If the dictator signs off with only a first name, key his or her complete name *(and title, if there is one).*

Yours very truly,

Samuel R. Wong, MD
Dean of Admissions
or
Sincerely,

Carla B. Black, MD, Medical Director *(note the punctuation)*

✓ **DO** list the full name followed by a comma and branch of military service *(abbreviated)* with no punctuation for the signature line of persons in the military.

Robert B. Hughes, CDR, USN *(commander)*
Mark J. Evans, WO, USAF *(warrant officer)*

NOTE: *If the rank or rating is spelled out in full, it should appear one line below the full name. The rank or rating should be followed by a comma and the abbreviation for the branch of service.*

Phillip M. McDougal
Captain, USAF

✓ **DO** identify an office employee's position in the firm and provide a courtesy title. The courtesy title for women *(Miss, Ms., Mrs.)* enables the correspondent to have a title to use in writing or telephoning. Enclose the courtesy title in parentheses or use it without parentheses.

(Ms.) Lynmarie Myhre, CMT, Supervisor
Department of Risk Management

(Mrs.) Elvira E. Gonsalves
Quality Control Manager

Miss Paula de la Vera, CMA
Assistant to Dr. Bishop

✓ **DO** place two signature blocks side by side or one beneath the other when two people are to sign a letter.

22–28 SPACING

✓ **DO** type all letters single spaced.

✓ **DO** lengthen a short letter by increasing the width of the margin.

22–29 *SUBJECT LINE*

See 22–24, Reference or Subject Line, and Figures 22–3 and 22–4, pp. 254 and 255.

22–30 *TABLES*

✓ DO   center a table between the right and left margins when it occurs in the text of a letter.

✓ DO   indent a minimum of one tab stop *(five spaces)* from each side margin.

✓ DO   allow from two to six spaces between columns.

✓ DO   leave one to three blank lines above and below the table to set it apart from the rest of the text.

22–31 *TABULATED COPY*

✓ DO   use tabulated copy when it is appropriate. It adds emphasis, makes the letter easier to read, and adds visual interest.

✓ DO   indent at least one tab stop *(five spaces)* from each margin to begin tabulated copy. *(See Figures 22–2 and 22–5 at the end of the chapter.)*

✓ DO   prepare a list single spaced with double spacing above and below the list. The list may be keyed the full width of the letter or indented one tab stop *(five spaces)* from each side margin. If an item in the list needs more than one line, leave a blank line between all items in the list. Align each line with the line above.

NOTE: *Use the word processing software indent feature to align any turnovers with the first word in the line above.*

✓ DO   use bullets *(circles, squares, triangles)* before items in a short list.

NOTE: *Use the automatic bullet insert feature. Set a tab wherever the first line of text is to begin after each bullet.*

To further evaluate your condition, we need to perform the following tests:

- *Electrocardiogram*
- *Stress test*
- *Twenty-four-hour Holter monitor*

KARL ROBRECHT, MD   ADRIANNA SACHS, MD
    Internal Medicine   Cardiology

Gulf Medical Group, Inc.
                    800 Gulf Shore Drive
                    Naples, FL 33940
Telephone 813 649-1111   FAX 813 987-5121

Approximately 3
blank lines
below letterhead   _____ Date line

Second line below   Confidential or
date line   _____   Personal notation

Fifth line below   _____
date line   _____   Inside address
                            _____

Double-space after
last line of address   _____: Salutation

Double-space after   _____
salutation   _____   Body
Single-spaced, with   _____.
double-space   _____
between paragraphs   _____

Double-space after   _____, Complimentary
last paragraph   close

4 blank lines   Signature
                                              area
                            _____ Typed signature line
                            _____ Title

Double-space   _____   Reference initials
Double-space   _____   Enclosure notation
Double-space   _____   Distribution
Double-space   _____   Postscript (P.S.)

Figure 22–1   Business letter setup mechanics illustrating spacing and each
part of the document. (See text for a description of each item illustrated.)

Kenneth A. Berry, MD

5933 Doheny Drive Suite 214
Beverly Hills, California 90210

310 555-0000   FAX 310 555-0001

July 3, 200X

Miss Goldie Hall
1956 Sunnyvale Drive
Twentynine Palms, California 92277

Dear Miss Hall:

This is in reply to your letter concerning the results of your tests that
were done here and by Dr. Sullard.

 1. Intestinal symptoms, secondary to a lactase deficiency.
 2. Generalized arteriosclerosis.
 3. Mitral stenosis and insufficiency.
 4. History of venous aneurysm.

You were seen on June 27, at which time you were having some
stiffness at the shoulders which I felt was likely to be due to a
periarthritis. (This is a stiffness of the shoulder capsule.)
What we may want . . .

Figure 22–2   Letter illustrating use of tabulated copy.

KARL ROBRECHT, MD   ADRIANNA SACHS, MD
Internal Medicine   Cardiology

Gulf Medical Group, Inc.

800 Gulf Shore Drive
Naples, FL 33940

Telephone 813 649-1111   FAX 813 987-5121

October 3, 200X

Matthew R. Bates, MD
7832 Johnson Avenue
Denver, CO 80241

Dear Dr. Bates:

RE: Leah Hamlyn

_____
_____
_____.

_____
_____
_____
_____.

_____
_____.

Sincerely yours,

Adrianna Sachs, MD

mlo

cc: Eric T. Myhre, DPM

Figure 22–3   Letter illustrating full block format with mixed punctuation and placement of reference or subject line.

KARL ROBRECHT, MD
Internal Medicine

ADRIANNA SACHS, MD
Cardiology

Gulf Medical Group, Inc.

800 Gulf Shore Drive
Naples, FL 33940

Telephone 813 649-1111

FAX 813 987-5121

October 3, 200X

Matthew R. Bates, MD
7832 Johnson Avenue
Denver, CO 80241

RE: Leah Hamlyn

Dear Dr. Bates:

_____
_____
_____
_____.

_____
_____
_____
_____.

_____
_____.

Sincerely yours,

Adrianna Sachs, MD

mlo

cc: Eric T. Myhre, DPM

Enclosure: Operative report

Figure 22–4 Letter illustrating modified block format with mixed punctuation at the salutation and placement of subject or reference line.

Jon L. Mikosan, MD
6244 Applegatge Road
Round Valley, XX 12345
555 921-8934

January 20, 200X

Wood County Medical Association
Committee on Insurance Review
1925 Mt. Woodsen
Round Valley, XX 12345

Dear Doctors:

RE: Balboa Health Program
     William R. Sylvan, MD
     Josephine Chow, patient

We have been asked to consider the total insurance liability in the above case. Our recommendations are as follows:

- Consultation fee of $150 is appropriate.
- Bilateral angiogram: The range in fees is $500 to $800. We would not recommend any change in the charged fee, $600.
- Surgical procedure: Excision of metastatic tumor and frontal lobectomy. We would recommend that a fee of $3000 be considered reasonable.

It would be my final recommendation. . . .

Figure 22–5   Letter illustrating use of tabulated copy and bulleted items.

23

Manuscripts

23–1   ABSTRACTS

 DO   sequence the content of an abstract to follow that of the article. It should be double spaced and should contain the title, summary, and bibliographic information.

 DO   use abbreviations and standard scientific symbols that are understood when used alone, such as pH and DNA.

Incorrect:
The patient received HCT 250.
Correct:
The patient received hydrocortisone 250 mg.
Correct:
The pH of the urine was 4.5.

✓ **DO**   end the abstract with a complete bibliographic reference.

> . . . intravascular coagulation played a significant role in the patient's death. In the second case prompt therapeutic maneuvers led to eventual recovery. (Wolfe BM, et al. Malignant hyperthermia of anesthesia. Am. J. Surg. Dec. 200X;126:717–721.)

🚫 **DON'T**   list citations of references cited in the text of the article.

🚫 **DON'T**   include tables or figures in abstracts.

23–2   BIBLIOGRAPHY

✓ **DO**   list all works consulted in the preparation of the manuscript as well as all the material that was cited in the notes. List authorship, title, edition, place of publication, publisher, date of publication, and physical description *(pages, illustrations, tables)*.

✓ **DO**   arrange the bibliography in alphabetical order by the surnames of the authors.

✓ **DO**   begin the bibliography on a new page, with the title *BIBLIOGRAPHY* in all capital letters and centered.

✓ **DO**   use the same margins as used for the other pages in the body of the manuscript, and number the pages. *(See 23–11 and 23–12.)*

✓ **DO**   key each entry single spaced at the left margin. Use double spacing if the manuscript is to be set in type. Indent the second line of each entry so the first word in each entry is easily visible.

✓ **DO**   double-space between entries.

✓ **DO**   follow the usual rules for capitalization.

✓ **DO**   use periods at the end of each bibliographic entry, and use commas to separate the elements within each entry, except for the title group. If the elements are not closely related, use a semicolon. Separate a title from a subtitle with a colon.

> Thomson WA, Denk JP. Promoting diversity in the medical school pipeline: a national overview. Acad Med 1999;74:312-314

NOTE: *Bibliography format and punctuation can vary, depending on the publisher's house style.*

23–3 BOOK REVIEW

✓ DO include the review heading *(title)*, the text of the review, the author statement, and the author affiliation.

✓ DO format the review heading with the same components as a bibliographic reference, and, in addition, list the number of pages, illustrations, and tables; the price; the International Standard Book Number (ISBN); and where the book can be purchased *(list an address)*. The ISBN is given on the book's copyright page.

✓ DO list the authors' names exactly as the names appear on the publication, and abbreviate authors' names only if that is how the names appear on the publication.

How 10: A Handbook for Office Professionals. James L. Clark, Lyn R. Clark, Thomson Learning South-Western, 5191 Natorp Boulevard, Mason, Ohio 45040, 2004, 10th edition. 540 pages. ISBN: 0-324-17882-4, $34.95.

23–4 CITATIONS
See Endnotes, 23–6.

23–5 COPYRIGHT

✓ DO place a copyright notice on the first page of the manuscript if the writer wishes to call attention to ownership of the material.

✓ DO include the following elements in the copyright notice: copyright ©, current year, the word *by*, and the author's name.

Copyright © 2004 by Health Professions Institute.

23–6 ENDNOTES

✓ DO type the endnotes *(words or ideas of a person other than the author that appear in a manuscript)* on a separate sheet. List them together at the end of each chapter or at the end of a complete report or manuscript. Type *NOTES* in all capital letters, centered on line 13. Double-space and begin numbering and typing the first endnote. Single-space each endnote unless the manuscript is to be typeset, in which case use double spacing to allow room for editing. Leave one blank line between endnotes. Indent the first line of each endnote five spaces. *(See also 23–7, Footnotes, and 23–17, Text Notes.)*

↓ 13

NOTES

↓ 3

1. James L. Clark, Lyn R. Clark. HOW 10: A Handbook for Office Professionals. Thomson Learning South-Western, Mason, Ohio, 2004, pp. 400-404.

↓ 2

2. Ibid. p. 405.

NOTE: *Endnote format and punctuation can vary, depending on the publisher's house style.*

23–7　FOOTNOTES

Footnotes are positioned at the bottom of a page. They are used to document direct quotes, paraphrase written works, state opinions of persons other than the author, list statistical data not compiled by the writer, present visuals such as photographs, tables, or charts not constructed by the author, and cite a reference.

✓ DO　　key a footnote that refers to a book. Include the footnote number, the author's name, the title *(underscored)*, the edition *(if not the first)*, the publisher, the place of publication, the year of publication, and the page reference. If the organization is more important than the contributors, list the organization's name *(rather than the contributors)* as author. *(See also 23–6, Endnotes, and 23–17, Text Notes.)*

✓ DO　　allow ½ inch for each footnote to be keyed at the bottom of a page on which a reference is made.

NOTE: *Use the word processing software feature for inserting a footnote with superscript references.*

✓ DO　　key an underscore 2 inches long at the bottom of the page to separate footnote material from the main text above. Key the underscore a double space below the last line of text, flush with the left margin.

✓ DO　　double-space below the underscore to key the first footnote.

✅ **DO** number and single-space each footnote and indent the first line five spaces *(one tab)*. If the manuscript is to be typeset, use double spacing to allow for editing. Leave one blank line between each footnote.

1. The AAMT Book of Style, 2nd ed., American Association for Medical Transcription, Modesto, California, 2002, p. 248.

2. Dorland's Illustrated Medical Dictionary, 30th ed., W. B. Saunders Company, Philadelphia, Pennsylvania, 2004, p. 1940.

NOTE: *Footnote format and punctuation can vary, depending on the publisher's house style.*

23–8 GALLEY PROOFS

✅ **DO** use formal proofreading marks to indicate corrections on galley proofs. The marks should appear at the site of the error in red pen as well as in right and/or left margins to draw the editor's eye to the line. *(See also Chapter 34, Proofreading and Revisions.)*

23–9 HEADINGS
See Figure 23–1 at the end of the chapter.

✅ **DO** key headings in all capital letters, centered on line 13. On the third line below the heading, begin keying the actual text.

✅ **DO** use three levels of text headings and subheadings. Centered headings may be keyed in all capital letters. Side headings begin flush with the left margin on a separate line and may be in all capital letters or in capital and lowercase letters that are underscored. Run-in or paragraph headings begin indented one tab stop *(five spaces)* from the left margin and are immediately followed by text on the same line. Run-in headings should be keyed in uppercase and lowercase letters, underscored, and followed by a period. The text begins two spaces after the period.

23–10 LEGENDS
Legends are captions that describe illustrations *(called figures)* that appear in the manuscript.

DO key legends on a separate sheet, double spaced, and numbered to correspond with each figure in the manuscript. Place the author's name, the title of the manuscript, and the number of the figure on the back of each illustration *(photograph, chart, drawing, and so forth).*

23–11 MARGINS
See Figure 23–1 at the end of the chapter.

 DO key double spaced on 8½ × 11 inch paper with 1-inch top, bottom, and side margins, except for a 2-inch top margin on the first page. If the manuscript is to be bound, the left margin should be 1½ inches. Indent the first sentence of each paragraph one or two tab stops *(five or ten spaces).*

 DO try to keep the right margin as even as possible, and divide words according to proper word division guidelines. You may key two or three spaces beyond the desired right margin to avoid word division.

🚫 **DON'T** have two consecutive end-of-line hyphenations.

🚫 **DON'T** end a page with a hyphenated word.

23–12 NUMBERING PAGES

 DO Use the word processing computer software feature for placing page numbers automatically and customize them to your document.

23–13 PROOFREADING

 DO proofread the entire manuscript several times to check for clarity of meaning, spelling, punctuation, grammar, and other mechanics before it is submitted for publication. Use a red pen to insert formal proofreading marks at the site of the error.

23–14 SUMMARY
See discussion under 23–1, Abstracts.

23–15 SYNOPSIS
See discussion under 23–1, Abstracts.

23–16 TABLE OF CONTENTS

✓ DO   center the words *Contents* or *Table of Contents* in all-capital letters 2 inches from the top edge of the paper.

✓ DO   list the major and minor headings with page numbers of the manuscript double or single spaced. Use leaders (. . . . .) to guide the reader from the topic *(on the left side of the page)* to its page number *(at the right)* unless there are fewer than five entries. *(See Figure 23–2 at the end of the chapter.)*

✓ DO   include supplemental parts of the manuscript *(appendix, bibliography, index)* with their page numbers.

23–17 TEXT NOTES

Text notes are used to document direct quotes, paraphrase written works, state opinions of persons other than the author, list statistical data not compiled by the writer, and present visuals such as photographs, tables, or charts not constructed by the author. These notes are written within the body of the material itself rather than being placed at the end of a report *(i.e., endnotes)* or at the bottom of a page *(i.e., footnotes)*.

✓ DO   key the text note directly below the statement referred to and separated by two solid lines. Number and indent each text note five spaces. Text notes may be single or double spaced. *(See also 23–6, Endnotes, and 23–7, Footnotes.)*

A manuscript submitted to an editor, publisher, or printer should be carefully and attractively typed.[1]

---

1. Sarah Augusta Taintor and Kate M. Munro. <u>The Secretary's Handbook,</u> The Macmillan Company, New York, New York, 1969, p. 435.

NOTE: *Text note format and punctuation can vary, depending on the publisher's house style.*

23–18 TITLE PAGE

✓ DO   include the title of the report in all-capital letters, as well as the name and title of the author, the group or organization of the intended reader, and the date. It is optional to precede the name with the words *prepared for* or *submitted by* (Figure 23–3). Some word processing software programs provide a template for a title page.

1 or 1½
inch margin   2 inches   1 inch
                                                   margin

Main Heading A MEDICAL PROFESSIONAL REPORT

Triple-space

This is your manuscript guide, which will help you
                                    Double-space
prepare a manuscript for your physician. Always double-space the
body of the manuscript and indent one or two tab stops (five or
ten spaces) at the beginning of each paragraph. Make a photocopy
of each page and retain it for your records. The left margin should
be 1 or 1½ inches, and the right margin should be 1 inch.

Title Page (underline)
        A title page is not necessary for most manuscripts
submitted for publication. Refer to Figure 23-3 for proper format.

Table of Contents (Underline)
        The table of contents is a list of headings of the major parts
of the manuscript. It is required by some, but not all, publishers.
When required, it is composed after the entire manuscript has
been completed so that correct page numbers can be inserted.
Notice that the entire table of contents has been centered vertically
in Figure 23-2.

1-inch
margin

Figure 23–1   Illustration of page one of a manuscript showing format and headings.

TABLE OF CONTENTS

TITLE PAGE.. 0
TABLE OF CONTENTS... 0
BODY OF MANUSCRIPT.. 0
Margins... 0
Footnotes.. 0
BIBLIOGRAPHY... 0

↑
Three spaces

Figure 23–2   Illustration of a table of contents for a manuscript.

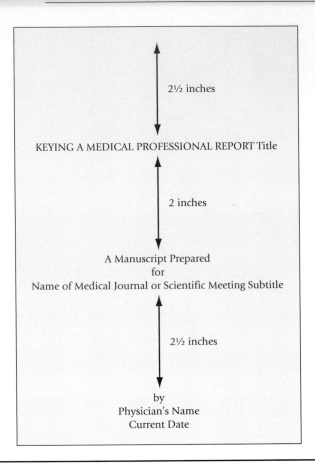

Figure 23–3 Title page of a manuscript.

24

Medical Reports

INTRODUCTION

This chapter gives information for preparing the "Big Four": the history and physical examination, operative report, consultation report, and discharge summary. In addition, information is given for a variety of other medical reports: autopsy protocols, medicolegal reports, pathology reports, radiology reports, and radiotherapy reports.

Use the formats and standard outlines preferred in your locality and/or hospital facility. Accuracy, appearance, and ease of readability are important factors in choosing a format. Examples of a variety of formats are at the end of the chapter so you can see how many different styles appear.

24–1 AUTOPSY PROTOCOLS

 DO   refer to your medical examiner's or county coroner's office and state board of medical examiners for the legal requirements when typing and reporting autopsy protocols, since only general guidelines are stated here.

✓ **DO**   prepare an autopsy protocol in one of the five pathology forms: the narrative *(in story form)*, the numerical *(by the numbers)*, the pictorial *(hand drawings or anatomic forms)*, protocols based on sentence completion and multiple-choice selection, or problem-oriented protocols *(a supplement to the problem-oriented medical record system). (See Figure 24–1 at the end of the chapter; this figure is a brief autopsy report just so you can examine one style, p. 282.)*

✓ **DO**   spell out abbreviations or keep them to a minimum because clarity is the essential element in an autopsy protocol. Interpretation of typed material must be accurate.

✓ **DO**   use military time if required by state law when documenting the time a body is brought in for autopsy.

     1420 hours

✓ **DO**   abbreviate when typing metric terms.

     0.5 cm   200 ml   3 × 3 mm

     NOTE: *Many facilities may prefer that transcriptionists spell out the word grams in hospital autopsy reports and forensic autopsy reports when reporting the weights of organs.*

     The heart weighs 330 grams.

 DO   spell out pounds and inches.

     The body weighs 160 pounds, and the body length is 65 inches.

🚫 **DON'T**   use quotation marks to indicate inches.

> **Incorrect:**
> 65"
> **Correct:**
> 65 inches

✓ **DO**   spell out all words when typing the body temperature.

> 88 degrees Fahrenheit

✓ **DO**   spell out numbers and put the figure in parentheses indicating how much or how many whenever clarity needs to be emphasized.

> two (2) stab wounds

✓ **DO**   use quotation marks when indicating a marking on the body.

> A superficial suture wound shaped like a "V" is present on the left cheek.

✓ **DO**   include the following in a *hospital autopsy protocol:*

> Clinical history *(a brief resume of the patient's medical history and course in the hospital before demise)*
> Pathologic diagnosis *(at autopsy)*
> External examination
> Evidence of injury
> Macroscopic examination
> Internal examination
> Gross findings *(visual examination of the organs of the body before any tissues are removed for preparation and examination)*
> Special dissections and examinations
> Microscopic examination *(an examination of the particular organs through the microscope)*
> Epicrisis or final pathologic diagnosis *(critical analysis or actual finding or discussion of the cause of disease after its determination)*
> Report of final summary or discussion
> Signature of pathologist

✓ **DO**   include the following in a *forensic pathology autopsy protocol:*

> External description
> Evidence of injury *(external and internal)*

Systems and organs *(cavities and organs)*
Special dissections and examinations
Brain *(and other organs)* after fixation
Microscopic examination
Findings *(diagnoses)*, factual and interpretative
Conclusion, interpretative and opinion
Signature of medical examiner/pathologist

NOTE: *Forensic dentists describe bite marks by size, shape, and location. They swab for saliva to determine blood type, make impressions or molds of the bite mark, and photograph and make impressions of the suspect's dentition.*

✓ **DO**   use both reference initials, as well as your own, when two medical examiners are involved.

RT:LOR:CRD
or
rt/lor/crd

24–2   CHART NOTES OR PROGRESS NOTES
See Chapter 33, Progress Notes or Chart Notes, p. 397.

24–3   COMPUTER FORMAT

✓ **DO**   use full block report style to reduce the number and complexity of machine manipulations required. Use of this style will save time and reduce errors.

✓ **DO**   use single spacing when keying a report. Double-space between paragraphs or topics.

24–4   CONSULTATION REPORTS

✓ **DO**   use letter form or report form, single spaced, with content similar to a history and physical medical report. Headings may or may not be included. These reports are sent to the attending physician who requested the consultation. The report should be signed by the examining physician. *(See Figures 24–2 and 24–3 at the end of the chapter; see also Chapter 19, History and Physical Format, and Chapter 22, Letter Format.)*

24–5 CONTINUATION SHEETS

☑ DO   key headings for page 2 and subsequent pages; use the format preferred by your employer and/or hospital facility. These headings include the patient's name, medical record number, page number, and other optional statistical information *(e.g., name of attending physician)*.

NOTE: *If you are using a template, the software program may automatically insert a heading on a continuation page and correctly number each subsequent page.*

☑ DO   key flush with the left margin or use a horizontal format.

Maria J. Valdez, #6893z
August 14, 200X
Page 2
or
Maria J. Valdez   #6893   August 14, 200X   Page 2

☑ DO   key *continued* on the bottom of all incomplete sheets, beginning with the first page, when the report includes more than one page.

🚫 DON'T   carry just one line of a medical report to a continuation sheet.

🚫 DON'T   carry only the signature line to a continuation sheet.

NOTE: *Some word processing programs have a feature that prevents the creation of orphans (printing the first line of a new paragraph as the last line on a page) and widows (printing the last line of a paragraph as the first line of a new page).*

24–6 CORRECTIONS

☑ DO   retain the original transcript when corrections necessitate retyping a medical report in hospital transcription. The physician should insert omitted words, correct all errors, and initial each correction directly on the original transcript. On the second draft, type *corrected for errors*. The physician should sign both copies, and they should be stapled together.

24–7 DATES

 DO   use the date the material was dictated, not the day it was transcribed.

 DO   spell out the date in full in either the traditional or the military style.

November 14, 200X *(traditional)*
22 December 200X *(British and military)*

 DO   key the dates of dictation and transcription at the end of the medical report on two lines below the reference initials. Use figures for the dates.

pod
D: 11-24-0X
T: 11-25-0X

rlp
D: 11/24/200X
T: 11/24/200X

NOTE: *Some facilities key in the time of day and/or a code number for the transcriptionist.*

D: 11/24/0X 1785
T: 11/25/0X 1015 #1642

24–8 DIAGNOSIS

DO   spell out any terms dictated as abbreviations in the diagnosis part of any medical report.

Incorrect:
DIAGNOSIS: ASHD
Correct:
DIAGNOSIS: Arteriosclerotic heart disease

DO   use numbering if dictated; it is optional if not dictated.

DIAGNOSES: Gastritis.
                 Pancreatitis.
or
DIAGNOSES
1. Gastritis.
2. Pancreatitis.

24-9 DISCHARGE SUMMARIES, CLINICAL RESUMES, AND FINAL PROGRESS NOTES

See Figure 24-4 at the end of the chapter, p. 286.

✓ **DO**   key single spaced with main headings, whether dictated or not, and insert subheadings as dictated:

Admission date
Discharge date
History of present illness
Pertinent past history
Physical examination on discharge
Admitting diagnosis
Laboratory and/or x-ray data on admission
Hospital course and treatment
Surgical procedures
Consultations
Discharge diagnosis
Disposition
Prognosis
Condition of the patient on discharge *(medications on discharge, instructions for continuing care, therapy, and followup postoperative office visit date)*

NOTE: *In the case of death, a summary statement should be added to the record either as a final progress note or as a separate resume. This final note should give the reason for admission, the findings and course of illness in the hospital, and the events leading to death.*

✓ **DO**   send a copy of the discharge summary to any known medical practitioner and/or medical facility responsible for followup care of the patient if authorized in writing by the patient or the patient's legally qualified representative.

24-10 FORMAT STYLES

Statistical Data: As determined by the medical facility, (e.g., patient's name, ID number, referring physician, and so on).

Title: Centered on the page or flush with left margin.
All capital letters.

Main Topics: All capitals.
May be underlined or not.
On a line by itself or introducing data on same line.
Begun on edge of left margin.

Subtopics:	First letter only capitalized or all caps.
	Begun on left margin.
Data:	Begun on the *same* line as subtopic.
	or
	Begun on left margin, double-spaced down.
	Single spaced.
	All lines return to the left margin.
	Double space between the last line of one heading and the next heading.
Margins:	Narrow (½ inch is appropriate).
Close:	Keyed line for signature.
	Author's typed name.
	Transcriptionist's initials.
	Date of dictation (D).
	Date of transcription (T).
Variations:	1. No space below main topic.
	2. Subtopics grouped after main heading in paragraph format.
	3. Subtopics indented and blocked.

See 18–3, Format Styles, for full information for keying full block, modified block, indented, and run-on format styles with many variations. The author or institution may prefer a certain style or variation. One goal is less formatting. Some authors, however, prefer the ease of readability and some of the more "fussy" indented or blocked styles. *(See also 24–3, Computer Format.)*

24–11 HEADINGS

 DO   key major headings in all capital letters followed by a colon. Place major headings on a line alone and underline depending on your format style choice. *(See 19-3, Format Styles.)* If the author moves in and out of paragraphs and does not dictate complete paragraphs, omit or add headings, depending on your employer's preference.

24–12 HISTORY AND PHYSICAL FORMAT
See Chapter 19, History and Physical Format.

24–13 MARGINS

 DO   use the default *(preset)* feature of the word processing software or use ½ inch to ¾ inch right and left and top and bottom margins.

24-14 MEDICOLEGAL REPORTS
See Figure 24-5 at the end of the chapter, p. 287.

✓ DO — use the physician's letterhead stationery and letter format, with or without headings and/or subheadings, for medicolegal reports. These detailed documents include the following information:

Patient's name
Date of the accident or work-related injury
Employer's name, if work injury
History of the accident, injury, or illness
Present complaint(s)
Past history and preexisting conditions
Physical findings on examination
Laboratory and/or x-ray findings
Diagnosis
Prescribed therapy
Disability
Prognosis

24-15 NUMBERING

✓ DO — be consistent in using arabic numbers to number vertically or horizontally all or none of the entries if the author numbers some but not all terms in a series. Capitalize the first letter of each numbered entry, and place a period at the end of each statement.

DISCHARGE DIAGNOSES
1. Ectopic tubal pregnancy delivered by repeat cesarean section.
2. Postoperative lower segment placental bed sinus hemorrhage of the uterus.

ADMITTING DIAGNOSES. (1) Left pleural effusion, (2) Left otitis media, (3) Procaine-induced lupuslike syndrome.

DIAGNOSES
1. Diabetes out of control.
2. Acute alcohol intoxication.
3. Peripheral neuropathy.
4. History of thyroidectomy.

24-16 OPERATIVE REPORTS
See Figures 24-6 and 24-7 at the end of the chapter, pp. 288 and 289.
See also 27-25, Suture Materials, on how to key information about suture materials.

DO key into a macro or preset form the name of the patient, the room number, the hospital number, the surgeon's name, the assistant surgeon's name, the anesthesiologist's name, the type of anesthesia, and the date of the operation.

 DO use single spacing with main headings, whether dictated or not, and insert those subheadings *(incision, sponge count, closure, and so forth)* as dictated.

Include the following headings in the report:
Preoperative diagnosis
Postoperative diagnosis
Reason for operation
Operation performed

NOTE: *Many hospitals break down the operative description into three sections: (1) positioning, prepping, and draping and opening the incision; (2) the internal operation; and (3) the closing.*

Indications for procedure
Findings
Procedure
Complications
Specimens
Estimated blood loss
Instrument and sponge counts
Signature of the surgeon

NOTE: *Some hospital policies require that if there is a dictation/transcription and/or filing delay, a comprehensive operative progress note must be entered in the medical record immediately after surgery in order to provide pertinent information for other physicians who may be attending the patient.*

 DO repeat the preoperative diagnosis for the postoperative diagnosis when "same" is dictated.

 DON'T use an abbreviation when keying the preoperative diagnosis, postoperative diagnosis, or procedure.

24-17 *OUTLINE*

For outline rules, see Autopsy Protocols; Consultation Reports; Discharge Summaries, Clinical Resumes, and Final Progress Notes; Medicolegal Reports; Operative Reports; Pathology Reports; and Radiology and Imaging Reports in this chapter.

See Chapter 19, History and Physical Format, for history and physical examination outlines.

24-10 PATHOLOGY REPORTS

See Figure 24-8 at the end of the chapter, p. 290.
See also 24-1, Autopsy Protocols.

 DO   key into a macro or preset format the pathology identification number, the name of the patient, the room number, the hospital number, and the date of the surgical procedure.

 DO   use single spacing with main headings whether dictated or not.

> Gross or macroscopic description
> Microscopic description
> Comment
> Recommendation
> Conclusion(s) and/or diagnosis
> Signature of the pathologist

 DO   use all capital letters and/or underline the section of the pathology report detailing benign or malignant lesions.

> A frozen section consultation at the time of surgery was delivered as NO EVIDENCE OF MALIGNANCY on frozen section, to await permanent section for final diagnosis.

 DO   use the past tense if a history is dictated for a pathology report.

> CLINICAL SUMMARY
> This baby was born at 2:30 p.m. on 9-23-XX and died at 6:25 p.m. the same day. The baby was quite pallid at birth. Respirations and cry were delayed and not heard until five and a half minutes had passed.

 DO   use the present tense when the pathologist is interpreting the findings.

> MICROSCOPIC DIAGNOSIS
> Cervical biopsy, 6 o'clock
> Endocervical mucosa shows squamous metaplasia with condylomatous atypia and coexisting mild dysplasia (CIN I or low-grade squamous intraepithelial lesion). There is involvement of endocervical glands, and moderate acute and chronic endocervicitis is demonstrated.

24–19 RADIOLOGY AND IMAGING REPORTS

See Figures 24–9, 24–10, 24–11, and 24–12 at the end of the chapter.

Some of the types of radiology reports dictated are the following: aortogram, barium enema, bronchogram, cardioangiogram, cholangiogram, cholecystogram, cineradiogram, computed tomogram (*CT scan*), cystogram, echogram, encephalogram, esophagogram, fluoroscopy (*chest, colon, gallbladder, stomach*) hysterosalpingogram, intravenous cholangiogram (*IVC*), intravenous pyelogram (*IVP*), laminagram, lymphangiogram, magnetic resonance imaging (*MRI*), myelogram, spinal, nephrotomogram, nuclear magnetic resonance (*NMR*), pneumoencephalogram, retrograde pyelogram, sialogram, single-photon emission computed tomography (*SPECT*), sonogram, stereoscopy, thermogram, tomogram, ultrasonogram (*bile ducts, gallbladder, kidneys, liver, ovaries and uterus*) upper and lower gastrointestinal series, venogram, ventriculogram.

✓ **DO**   use a macro or preset format and key in the name of the patient, the name of the attending physician, the radiology identification number, the patient's age, the date, and the type of examination. In addition, in a hospital case, insert the room number and the hospital number.

✓ **DO**   use single spacing with main headings, whether dictated or not.

         Name of the x-ray examination, scan, xeroradiography, thermography, nuclear magnetic resonance, ultrasound, and so forth.
Findings or interpretation
Impression or diagnosis
Conclusion
Recommendations
Signature of the radiologist

✓ **DO**   use the present tense when the radiologist is interpreting the findings.

✓ **DO**   use the date of radiologic service rather than the date of dictation when inserting the date in the heading of the radiology report.

24–20 RADIOTHERAPY REPORTS

✓ **DO**   key into a macro or preset format the name of the patient, the date, and the name of the physician requesting the consultation. If a hospital case, put in the room number and hospital number.

✓ **DO**   use single spacing with main headings, whether dictated or not.

> X-ray interpretation
> Consultation
> Therapy *(specific preparation of the patient, identity, date, and amount of radiopharmaceutical medications used)*

24–21   *REFERENCE INITIALS*

✓ **DO**   use a double space below the typed signature line and type flush with the left margin.

✓ **DO**   key the author's, signer's, and the typist's initials when the author differs from the person who signs the document.

> mjp/lrc/wpd *or* mjp:lrc:wpd
> Here, *mjp* stands for the dictator, *lrc* stands for the signer, and *wpd* stands for the typist.

✓ **DO**   use either all capitals or all lowercase letters for both sets of initials, with a colon or virgule between them.

⊘ **DON'T** use humorous or confusing combinations of reference initials.

> crc *(rather than cc)*
> db *(rather than dmb)*
> dg *(rather than dog)*
> mod *(rather than md)*

✓ **DO**   Refer to 24–1, Autopsy Protocols, when two medical examiners are involved in an autopsy protocol.

> mjp/lrc/wpd *or* mjp:lrc:wpd
> Here, *mjp* stands for the author, *lrc* stands for the signer, and *wpd* stands for the transcriptionist.

✓ **DO**   code your documents for ease of retrieval. *(Some institutions automatically format this information on all documents.)*

24–22   *SIGNATURE LINE*

✓ **DO**   leave four to six lines between the end of the report and the signature line.

✓ **DO**   key the author's name. It is optional to insert a line for the signature.

Dwayne B. Stamford, MD
Han S. Ling, MD

24–23   SPACING OF HEADINGS

✓ **DO**   use double spacing or a space and a half between the last line of one heading and the next heading. It is optional to use no space below the main topic. Headings not dictated should be inserted.

24–24   STATISTICAL DATA

✓ **DO**   include the information and use the format preferred by your employer and/or hospital facility.

✓ **DO**   give each document a unique file name. This way transcribed documents may be retrieved easily and quickly when needed. You may be able to use your own file name; however, the dictator or organization may prefer that you use their unique codes. If you are able to use your own codes here are some hints to make it simple.

Use minimum data: ID # for the dictator; patient name; date.
Use letters and numbers: for dates, use just the last digit of the year; use 1-9 for the first nine months and *o, n, d* for the last three.
Use a period for a separation mark.
Place it as the last entry on the page.
Decrease the font size to 8 or 9.
Use the identical code as your "save."
Use on your file copy and computer copy only.
Example
(using Figure 24-6)
(Your ID # for Dr. Stanford is S1)
S1.Levin72X
Uncoded: Dr. Stanford dictated a report on patient Levin on July 2, 200X.

24–25   SUBHEADINGS

✓ **DO**   use all capitals or uppercase and lowercase followed by a colon. It is optional to begin each subtopic on a separate line. Headings needed but not dictated may be inserted, but this, too, is optional.

24–26   TITLES OR MAJOR HEADINGS

✓ DO   begin titles or major headings centered or at the left margin, depending on the preference of your employer and/or hospital facility. Use all capital letters. It is optional to underline the title. Titles might be Autopsy Protocol, Consultation, Discharge Summary, Operative Report, Pathology Report, Radiology Report, and so forth.

AUTOPSY PROTOCOL

Chan, Marylou Foster

September 2, 200X

CLINICAL DIAGNOSIS:
Congenital heart defect.

GENERAL EXAMINATION:
The body is that of a well-developed and well-nourished newborn female infant, having been embalmed prior to examination through a thoracic incision and cannulization of the heart. The recorded birth weight is 7 pounds 2 ounces.

THORAX OPENED:
Considerable blood is present around the heart incident to the embalming procedure, and two incisions in the cardiac muscle are evident; but the valves and great vessels do not appear to have been injured by the embalming procedure. Examination discloses a massive heart, lying transversely in the midanterior thorax, the distended right ventricle exceeding in volume the ventricular mass. Examination discloses no enlargement of the ductus arteriosus or any significant deviation of the size of the great vessels. On exploration of the heart, there is found to be a completely imperforate pulmonary artery at the level of the pulmonary valve, all three cusps of which appear to be adequately formed but fused by scar tissue slightly proximal to the free margins of the cusps. It is impossible to prove the existence of any opening in this area. The right heart is markedly hypertrophic, approximating three times the muscle mass of the normal infant heart. There is no evidence of an interventricular defect. There is a sacculation adjacent to the valve of the inferior vena cava as it enters the inferior right auricle; and in the dome of this sacculated area, the foramen ovale is demonstrated. The foramen is unusually small in diameter (estimated to be no more than 4 mm in diameter) and this is covered by a plica. It would appear that the pressure of the distended right auricle would further compromise the capacity of the foramen to transmit blood. In the absence of any interventricular defect, this would be the only way that blood could get from the right to the left side of the heart. The lungs are heavy and poorly serrated, and the bronchial tree contains some yellowish fluid which, in the absence of feeding by mouth, must be assumed to be aspirated vernix.

Figure 24–1 County coroner's autopsy protocol, keyed in narrative report form and in full block format, p. 1.

Chan, Marylou Foster
September 2, 200X
Page 2

ABDOMEN OPENED:
The stomach contains some bloody mucus but no evidence of
formula. The liver and abdominal viscera appear entirely negative
throughout.

HEAD:
Not opened.

CAUSE OF DEATH ON GROSS FINDINGS:
Massive chylous pericardial effusion, etiology not established but
presumptively related to defect in formation of thoracic duct tissue.

MICROSCOPIC:
Sections of the thymus gland reveal a generally normal histological
architecture for the thymus of the newborn, epithelial elements still
being distributed through the lymphoid tissues. Certainly no tumor
is present in the thymic tissue. The pulmonary tissues are poorly
expanded although the bronchi appear open. There is a general
vascular congestion of pulmonary tissue and some apparent
extravasation of blood into the poorly expanded alveoli. In
addition, there are deposits of hyaline material on the surfaces of
some of the air spaces that would indicate the existence of hyaline
membrane disease. The liver shows marked congestion and a rather
active hematopoiesis. The heart muscle is not remarkable and the
epicardial surface does not appear thickened or unusual. The kidney
tissue exhibits some punctuate hemorrhages in the parenchyma
consistent with anoxia.

MICROSCOPIC DIAGNOSIS:
Renal hemorrhages incident to anoxia.

Chief Pathologist _____
Susan R. Foster, MD

lao
D: 09/03/0X
T: 09/03/0X

Figure 24–1   Cont'd

KARL ROBRECHT, MD
Internal Medicine

ADRIANNA SACHS, MD
Cardiology

Gulf Medical Group, Inc.
800 Gulf Shore Drive
Naples, FL 33940

Telephone 813 649-1111

FAX 813 987-5121

February 19, 200X

Franklin J. Croydon, MD
8754 Gulf View Parkway
Naples, FL 33940

Dear Dr. Croydon:

RE: Loren Cavara

I saw this 71-year-old man this morning at Gulf General Hospital. He was admitted yesterday with a 10-day history of chills, sweats, rash, and malaise. He had a distant history of Hodgkin disease treated with radiation therapy in 1999. He does have a history of multiple lipomas.

On admission he was noted to have enlarged left inguinal nodes and possible enlarged axillary nodes. CT scan was performed which showed possible densities in the duodenum and distal small bowel which were felt to possibly represent lymphoma.

There is a macular rash of the trunk. There are multiple subcutaneous nodules of the back and abdominal wall consistent with lipomas or fibrolipomas. There is no cervical or axillary adenopathy. There is no right axillary adenopathy. There are several nodes palpable and enlarged in the left groin, especially laterally.

Assessment: Adenopathy, rule out lymphoma.

CT findings are consistent with possible lymphomatous or other malignant process.

Plan: I feel that node biopsy would be an appropriate diagnostic step. Excision of the largest inguinal node under local anesthesia with monitored anesthesia care. (This will be sent for lymphoma studies.) This has been scheduled for this evening.

Thank you for permitting me to assist you in the care of this patient.

Sincerely yours,

Karl Robrecht, MD

wpd

Figure 24–2   Consultation report in letter form and in full block format.

DATE OF CONSULTATION: 7/23/0X

REASON FOR CONSULTATION: Facial deformity secondary to dog
bite injuries.

HISTORY OF PRESENT ILLNESS: This is a 9-year-old little girl who
13 months ago was bitten in the face by a friend's dog. The wounds
were evaluated and closed at a local hospital. The patient now
presents to the clinic for evaluation of significant facial deformities
due to the dog bite injury.

PHYSICAL EXAMINATION.
Extensive dog bite scars which are depressed involving the lower lip
measuring 1.5 cm, several of the cheek measuring between 3-4 cm,
and numerous ones of the left lower lip/chin junction, cheek
measuring 4 cm. All are distorted and tethered producing a
significant cosmetic deformity to the patient's facial appearance.

IMPRESSION:
Extensive scarring of the face secondary to dog bite wounds.

PLAN:
Revision of dog bite wound scars. This was discussed with the
parents.

Daniel E. Ansted, MD

dee
DD: 7/23/0X 1441
DT: 7/24/0X
Doc. #C202R007.VCM
    [131006]

PITMAN COUNTY MEDICAL CENTER   PT: Shelly Rose Dexter
                                      MR#: 762962B
PLASTIC SURGERY CONSULTATION   Abbott Sheltland, D.O.

Figure 24–3   Plastic surgery consultation report in full block format, generated
in a clinic setting.

ADMITTED: 6/27/0X   DISCHARGED: 7/1/0X

ADMITTING DIAGNOSES:
1. Term pregnancy.
2. Labor.

DISCHARGE DIAGNOSES:
1. Term pregnancy.
2. Cephalopelvic disproportion.
3. Status post primary cesarean section with lower uterine segment transverse incision.

ATTENDING PHYSICIANS:
Barry Templeton, M D
Randolph T. Day, M D

RESIDENT PHYSICIANS:
Holly Pabarue, M.D.
Aaron Sklar, M.D.

HOSPITAL COURSE: The patient presented to the labor and delivery floor on 6/27/0X with the chief complaint of a gush of fluid at 4:30 p.m. with the subsequent onset of uterine contractions, which were increasing in frequency and intensity. The patient continued in labor. She was found to have some very low decelerations, but with prompt return. The patient was noted to have some variable decelerations that were persisting, with some decreasing variability. She had not dilated for greater than four hours. Therefore, the patient was prepared and readied for a cesarean section. The patient underwent the cesarean section and delivered a male infant.

The patient did well postoperatively. She was ambulating and tolerating clear liquids. She remained afebrile. She was tolerating a general diet on discharge. At the time of discharge, her temperature was 97.8 F, blood pressure 140/76, pulse rate 67, respiratory rate 16. Her breasts were not engorged. Her lungs were clear to auscultation bilaterally. Her cardiovascular examination revealed a regular rate and rhythm. The S1 and S2 were normal. There were no murmurs or rubs. On abdominal examination, her fundus was firm. She had minimal lochia. Her feet revealed 2+ pitting edema bilaterally, but her extremities were otherwise within normal limits.

DISPOSITION: The patient was diagnosed status post cesarean section, which was performed secondary to cephalopelvic disproportion. The patient will follow up with Dr. Ford in one week for removal of the staples. She will continue to take her iron and prenatal vitamins for the next month. She was also prescribed Colace and Tylenol No. 3 p.r.m. The patient has a followup appointment at the Holly Avenue Clinic on 7/2/0X at 10 a.m.

AS:yre/vo
DD: 7/13/0X 1532
DT: 7/16/0X   _____
Doc. #D124VO14.VCM   Aaron Sklar, M.D.

_____   _____
       PITMAN COUNTY MEDICAL CENTER   PT: Aisha Storm
          DISCHARGE SUMMARY   MR # 14-96-97
                                                    DR: Aaron Sklar, M.D.

Figure 24–4   A hospital discharge summary, keyed in report form and full block format.

William A. Berry, MD

Suite 10B
759 West Mountain Meadow Road
White Oaks, XX 00990

555 982-3483   Orthopaedic Surgery

January 8, 200X

Ms. Mary M. O'Shaunessy
5588 Maryland Avenue
Whiteoakes, XX 99900

Dear Ms. O'Shaunessy:

RE: O'SHAUNESSY, Mary Maude
        Breast implant claims #655-86-7777

Thank you for coming to my office for reevaluation and review of your
medical records with regard to the Claims Administrator's Office letter of
12/23/0X. I would like to submit the following information to help clarify the
medical records.

Your diagnosis is symmetrical polyarthritis, not classical rheumatoid arthritis.
Classical rheumatoid arthritis requires more diagnostic criteria than you
presented, in accordance with the revised 1958 ACR criteria.

You have demonstrated symmetrical polyarthritis of a number of different
joint groups: certainly the wrists, shoulders, elbows, hands and feet. This
represents more than two joint groups. I have noted swelling of the wrists and
MCP joints, specifically the second and third MCP joints have been noted to be
swollen and the left wrist. Other rheumatologists have noted swelling of the
shoulders.

Concerning your sicca syndrome, I found no evidence that you had symptoms,
sought medical care or took medication for sicca syndrome prior to your
breast implants. There is no secondary cause for sicca syndrome noted on my
examination.

A positive antinuclear antibody (ANA) 1:80 homogeneous pattern was
collected 12/15/XX. There was also an anticentromere antibody found positive
1:40 dilution.

Sincerely,

William A. Berry, M.D.

ref

Figure 24–5   Medicolegal report generated from a medical office and typed in
modified block format.

OPERATIVE REPORT

PATIENT NAME:	LEVIN, ORA
DATE:	07-2-0X
PREOPERATIVE DIAGNOSIS:	Left lower quadrant pain.
POSTOPERATIVE DIAGNOSIS:	Normal gynecological examination.
SURGEON:	RAYMOND M. STANFORD, MD
ASSISTANT:	JENNI R. DEVON, MD
ANESTHETIC:	General with LMA
ANESTHESIOLOGIST:	HELEN DAVIDSON DORUNDA, MD
PROCEDURE:	Diagnostic laparoscopy.

INDICATIONS FOR PROCEDURE: The patient is a 22-year-old gravida 3 para 2 ab 1 who had a history of left lower quadrant pain and an ultrasound suggesting a left adnexa mass. The patient was admitted to the hospital for diagnostic laparoscopy.

DESCRIPTION OF PROCEDURE: The patient was taken to the operating room where she was administered a general anesthetic. She was then placed in the dorsal lithotomy position and prepped and draped for a laparoscopic procedure.

Examination under anesthesia revealed the uterus to be anterior and mobile. No specific adnexal masses were felt.

A speculum was placed. The anterior lip of the cervix was then grasped with a tenaculum. A uterine mobilizer was placed to help move the uterus during the procedure. The bladder was then drained with a Robinson catheter. A small incision was then made in the inferior aspect of the umbilicus. A Veress needle was inserted into the abdomen and the abdomen inflated with 4 L of carbon dioxide. The laparoscope trocar was then placed and then the operating laparoscope. A small suprapubic incision was made so a probe could be placed to help completely evaluate the pelvic organs. The patient was noted to have some adhesions of the omentum to the anterior abdominal wall probably from her previous cesarean section. The uterus itself, however, was normal in appearance. It was smooth in contour. There were no adhesions involving the anterior posterior cul-de-sacs. The posterior cul-de-sac was carefully visualized and no evidence of endometriosis was noted. The left tube and ovary were entirely normal. There were no cysts noted in the ovary and no peritubal or periovarian adhesions. There was a small area of adhesion of the omentum into the right lower quadrant; however, the right tube and ovary also appeared to be quite normal without any evidence of a cyst or periovarian or peritubal adhesions. The procedure was terminated, determining that the patient's pelvic organs were normal. The accessory probe and laparoscope were removed allowing the gas to escape from the abdomen. The small incisions were repaired with interrupted subcuticular sutures of 4-0 Dexon.

ESTIMATED BLOOD LOSS: Negligible.

The sponge and needle count was correct.

The patient was taken to the recovery room in good condition.

LRT

D: 7-2-0X
T: 7-2-0X

RAYMOND M. STANFORD, MD

Figure 24–6 A hospital operative report, prepared in block format.

OPERATIVE REPORT

Patient: Jonah Fraenkel   Date: September 7, 200X

PREOPERATIVE DIAGNOSIS:
Bright red blood per urethra.

POSTOPERATIVE DIAGNOSIS:
Probable urethral catheter trauma, secondary to incomplete Foley catheter insertion.

PROCEDURE:
Difficult catheter insertion.

SURGEON:
Ralph M. McMurray, MD

ANESTHESIA:
Local, by surgeon.

SITE:
In Surgical ICU bed #4.

INDICATIONS:
This gentleman is status post coronary artery bypass with bright red blood per urethra and difficult Foley catheter management. Consultation was requested to control both. The existing Foley catheter was removed at my direction on consultation.

DESCRIPTION OF PROCEDURE:
The patient was routinely prepped and draped in the supine position while in bed. The urethra was instilled with viscous 1 % Xylocaine gel. At that point, a 24 French Foley with a 30 cc balloon, 2-way, was advanced up the urethra with the intention of placing this in the bladder. It was able to pass through the prostatic fossa and significant bleeding was encountered when the catheter entered into the prostatic fossa. At this point, a catheter guide was employed in the routine fashion and subsequently the appropriate tract to the lumen of the bladder was obtained using a catheter guide. Then, 30 cc was placed in the 30 cc balloon and set to gravity drainage. A small amount of relatively light urine was obtained. There was still some mild bleeding around urethra. IBI was set up, and intermittent bladder irrigation was basically clear, indicating that the bleeding and site of the difficulty was in the prostatic fossa and not in the bladder. Therefore, the large Foley catheter should tamponade the bleeding and ultimately correct the difficulty. The Foley catheter was left indwelling and the urine culture was asked to be sent from the Foley. The patient tolerated the procedure well.

_____
Ralph M. McMurray, MD

wgs
D: 09/07/200X
T: 09/07/200X

Figure 24–7   A hospital operative report, prepared in full block format.

SONORAN DESERT HOSPITAL
La Mirage, XX 99999
555 644-4492

Director of Pathology:
A. T. Hiep, MD

Patient: Victoria McMurray
HC#: 010568945
Admit #: 078934-22Ptype: H
DOB: 40/30/19XX Age: 70 Sex: F
LOC: 3EST -322-01
Reg Date: 07/20/XX
Req Dr: BARRY, DAVID
Path #: 11-SP-00-004532

SURGICAL PATHOLOGY REPORT

CLINICAL HISTORY
Right upper lobe mass, history of cigarette smoking.

GROSS
The specimen consists of a CT-guided needle aspiration of right upper lobe lung mass. The procedure is performed by Dr. Keith Broyard of Interventional Radiology. A single pass is made. Three smear preparations are made for immediate evaluation and the remaining material is submitted in formalin for cell block preparation.

IMMEDIATE EVALUATION: CARCINOMA. (OAA)

Iro

Date: 07/20/0X

MICROSCOPIC
Three direct smear preparations and one cell block are examined.
Immunocytochemical stains pending.

Iro   DATE: 07/21/0X

DIAGNOSIS
Lung, right upper lobe region, image-guided fine needle aspiration and cytologic preparation.
Small-celled carcinoma.
Small-cell undifferentiated carcinoma ("oat cell carcinoma") versus small-celled squamous carcinoma.
Favor small-cell undifferentiated ("oat cell") carcinoma.
Confirmatory-immunocytochemical stains pending. A separate definitive report will follow.

_____
Delease Gunder, MD

07/21/0X
Irm

Figure 24–8   A pathology report, prepared in full block format.

College Hospital

4567 College Park Boulevard
Wood Creek, XY 12345

RADIOLOGY REPORT

Examination Date:	June 14, 200X	Patient:	Nora Benehamn
Date Reported:	June 14, 200X	X-ray No.:	43200
Physician:	Harold B. Cooper, MD	AGE:	19
Examination:	PA Chest, Abdomen	Hospital #	19 80-32-11

Findings:

PA CHEST: Upright PA view of chest shows the lung fields are
                  clear, without evidence of an active process. Heart size
                  is normal.

                  There is no evidence of pneumoperitoneum.

IMPRESSION: NEGATIVE CHEST.

ABDOMEN: Flat and upright views of the abdomen show a normal
                  gas pattern without evidence of obstruction or ileus.
                  There are no calcifications or abnormal masses noted.

IMPRESSION: NEGATIVE STUDY.

                  Radiologist _____
                                    Marian B. Skinner, MD

nar
D: 6-14-0X 1430
T: 6-14-0X 1735
<23-CPH-94>

Figure 24–9   A hospital radiology report, prepared in modified block format.

VILLAVIEW COMMUNITY HOSPITAL
5550 University
Grand View, XX 99999

ELECTROENCEPHALOGRAPH REPORT

PATIENT: Theo Stupin   MR#: 876-43

DATE OF PROCEDURE: 05/31/XX   DOB: 09/20/1958

REFERRING PHYSICIAN: François Bettencourt, M.D.

REASON FOR STUDY
Chronic headaches and weakness on the right side of the body,
previous abnormal EEG.

DISCRIPTION
This record shows a posterior 9 to 10 Hz alpha rhythm with an
amplitude of approximately 35 microvolts. The alpha activity is
mixed with some theta and occasional intermittent delta activity.
Sharp waves are noted in the frontal regions bilaterally, but these
may be in some way due to eye movement artifact. Hyperventilation
increased the background slow activity. As the record progresses,
there are intermittent episodes of sharp and slow waves activity
mostly in the bifrontal central region and essentially symmetrical.

IMPRESSION
Mildly abnormal EEG due to episodes of bilateral paroxysmal sharp
and slow wave complexes seen intermittently throughout the record.

COMMENT
This record shows similar abnormalities that were noted previously.

_____
Ellen Rifter, M.D.

MQ73
D: 06/01/200X
T: 06/05/200X

Figure 24–10   Electroencephalograph report, prepared in full block format.

ECHOCARDIOGRAM REPORT

Date: November, 26, 200X   Patient: Marie A. Friedman
Physician: Maureen J. Smith, MD   Hospital No.: 534981
Room: 507A

PROCEDURE

Echocardiogram is recorded with Smith-Kline Echoline 20 apparatus, electronics for medicine strip-chart recorder. The following normal values are obtained:

    1. Aortic root: 2.6 cm
    2. Left atrium: 3.2 cm
    3. IV septal thickness: 0.9 cm
    4. LV posterior wall thickness: 0.9 cm

The anterior mitral leaflet shows increased excursion, 3.8 cm. The posterior leaflet is partially visualized. In early systole, there is a hammock configuration to the signal of the junction of the posterior and anterior leaflets, typical of prolapsed mitral leaflet. The left ventricle shows good contractility with normal interventricular septal motion. There is no hypertrophy, but the left ventricle shows mild dilation, internal dimension 6.1 cm at end-diastole (normal value up to 5.8 cm). The aortic valve is not well seen, but the aortic root appears normal, and there is no increase in the left atrial size as one would expect in mild mitral regurgitation.

CONCLUSION

1. No evidence of rheumatic mitral valve disease, but evidence of prolapsed posterior mitral leaflet syndrome, probably on a congenital basis.
2. Mild dilation of the left ventricle, consistent with mild to moderate mitral regurgitation.

The study is otherwise unremarkable. The left ventricle shows good contractility and no hypertrophy.

_____

William B. Waxman, MD

wpd
D: 11-26-0X
T: 11-27-0X

Figure 24–11   Echocardiogram report, prepared in full block format.

BONE MINERAL DENSITY (DEXA) ASSESSMENT REPORT
using the
Hologic 1000 Dual Energy X-ray Absorptiometry Unit (DEXA)

Patient Name: Hutchison, Phinecia

Age: 54

Referring Doctor: Stephen Julian, M.D.

Date of Examination: 05/17/XX

Clinical History: This is a right-hand-dominant woman, height 62 inches, weight 140 lb, fair complexion, small build, with a history of vertebral compression fracture. On Prempro 0.625 mg/day, calcium and vitamin A supplementation.

RESULTS

- TOTAL HIP is -0.3 deviations below peak bone mass.

- LEFT FEMORAL NECK is -2.9 standard deviations below peak bone mass.

- LUMBAR SPINE is averaged at -2.5 standard deviations below peak bone mass and has markedly low bone mass for her age group.

DISCUSSION/RECOMMENDATIONS: The patient is at marked increased risk for fracture and has markedly low bone mass for her age group. An aggressive management approach is suggested. Secondary causes for the development of osteoporosis should be sought as well, and a repeat bone density in one year should be done to determine the efficacy of management.

_____
Alexander Lord, MD

lhm

Figure 24–12 Bone density report, prepared in full block format.

Memos, Minutes, and Other Reports

25–1 AGENDA

The agenda is the first tool in minute taking. It is prepared before a meeting and establishes the order of business of the meeting and the items to be discussed or the plan of activities. It may be emailed or sent to the membership well before the meeting or distributed as the meeting begins. The secretary will be able to use a copy to assist in taking notes and preparing the minutes. The format of the agenda should be functional and easy to read. These goals are achieved by using layout techniques such as centered headings, columnar lists for agenda items, and white space between items.

✓ **DO**   use double spacing, and keep the agenda to one page if possible. Roman numerals are often used to number the items.

✓ **DO**   use the following information in a formal agenda:

1. The name, date, and time of the meeting (centered on the page).
2. The location of the meeting.
3. Call to order.
4. Roll call and/or introduction of members and/or board of directors.
5. Introduction of guests and/or new members.
6. Reading and approval of the minutes of the previous meeting. Often the minutes of the previous meeting are emailed or sent to the members to read before the meeting. This practice helps speed the meeting along.

7. Officers' reports. *Officers' Reports* is the main topic; the individual reports are listed as subtopics.
8. Committee reports. *Committee Reports* is the main topic; the individual committee reports are listed as subtopics.
9. Old business. Unfinished business from the previous meeting is included. *Old Business* is the main topic; the individual topics constituting old business are listed as subtopics.
10. New business. *New Business* is the main heading; the individual topics *(when known)* constituting new business are listed as subtopics. Additional space is allowed at this point so that new topics may be added shortly before the meeting *(at the president's discretion)* or during the meeting itself. When the agenda is emailed or sent out before the meeting, a request is often made for suggestions for new agenda items.
11. Announcements. The announcement part often includes when and where the next meeting will be held.
12. Adjournment.

Figure 25–1 provides a sample formal agenda, and Figure 25–2 provides a sample informal agenda. These figures are at the end of the chapter.

25–2 ELECTRONIC MAIL

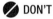 **DO** use email to assist in distribution of agendas and minutes whenever possible. *(See Chapter 12, Electronic Mail, and 25–3, Memorandums.)*

25–3 MEMORANDUMS

The purpose of the memorandum or memo is to send information to one or more persons within the office, company, division, department, or hospital quickly and economically in any situation in which written communication is appropriate. Memos are less formal than letters, and they also differ from letters in that they deal with routine information communicated between members of the same organization. Consequently, less background information is necessary.

 DON'T write a memo if it is about a confidential matter or a delicate subject.

 DO use preprinted forms or macros. Most word processing programs include them in the system.

 DO single-space memos.

✓ DO   set the tab stops two or three spaces after the longest guide word in each column so that the information is vertically aligned. This format is preferred when additional space is required for the list of the persons receiving the memo.

✓ DO   key in the date of origination. Sometimes this date is put in the position of the date line of a letter in modified block format, just to the right of the midline of the paper, as shown in Figure 25–4, rather than lined up with the other headings as you see in Figure 25–3.

NOTE: *To automatically insert the current day's date, use the date feature of the word processing program.*

✓ DO   list all of the names of the persons or departments for routing the memo after the *To* heading. A professional title may be used with the name, followed by the department, branch, and floor if deemed necessary. Generally, courtesy titles *(Mr., Miss, Mrs., Ms.)* are not used for either the addressee or the writer of memos. When sending a memo to persons who are on the same level, list the names in alphabetical order. If a memo is being sent to persons on various professional levels, list the names by rank. Indicate distribution by writing *please route* on a single copy of the memo with names listed or by making a copy for each person or department.

✓ DO   write the name of the author, or writer, of the document after the *From* heading. The originator usually does not sign the memo but may initial it next to his or her name or at the bottom of the memo.

✓ DO   write a specific and accurate topic for the memo after the *Subject* heading.

Headings

✓ DO   use the memo macro or key in the following headings in either the vertical or horizontal format, depending on the author's or preparer's preference.

Vertical format
DATE:
TO:
FROM:
SUBJECT:

Horizontal format
TO: DATE:
FROM: SUBJECT:

Vertical Setup
In the vertical format, the headings are keyed flush with the left margin in all cap letters followed by a colon. Begin keying the headings 2 inches from the top of the paper, and double-space between headings. Set a tab 12 spaces in from the left margin, and tab over to fill in the headings. Triple-space and then begin the body of the memo. The body of the memo is single spaced, with a double space between paragraphs. Use full block format. *(See Figure 25–3 at the end of the chapter for a sample of the vertical-style memo.)*

Horizontal Setup
The horizontal format takes up less space but is not as easy to use as the vertical format. Key the first two headings flush with the left margin, and double-space between the headings. Tab over eight spaces from the left margin to fill in the name of the recipient(s) of the memo, and repeat to fill in the name of the author. Key *DATE* and *SUBJECT* just to the right of the center of the page. From the first letter of *DATE*, tab over 12 spaces to begin keying the date, and repeat to fill in the subject. You can see that this format is not as easy to do as the more popular vertical style and could be inappropriate if the subject line is lengthy. Triple-space down to the body of the memo and complete as described for the vertical style. *(See Figure 25–4 at the end of the chapter for a sample of a horizontal-style memo.)*

✓ **DO**   prepare a memo macro on your computer that you can recall anytime you need to compose or transcribe a memo. If you use plain paper and prepare memos often, it is worth the time to make a macro.

    HINT: *When preparing these macros, do not forget to insert the "pause" feature after each heading so you are able to insert the variables when you play it out.*

Electronic Mail

✓ **DO**   use email to send memos whenever possible. You need only insert the names of the recipients, with their email addresses and the subject, because the date and your name will appear as a regular part of the email message.

✓ **DO**   keep email messages simple *(no bullets, fancy symbols, or sophisticated format)* because the body is often reformatted during transmission and may not appear as neat or as attractive when received.

Lists

The following rules apply to listing in memos, reports, minutes, and policies.

✓ DO   introduce lists with serial numbers or letters of the alphabet followed by a period or parentheses. Bullets *(which may be solid circles, squares, or triangles)* are also appropriate substitutes for numbers or letters.

✓ DO   key lists in block format under the beginning of each line, and align overrun lines with the first word, not the number, letter, or bullet.

✓ DO   compose lists by using parallel construction; be grammatically consistent. For example, each line begins with a verb *(type, list, spell, space)*, or each line begins with a noun or pronoun *(who, what, when, where)*, or each line is a complete sentence. *(See 17-6, Parallel Structure.)*

✓ DO   omit punctuation in a list that does not form complete sentences.

The following activities should be listed in the job description
- *Daily duties*
- *Weekly duties*
- *Monthly duties*

Closing Elements

✓ DO   complete the memo with the preparer's initials a double space after the last line of the body of the memo. It is not necessary to key the author's initials, but one should do so if it is the custom in the organization. A signature line is not used, and the author does not sign the memo. Even though the memo is not signed by the author, it should always be submitted to him or her for approval before being distributed. Some writers will initial their memo after their name on the *FROM* line.

✓ DO   handle reference initials, enclosures, and copy notations exactly as they are in a letter. Reference initials are keyed two blank lines below the closing, followed by the enclosure line, the copy notation, and the postscript, in that order, with one or two blank lines between each one.

Continuations

✓ DO   begin subsequent pages by keying 1 inch down from the top of the page and key in your headings: name of the addressee, date, and page number. Triple-space and continue with the body of the memo.

NOTE: *Avoid having more than one page to a memo. If there is more than one subject, make a separate memo for that subject. Memos, by their very nature, concern matters that are brief and uncomplicated.*

25–4 MINUTES

Minutes are the formal or informal records of an organization's meeting and become the official documentation of what transpires during a meeting. They are usually taken by the recording secretary, although anyone attending the meeting may take minutes. It is helpful for the secretary to have the minutes of the previous meeting, a list of the membership, and the agenda for the meeting. The detail with which the notes are taken *(or tape recorded)* will be determined by the organization itself and the business conducted. It follows then that the content of the minutes will reflect the necessary detail. Whether the recorder merely summarizes the discussions or cites the speakers by name will be determined by the policy of the organization itself. Minutes may be formal or informal but are the important means of conveying information to people who were unable to attend the meeting, a reminder of future actions expected, and a background for the decisions made by the group.

✓ DO   set up a prepared standardized form that can be used to fill in information as the meeting is conducted. The form also serves as a reminder to the note taker to be certain that important data are recorded. These forms are fairly easy to format and reflect the items found in the agenda. *(See Figure 25–5 at the end of the chapter for a sample prepared form.)*

✓ DO   prepare an attendance list.

✓ DO   make an outline of how the finished minutes will look, leaving a space to fill in the information from the meeting, or make a notebook with each page listing an agenda item.

✓ DO   transcribe your minutes as soon as possible after the meeting.

DO include the following in the minutes:

- *Title. The heading is usually centered on the page and keyed in full capital letters. It may be underlined as well.*
- *Date, time, and place. Date, time, and place of the meeting may be part of the heading or part of the report itself. The presiding officer is identified with the call to order or adjournment notation.*
- *Names of the members. Names of the members present as well as those of members absent are listed in the minutes. If roll is taken, that sheet may be attached to the minutes. The names are usually listed in alphabetical order. List the names and include appropriate titles and other identifying information of any ex officio members or guests in attendance.*
- *Approval of minutes of previous meeting.*
- *Records of all officer and committee reports.*
- *Unfinished business agenda topics with decision on the topic, action required, and who will do what and when.*
- *New business with action details.*
- *Announcements, including the date, time, and place of the next meeting.*
- *Time of the adjournment.*

The format should be consistent from meeting to meeting and secretary to secretary. The events should be reported in the order in which they occurred during the meeting. Outline format should be followed, and the full block, modified block, or indented style should be used. The titles of the sections follow those of the agenda used at the meeting itself. Roman numerals are often used to introduce the titles of each section. Generally, headings *(with or without numbers)* should be flush with the left margin. Single-space the material under the headings and double-space between headings. The headings are either in all capital letters and underlined or with just the initial letter of the main words capitalized and the entire heading underlined.

 DO type the word *continued* at the bottom of the completed page if the minutes continue to more than one page. The subsequent page or pages begin an inch from the top of the page with the title of the minutes, the page number, date, and any other important data.

See Lists (under 25-3, Memorandums) for rules on listing.

 DO type the originator's name a triple space after the close of the minutes. The transcriptionist identifies the preparation of the document with a two- or three-letter identification *(i.e., initials)*, a double space after the originator's name, flush with the left margin.

✓ **DO**   complete the minutes as soon as possible after the meeting and send a copy to all members *(those present at the meeting and those absent)* unless it is the custom to read the minutes at the following meeting. Some committees or organizations have a special distribution list that will include anyone who needs to be aware of the proceedings. At the next meeting, the minutes are read aloud and amended, if necessary, either on the page or, if lengthy, typed and attached as an addendum.

Figures 25–6 and 25–7 at the end of the chapter provide samples of informal minutes.

25–5   OUTLINES

✓ **DO**   prepare outlines in the traditional method as shown in Figure 25–8 at the end of the chapter.

✓ **DO**   have at least two divisions or subdivisions in each set; otherwise a set cannot be made.

✓ **DO**   use roman numerals, arabic numerals, and letters of the alphabet or a combination to identify different heading levels.

✓ **DO**   use a period and a double space after each number or letter of the alphabet except at the levels where the parentheses are used, at which point you double-space after the closing parenthesis.

✓ **DO**   indent the outlines so that successive levels are obvious. Leave space to backspace from the main topics in order to accommodate the width of the roman numerals. It is helpful to use the decimal tab set to align these numerals properly.

25–6   REPORTS AND POLICIES

See also Chapter 19, History and Physical Format, and Chapter 24, Medical Reports.

Reports and policies, just like minutes, have individual headings for the topics and titles. Unlike minutes, in reports these headings will vary just as the nature of the report will vary. The originator of a report may or may not formulate the title for the transcriptionist, so you should be able to extract the title from the paragraph itself by pulling out the main idea and composing a brief heading for that section. The hospital or institution will usually have a special format, often special paper, for recording these documents.

✓ DO   keep headings consistent throughout the report and follow simple guidelines:

- *Title: all capital letters followed by 2 blank lines.*
- *Main topics: all capital letters underlined.*
- *Subtopics: all capital letters not underlined.*
- *Minor topics: uppercase and lowercase letters underlined.*

✓ DO   see Lists (under 25-3, Memorandums) for rules on listing.

✓ DO   type the word *continued* at the bottom of the completed page if a report continues to more than one page. The subsequent page or pages begin 1 inch from the top of the page with the title of the document, the page number *(the second page might be shown as ED-2 for emergency department, RD-2 for radiology department, and so on),* and any other important data *(e.g., the policy number).*

✓ DO   see Figures 25–9 and 25–10 at the end of the chapter, which illustrate a closing format for a policy and a format for a hospital procedure or policy. Preparers should identify every report or policy they complete with a two- or three-letter identification *(i.e., initials).* Hospital protocols or policies are approved by hospital committees and are revised from time to time.

AGENDA
TEAM MEDICAL MANAGEMENT PROGRAM
May 9, 20XX

I.   Call to order

II.   Roll call and introduction of guests

III.   James Morgan, MD, representative from Bayview Hospital

IV.   Approval of minutes of April 14, 20XX

V.   Committees
      1. Bylaws Committee
      2. Membership Committee
      3. Nominating Committee
      4. Credentials Committee

VI.   Old business
      1. Attendance
      2. Proposed changes to meeting time or day
      3. Special project funding

VII.   New business
      1. Health Fair (Dr. Dunn)
      2. Evaluation of treadmill (Dr. Patton)
      3. Discussion of 20XX vacation schedules (Dr. Majur)

VIII.   Announcements

      Position open at Desert View Community (See Ron Miller)

      Next meeting: June 18, 3 p.m., Board Room
         (subject to approval today)

IX. Adjournment

Figure 25–1   Sample of a formal agenda.

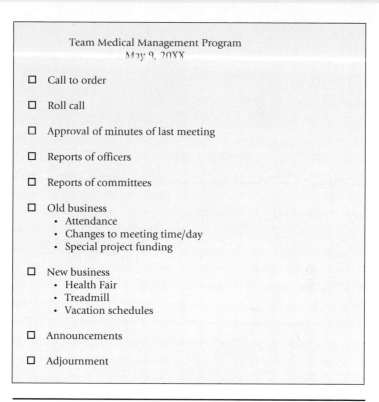

Figure 25–2 Sample of an informal agenda. Boxes (□) introduce main headings, and bullets (•) introduce subheadings.

MEMORANDUM

DATE: January 14, 200X

TO: Joan M. Abbott
                 Shirley N. Andrews
                 Martin P. Dorley

FROM: Michael Jones, MD

SUBJECT: Office Procedure Manual

It has come to my attention that when someone is sick or leaves on vacation, it is difficult to know how to complete certain tasks in the office. Therefore, I would like for each of you to work on a procedure manual for your specific job in this office, outlining from A–Z exactly what tasks you perform and how to carry them out.

The following activities should be listed:

1. Daily duties
2. Weekly duties
3. Monthly duties
4. Quarterly duties
5. Yearly duties
6. Job attitudes
7. Skills required for the job
8. Clothing requirements

Please have this ready by April 1. Thank you.

sna

Figure 25–3   Sample of the vertical-style memo.

MEMORANDUM

TO: Joan M. Abbott   DATE: January 14, 200X
          Shirley N. Andrews
          Martin P. Dorley

FROM: Michael Jones, MD   SUBJECT: Office Procedure
                                    Manual

It has come to my attention that when someone is sick or leaves on vacation, it is difficult to know how to complete certain tasks in the office. Therefore, I would like each of you to work on a procedure manual for your specific job in this office, outlining from A–Z exactly what tasks you perform and how to carry them out.

The following activities should be listed:

1. Daily duties
2. Weekly duties
3. Monthly duties
4. Quarterly duties
5. Yearly duties
6. Job attitudes
7. Skills required for the job
8. Clothing requirements

Please have this ready by April 1. Thank you.

sna

Figure 25–4   Sample of the horizontal-style memo.

Form for Recording Minutes

Name of organization _____

Date _____ Time _____ Place _____

Present _____

_____

_____

Absent _____

Guests _____

Minutes _____

Officers' reports _____

Committee reports _____

_____

_____

Old business _____

_____

_____

New business _____

_____

_____

Announcements _____

Next meeting _____

Figure 25–5   Sample form for recording minutes.

CUYAMACA WOODS FIRE SAFE COUNCIL
MINUTES

DATE
Rita Hardin, presiding chair, called the meeting to order at 9:45 a.m. on
February 8, 200X. Agendas were distributed, as were the minutes of the last meeting.
No additions were made to the agenda.

MEMBERS PRESENT
There were 18 members present. The roll sheet is attached.

GUESTS
There were two guests present. Mr. Roland Wolf, president, and
Mr. Jonathan Hebert, general manager, of LANE Tree Service and Land Clearing.

PRESENTATION
The guests were asked to make their presentation out of agenda order so they
would be able to leave the meeting before other business was discussed.

- Mr. Wolf gave the group a brief history of his 17-year land clearing,
  brushing, chipping, and tree felling service in this area. He and his employees
  are licensed and insured. (A list of clients in the area was provided.) He
  has a several-man crew, numbers of which are used depending on the job
  requirements. Both large and small jobs are accepted with a 2-hr. minimum.
  He introduced his project manager, Mr. Hebert, who is also a highly
  qualified and experienced crew member with intimate forest knowledge.

- Fees for services are $75/hr for a 2-man crew. There is a $35/hr charge for
  each additional crew member needed on the job site. Detailed written
  estimates are given for all major jobs.

- He acknowledged that only a short lead-in time would be required and
  that delayed response to invoice billing was understood and acceptable
  from nonprofit groups such as ours.

MINUTES
Minutes of the January 11, 200X, meeting were distributed. A correction was made to
the spelling of Carolyn Roth's name. The minutes were then approved as corrected.

CHAIR REASSIGNMENTS
Rita Hardin asked for a reassignment of meeting leadership. She agreed to continue
as Vice Chair, and Carolyn Roth agreed to accept the responsibility as Chair.
(The meetings will continue to be held in the Hardirs' home.) The meeting
continued with Carolyn as Chair.

BUSINESS CARDS
Mary Harreld distributed business cards so that members would have details
concerning tax receipts and mailing addresses for potential donors to the Fire Safe
Council funds. Individuals may write their name in the place provided. Additional
cards may be obtained from Mary.

Figure 25–6   Sample of minutes.

Continued

INFORMATION LETTER
Jim Yubetta, who has been drafting an information letter for CW property owners to raise the awareness of the fire dangers, distributed a rough draft of his document. He asked the group to review it and to make editing suggestions before it is finalized and sent to the CW property owners. Several suggestions were made, and Terri Germano and Mary Harreld agreed to help him with the final draft.

GRANT WRITING
Mary is still gathering information for our proposed grants for both state and federal funds. Terri suggested that we apply for funds to hire a forest management consultant to help decide which trees should be eliminated, pruned or thinned to keep a healthy forest as there isn't enough water to support all the trees, even after eliminating those that have died.

FORREST COUNTY FIRE SAFE COUNCIL
Mary Harreld told us how the FS Council in Forrest County was able to obtain a $200,000 state grant for work done by property owners in their area who documented their work efforts and received matching funds. Members were asked to begin making a list of the hours they have donated to FS Council business.

BRUSH CLEARING/CHIPPING
No action at this time. The committee will continue to work on it. Paul, Frank, and Marijane agreed to telephone people they know on the reference list given us by LANE Tree Service. They will report their findings at the next meeting.

BY-LAWS COMMITTEE
The by-laws committee has met twice and will be ready to present the changes to the by-laws at the next meeting.

CW FIRE MAP
* Ralph presented copies of a large fire map, which he had compiled to conform with the requirements for the fire fighters in the event of a fire. The map was put to the members for review over the next months for verification of correctness. It includes property addresses, locations of residences and habitable structures, driveway locations (including types of driveways), water tanks (including size of water tank), fire hose connections, fire hydrants, and fire truck turn-arounds. The group thanked Ralph for his volunteer efforts.

* It was recommend that the complete maps could be provided not only to all the local fire agencies and Department of Forestry, but copies should go to the road chairs so they are available for any visiting fire personnel in the event of a fire.

* All members who review the map should bring any changes or additions to the next FSC meeting.

ADJOURNMENT
The meeting was adjourned with confirmation of date of next full meeting: March 8, 200X, at 9:30 a.m.

Mary Harreld, Recording Secretary.

Figure 25–6   Cont'd

CUYAMACA WOODS FIRE SAFE COUNCIL
MINUTES
February 8, 200X

Rita Hardin, presiding chair, called the meeting to order at 9:45 a.m. on February 8, 200X. Agendas were distributed, as were the minutes of the last meeting. No additions were made to the agenda.

I. ROLL CALL
There were 18 members present. The roll sheet is attached.

GUESTS
There were two guests present: Mr. Roland Wolf, president, and Mr. Jonathan Hebert, general manager, of LANE Tree Service and Land Clearing.

II. PRESENTATION
The guests were asked to make their presentation out of agenda order so they would be able to leave the meeting before other business was discussed.

- Mr. Wolf gave the group a brief history of his 17-year land clearing, brushing, chipping, and tree felling service in this area. He and his employees are licensed and insured. (A list of clients in the area was provided.) He has a several-man crew, numbers of which are used depending on the job requirements. Both large and small jobs are accepted with a 2-hr. minimum. He introduced his project manager, Mr. Hebert, who is also a highly qualified and experienced crew member with intimate forest knowledge.

- Fees for services are $75/hr for a 2-man crew. There is a $35/hr charge for each additional crew member needed on the job site. Detailed written estimates are given for all major jobs.

- He acknowledged that only a short lead-in time would be required and that delayed response to invoice billing was understood and acceptable from nonprofit groups such as ours.

III. MINUTES
Minutes of the January 11, 200X, meeting were distributed. A correction was made to the spelling of Carolyn Roth's name. The minutes were then approved as corrected.

IV. CHAIR REASSIGNMENTS
Rita Hardin asked for a reassignment of meeting leadership. She agreed to continue as Vice Chair, and Carolyn Roth agreed to accept the responsibility as Chair. (The meetings will continue to be held in the Hardins' home.) The meeting continued with Carolyn as Chair.

V. REPORTS

BUSINESS CARDS
Mary Harreld distributed business cards so that members would have details concerning tax receipts and mailing addresses for potential donors to the Fire Safe Council funds. Individuals may write their name in the place provided. Additional cards may be obtained from Mary.

Figure 25–7   Sample of minutes.

Continued

FSC Minutes, continued
Page 2
February 8, 200X

INFORMATION LETTER

Jim Yubetta, who has been drafting an information letter for CW property owners to raise the awareness of the fire dangers, distributed a rough draft of his document. He asked the group to review it and to make editing suggestions before it is finalized and sent to the CW property owners. Several suggestions were made, and Terri Germano and Mary Harreld agreed to help him with the final draft.

GRANT WRITING

Mary is still gathering information for our proposed grants for both state and federal funds. Terri suggested that we apply for funds to hire a forest management consultant to help decide which trees should be eliminated, pruned or thinned to keep a healthy forest as there isn't enough water to support all the trees, even after eliminating those that have died.

FORREST COUNTY FIRE SAFE COUNCIL

Mary Harreld told us how the FS Council in Forrest County was able to obtain a $200,000 state grant for work done by property owners in their area who documented their work efforts and received matching funds. Members were asked to begin making a list of the hours they have donated to FS Council business.

BRUSH CLEARING/CHIPPING

No action at this time. The committee will continue to work on it. Paul, Frank, and Marijane agreed to telephone people they know on the reference list given us by LANE Tree Service. They will report their findings at the next meeting.

BY-LAWS COMMITTEE

The by-laws committee has met twice and will be ready to present the changes to the by-laws at the next meeting.

CW FIRE MAP

- Ralph presented copies of a large fire map which he had compiled to conform with the requirements for the fire fighters in the event of a fire. The map was put to the members for review over the next months for verification of correctness. It includes property addresses, locations of residences and habitable structures, driveway locations (including types of driveways), water tanks (including size of water tank), fire hose connections, fire hydrants, and fire truck turn-arounds. The group thanked Ralph for his volunteer efforts.

- It was recommend that the complete maps could be provided not only to all the local fire agencies and Department of Forestry, but copies should go to the road chairs so they are available for any visiting fire personnel in the event of a fire.

- All members who review the map should bring any changes or additions to the next FSC meeting.

VI, ADJOURNMENT

The meeting was adjourned with confirmation of date of next full meeting: March 8, 200X, at 9:30 a.m.

Mary Harreld, Recording Secretary.

Figure 25–7 Cont'd

TITLE CENTERED AND TYPED IN FULL CAPS

I. Main Topic (first item) (Capitalize the first letter of each important
            word.)
   A. Secondary heading (Capitalize the first letter and any
   B. . . .   proper nouns here and at all
   C. . . .   other levels.)
   D. . . .
      1. Third level heading
      2. . .
      3. . .
      4. . .
         a. Fourth level heading
         b. . . .
           (1) Fifth level heading
           (2). . . .
           (3). . . .
              (a) Sixth level heading
              (b). . . .
II. Main Topic (second item) (You will have to backspace once
   A. . . .   to allow for the roman numeral —
   B. . . .   for balance.)
   C. . . .
      1. . . .
      2. . . .
   D. . . .
      1. . . .
      2. . . .
      3. . . .
III. Main Topic (third item) (You will have to backspace twice on this
            line for balance.)

The major headings and subdivisions may be a single word or
phrase; long phrases or clauses; complete sentences; or any
combination of sentences, phrases, and single words.

Between-line spacing is as follows:
   After title: triple-space.
   Main topic: double-space before and after each one.
   Subdivision items: single-space.
   Very brief outline: double-space all.

Indenting is as follows:
   Roman numerals: align to the left margin
   Division under each topic: set tab stops for four-space indent
   Second line: begin the second line of an item directly under
            the first letter of that line

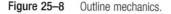

Figure 25–8   Outline mechanics.

Approved _____ (Name)	Policy Number _____
Effective date:	Revised:
Reviewed:	Revised:

Figure 25–9   Sample of closing format for a policy.

ALVARADO HOSPITAL MEDICAL CENTER

DEPARTMENT OF NURSING SERVICES   Date:

Approved:

Page: 1 of

PROCEDURE:

Reviewed/ Revised by:									
Date:									

Figure 25–10   Sample format for a hospital procedure or policy.

26

Metric System

INTERNATIONAL SYSTEM OF UNITS (SI) AND OTHER FORMS OF MEASUREMENT

26–1   ENGLISH UNITS OF MEASUREMENT

The use of abbreviations with the English form of measurement is optional. When you do abbreviate, follow these rules.

✓ **DO**   use the symbol for *foot* (′) and the symbol for *inches* (″) if desired in technical typing and tables only.

🚫 **DON'T**   use an abbreviation unless it is expressed with a number.

Incorrect:
There was about an oz left in the beaker.

✓ **DO**   use the following abbreviations for these common English measurements:

ft   foot
in.   inch *(punctuate this one)*
yd   yard
pt   pint

qt	quart
oz	ounce
fl oz	fluid ounce
gal	gallon
lb	pound
grain	grain *(do not abbreviate)*
dram	dram *(do not abbreviate)*
tsp	teaspoon
tbsp	tablespoon
cup	cup *(do not abbreviate)*
F	Fahrenheit

 DON'T make these abbreviations plural or use punctuation marks with them unless a word itself is formed when it is unpunctuated. For example, *in.* is the correct abbreviation for *inch*.

Correct
The patient is 57 in. tall.
The patient is 57 inches tall. *(preferred)*
The baby's birth weight was 7 lb 3 oz.
The baby's birth weight was 7 pounds 3 ounces.
 (preferred)
Incorrect
The baby's birth weight was 7 lbs 3 ozs.
See Chapter 27, Numbers, for further illustration of the use of measurements.

26–2 BASE UNITS, METRIC

Metric Unit	Symbol	Measures	English Equivalents
meter	m	length, thickness	inch, foot, yard, mile
kilogram	kg	mass (weight)	ounce, pound
liter	L	volume	cup, pint, quart, gallon
Celsius	C	temperature	Fahrenheit

There are other base units in the metric (SI) system, but they are not used frequently in daily life so they are not dealt with in this chapter.

The American spelling for all SI (metric) units is used throughout, since that is preferred in the United States. That is, *meter* is used rather than the French *metre* and *liter* rather than *litre*.

26–3 GENERAL RULES FOR SI MEASUREMENTS

✓ **DO** write all abbreviations in small letters except for *C* for Celsius and *L* for liter.

⊘ **DON'T** use abbreviations unless used with a number.

Incorrect:
There was only about a mm difference.
Correct:
There was only about a millimeter difference.

⊘ **DON'T** combine a name with a symbol. When two or more names or symbols are used together, they should be spelled out in full or used in abbreviated forms.

Correct
The temperature is 36° C.
The temperature is 36 degrees Celsius.
Incorrect
The temperature is 36 degrees C.
The temperature is 36° Celsius.
The temperature is 36° C. *(note spacing)*

⊘ **DON'T** use commas in large numbers expressing metric measurement.

Incorrect:
25,000
Correct:
25 000 *(notice space)* or 25000 *(preferred)*
Incorrect:
3,000 mL
Correct:
3000 mL

✓ **DO** use a zero in front of the decimal point if the number is less than 1.

Incorrect:
.5
Correct:
0.5
Incorrect:
.1
Correct:
0.1

⊘ **DON'T** add a trailing zero unless dictated

Incorrect:
5.50 mL
Correct:
5.5 mL

EXCEPTION: *Specific gravity is expressed with four digits and a decimal point between the first and second digit even though the value may be dictated as "one zero," "one oh," or "ten."*

Dictated:
Specific gravity ten twenty
Transcribed:
Specific gravity 1.020
Dictated:
Specific gravity one point zero three
Transcribed:
Specific gravity 1.030

 DON'T   use common fractions with the metric system.

Incorrect:
¼ cm
Correct:
0.25 cm
Incorrect:
1 ¾ L
Correct:
1.75 L *or* 1750 mL

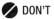 **DO**   leave a space between the number and the symbol or abbreviation.

Incorrect:
25mg
Correct:
25 mg
Incorrect:
0.4L
Correct:
0.4 L

EXCEPTION: *Temperature is properly written with no spaces between numbers, degree symbol, and abbreviation.*

37°C is normal body temperature.
or
37 degrees Celsius is normal body temperature.

 DON'T   make symbols plural, no matter how many.

Correct:
35 m *(35 meters)*
Incorrect:
35 ms

DON'T follow metric abbreviations with a period unless the abbreviation is the last item in a sentence.

Incorrect:
1000 mL.
Correct:
1000 mL
Incorrect:
36°C.
Correct:
36°C

DO use a hyphen to link a number and a unit when they are used as a modifier.

There is a 2-cm difference now.
We noticed a 2.5-kg weight gain.
He gained 2.5 kg.

26–4 MEASURING LENGTH, DISTANCE, THICKNESS: METER

DO use *meter* for measuring length, distance, or thickness. Large distances are measured in *kilometers (km)*, short lengths or distances are measured in *meters (m)*, small thicknesses are measured in *centimeters (cm)*, and very small thicknesses are measured in *millimeters (mm)*.

DO use the following abbreviations for meter and its components:

m for *meter*
km for *kilometer (1000 meters)*
cm for *centimeter (1/100 meter)*
mm for *millimeter (1/1000 meter)*

26–5 MEASURING MASS (WEIGHT): KILOGRAM

DO use the *kilogram* for measuring mass. A large mass is measured in *kilograms (kg)*, a small mass is measured in *grams (g)*, and a very small mass is measured in *milligrams (mg)*.

DON'T use *kilo* or *kilos* as an abbreviation for kilograms.

✓ **DO** use the following abbreviations:

kg	for *kilogram (1000 grams)*
g *or* gm	for *gram*
mg	for *milligram (1/1000 gram)*

26–6 MEASURING TEMPERATURE: CELSIUS

✓ **DO** use *degrees Celsius (°C)* for measuring temperature. Sometimes the term *centigrade* is used instead of *Celsius*. The two terms are equal to the same unit, and *Celsius* is preferred.

✓ **DO** use the abbreviation °*C* or write out *degrees Celsius* to express temperature.

26–7 MEASURING VOLUME: LITER

✓ **DO** use *liter* for measuring volume. Large volumes are measured in *liters (L)* and small volumes in *milliliters (ml* or *mL).*

✓ **DO** use the following abbreviations:

L	for *liter (the lowercase letter looks like the number one)*
mL *or* ml	for *milliliter (1/1000 liter)*

🚫 **DON'T** use *cc (cubic centimeter* or *cm³)* as a substitute for *ml,* even though the volumes are the same, unless "see-see" *(cc)* is dictated. *(The abbreviation* cc *is an incorrectly derived unit that has been substituted for* ml*.)*

26–8 METRIC CONVERSIONS
A metric conversion table (Table 26–1) is provided for your reference at the end of the chapter.

26–9 MISCELLANEOUS DERIVED SI UNITS

✓ **DO** use these abbreviations for these derived units.

Hz	hertz	frequency
J	joule	energy
W	watt	power
v	volt	electric potential

26-10 PREFIXES COMMONLY USED

	Prefix	Symbol	Relation	Example
More Than	kilo	k	1000 units	1 kilogram = 1000 g
One of a Unit	hecto	h	100 units	1 hectometer = 100 m
Less Than	deci	d	1/10th unit	1 deciliter = 0.1 liter
One of a Unit	centi	c	1/100th unit	1 centimeter = 0.01 m
	milli	m	1/1000th unit	1 milliliter = 0.001 L

Metric measurements can be expressed in more than one way. Thus, *1.5 m (meters)* is also expressed as *150 cm (centimeters)* or *1500 mm (millimeters)*. The least complex expression is usually chosen; however, tradition may also dictate which is chosen. *(Of course the transcriptionist transcribes exactly what is dictated, not making a "choice.")*

26-11 SUMMARY OF SI UNITS

Table 26–2, located at the end of the chapter, is a summary of the units you need to know.

◆ TABLE 26-1

METRIC CONVERSIONS

	When You Know	You Can Find	Symbol	If You Multiply by
Length	inches	millimeters	mm	25
	feet	centimeters	cm	30
	yards	meters	m	0.9
	miles	kilometers	km	1.6
	millimeters	inches	in.	0.04
	centimeters	inches	in.	0.4
	meters	yards	yd	1.1
	kilometers	miles	mi	0.6
Area	square inches	square centimeters	cm^2	6.5
	square feet	square meters	m^2	0.09
	square yards	square meters	m^2	0.8
	square miles	square kilometers	km^2	2.6

Continued

◆ TABLE 26-1

METRIC CONVERSIONS—cont'd

	When You Know	You Can Find	Symbol	If You Multiply by
Area—cont'd	acres	square hectometers (hectares)	ha	0.4
	square centimeters	square inches	sq in.	0.16
	square meters	square yards	yd²	1.2
	square kilometers	square miles	mi²	0.4
	square hectometers (hectares)	acres		2.5
Mass	ounces	grams	g	28
	pounds	kilograms	kg	0.45
	short tons (metric tons)	megagrams		0.9
	grams	ounces	oz	0.035
	kilograms	pounds	lb	2.2
	megagrams	short tons (metric tons)		1.1
Liquid Volume	ounces	milliliters	ml	30
	pints	liters	L	0.47
	quarts	liters	L	0.95
	gallons	liters	L	3.8
	milliliters	ounces	oz	0.034
	liters	pints	pt	2.1
	liters	quarts	qt	1.06
	liters	gallons	gal	0.26
	teaspoons	milliliters	mL	5
	tablespoons	milliliters	mL	15
	fluid ounces	milliliters	mL	30
	cups	liters	L	0.24
Temperature	degrees Fahrenheit	degrees Celsius	°C	0.556 (after subtracting 32)
	degrees Celsius	degrees Fahrenheit	°F	1.8 (then add 32)

◆ TABLE 26-2

THE METRIC (SI) SYSTEM

Unit	Symbol	Measures	Example
meter	m	length, distance, thickness	1 m
gram	g	mass (weight)	200 g
liter	L	volume	6.5 L
Celsius	C	temperature	36° or 36°C
Prefixes commonly used for more than one of a unit			
kilo	k	1000 of them	1 kg = 1000 g
*hecto	h	100 of them	1 hm = 100 m
Prefixes commonly used for less than one of a unit			
*deci	d	1/10th of a unit	1 dl = 0.1 L
centi	c	1/100 of a unit	1 cm = 0.01 m
milli	m	1/1000 of a unit	1 mL = 0.001 L

NOTE: *cc (cubic centimeter)* is a derived unit and is the same as *mL* (e.g., 2 cc = 2 mL.)

- *All units of measure are multiples or submultiples of ten.*
- *Commas are not used in large numbers.*
- *A zero precedes the decimal point if the number is less than 1 (e.g., 0.50).*
- *Symbols are not made plural, no matter how many.*

meter or meters	m
gram or grams	g *(gm is an alternative)*
liter or liters	L *(always a capital letter)*
milliliter(s)	mL *(ml is an alternative)*
milligram(s)	mg

- *Leave a space between the number and the symbol.*

  25 mg   0.5 mL
- *Symbols are not punctuated unless they occur at the end of the sentence.*

  75 kg   1000 mL
- *The zero (0) is used for the numbers and* not *the capital "oh" (O).*

  50 cm
- *Common fractions are not used with metric numbers.*

  5.5 m *not* 5 ½ m

*Not frequently used in ordinary medical documents.

27

Numbers

INTRODUCTION

We have the terms *numeral, arabic numeral, roman numeral, numeric term, cardinal number, ordinal number,* and *figure.* Each one describes a different way that numbers themselves are expressed or written. Numbers can be spelled out, written as figures, or written in a combination of a figure and a part of a word *(e.g., 3rd).*

Numeral and *arabic numeral* mean the *figures* and combinations of the figures 0, 1, 2, 3, 4, 5, 6, 7, 8, 9.

Numeric term refers to written-out numbers.

Roman numerals refer to the use of certain letters of the alphabet, most frequently the capital letters and combinations of the letters *I, V, X.*

Cardinal numbers refer to the quantity of objects in the same class. A cardinal number may be a whole number, a fraction, or a combination *(e.g., 3 days, $15).*

Ordinal numbers express position, sequence, or order of items in the same class. They can be spelled out or written as a figure plus a word part *(e.g., first, 1st, third, eleventh, 14th).*

27–1   ABBREVIATIONS

✓ DO   abbreviate *number* by using *No.* or *#.*

> A #14 Foley was used. . . .
> We used #3-0 silk sutures . . .
> Number 3-0 silk sutures. . . . *(Spell out at the beginning of a sentence.)*

NOTE: *It is optional to place the # symbol or No. before the suture size unless the dictator dictates it or prefers this style.*

✓ DO   use a capital *D:* (with colon) followed by a date to indicate the date a document was dictated, and place a capital *T:* followed by a date to indicate the date a document was transcribed. These follow your reference initials. *(See Chapter 24, Medical Reports.)*

> ref
> D: 3-8-XX   *or*   D: 03/08/XX
> T: 3-9-XX   T: 03/09/XX
>   *or*   ref
>   D: 03/08/20XX
>   T: 03/09/20XX

☑ **DO** use figures when numbers are directly used with symbols or abbreviations.

6 lb 7 oz	1 q.i.d.	99°F	2%
15 mmHg	$10	#14 Foley	8 × 3
pH 6.5	1200 mL	6 cm	3 a.m.
ICD-9	OM-2	AE-60-I-2	4+
T&A	−2	q.4 h.	

☑ **DO** leave a space between the number and the abbreviation.

EXCEPTION: *q.4 h.* (Abbreviations concerning "every so many hours" are written closed up after the abbreviation *q.* for *every* and with a space after the number for ease of reading.)

⊘ **DON'T** leave a space between the number and the symbol.

2%   99°F $10

EXCEPTION: *Leave a space on either side of the x when used to mean* times *or* by.

I used a 3 × 5 card.

⊘ **DON'T** combine a name with a symbol. When two or more names or symbols are used together, they should be spelled out in full or used in abbreviated form.

Correct
The temperature is 35° C.
The temperature is 35 degrees Celsius.
Incorrect
The temperature is 35 degrees C.
The temperature is 35° Celsius.
The temperature is 35° C. *(wrong spacing)*

☑ **DO** use figures with metric abbreviations.

1 mm	10 cm	0.5 mm	7 mL
20 kg	37°C	1 L	50 g

☑ **DO** use figures and symbols when writing plus or minus with a number.

pulses were 2+
presenting part was at a −2 station
use a +8.50 lens
a 2 to 3+ skin redundancy
1+ protein

✓ **DO** use a hyphen in a compound modifier.

> a 3-cm nevus
> a 2-mm × 4-mm lesion

DO abbreviate interleukins joined to their identifying number 1 through 16.

> IL-1 IL-1RA

27–2 ADDRESSES

DO spell out the house number and post office box number *one* and the ordinal (*first, second,* and so on) street numbers one through ten.

> One East Wacker Drive
> 5060 Ninth Avenue *(easier to read than 5060 9th Avenue)*
> PO Box One

✓ **DO** use figures for all other house numbers, post office box numbers, apartment numbers, suite numbers, unit numbers, space numbers, and street and route names.

> 1335 11th Street, Apartment 6B
> 704 Warford Drive
> PO Box 1178
> Star Route 4

See Chapter 2, Address Formats for Letters and Forms of Address, and Chapter 22, Letter Format, for further help with addresses.

27–3 AGES

DO use figures when expressing ages.

> She had her first menses at age 12.
> She is a 31-year-old police officer.
> He is a 25-day-old infant.
> He was 2 days 14 hours old.

DON'T separate parts of the age with a comma.

> **Incorrect:**
> He was 2 days, 14 hours old.

DON'T use figures when expressing an indefinite age.

> He was in his late fifties.
> She started school at age four or five.

27–4 DATES

 DO use figures for the day of the month and the year; *write out the month when used in narrative text and the date line of a letter.* Use figures separated by hyphens or slashes in other formats.

Date line for letter or report
November 3, 200X
3 November 200X *(military and foreign style; not used in text format)*
Text use
Correct:
The patient was first seen in the emergency department on March 3, 200X.
Incorrect:
The patient was first seen in the emergency department on 3-3-0X.
Incorrect:
The patient was first seen in the emergency department on 3/3/0X.
Correct:
The patient was first seen in the emergency department on 3 March 20XX. *(not correct in nonmilitary documents)*
Incorrect:
The patient was first seen in the emergency department on March 3 last year. *(Find out the correct year and insert it.)*
In reports
DOB: 03-03-93 *(date of birth)*
Office visit: 3 3 0X.
Office visit: 03-03-0X.
Office visit: 8/3/XX.
D: 11-3-XX. *(date of dictation)*
T: 11-4-XX. *(date of transcription)*
The double-digit dating system
D: 11-03-XX *or* 11/03/200X
T: 11-04-XX *or* 11/04/200X

 DO convert military style to conventional form in *text* formats.

Incorrect:
He was born on 27 July 200X.
Incorrect:
He was born on 7/27/0X.
Correct:
He was born on July 27, 200X.

☑ DO   use cardinal numbers *(1, 2, 3, and so forth)* for expressing the date after the month and ordinal numbers *(1st, 2nd, 3rd, and so forth)* for expressing the date before the month. The ordinal number is used with the date only before the name of the month.

Correct:
She was first seen on the 2nd of May.
She was first seen on May 2.
Incorrect:
She was first seen on May 2nd.
She was first seen on 2 May.

27–5   DECIMAL FRACTIONS

☑ DO   use figures in writing numbers containing decimal fractions.

There was a 3.5-cm cut above the left eyebrow.

☑ DO   express the pH of a substance *(from 0 to 14)* with a whole number and a decimal fraction. If there is no following fraction, this is indicated with a *zero* (0).

The pH was 5.2.
The patient had a pH of 7.0.

☑ DO   express specific gravity with four digits and a decimal point. Place the decimal between the first and second digits.

The normal range for specific gravity in urine is 1.015-1.025.

☑ DO   express temperature readings in decimal fractions when fractions are given.

98.6°F   35°C

☑ DO   place a zero before a decimal that does not contain a whole number. *(Be very careful with the placement of the zero and decimal. Incorrect placement could result in a 10- or 100-fold error.)*

The incision site was injected with 0.5% Xylocaine.

EXCEPTION: *He used a .22-caliber rifle.*

🚫 **DON'T**   add trailing zeros after a whole number unless dictated. *(pH is an exception)*

Incorrect:
4.0 cm tear
Correct:
4 cm tear

27–6 DIMENSIONS AND MEASUREMENTS
See also Chapter 26, Metric System.

 DO   use figures and symbols when writing dimensions. Leave a space each side of the *x*. Use lowercase *x*.

two 4 × 4 sponges
The burn scar was 60 mm × 4 cm.
12 × 14 ft area

 DO   use common fractions to express nonmetric measurements.

It had swollen to 1½ times its normal size.

27–7 DRUGS

✅ **DO**   use figures in all expressions pertaining to drugs, including strength, dosage, and directions.

He is to take Tofranil, 75 mg/d × 3 days, to be increased to 100-150 mg/d if there is no response.

The directions for her Motrin were 400 mg q.4 h. p.r.n. pain.

One generally gives 6.2 mg/kg to 9.4 mg/kg for those children 9 years old or younger.

27–8 ELECTROCARDIOGRAPHIC LEADS

✅ **DO**   use figures and abbreviations when writing electrocardiographic *chest* leads. *(These leads are V₁ through V₆ and aVₗ, aVᵣ, and aVբ.)* They may be written properly with subscripts or on line when the subscript format is unavailable.

✅ **DO**   use roman numerals for standard leads and intercostal spaces.

lead I   lead II   lead III   V3III

✓ **DO** use capital *V* for central terminal chest leads with a number for the chest electrode.

V1 through V9 *or* V_1 through V_9

✓ **DO** use a letter for right arm, left arm, or foot.

aVR   aVL   aVF
or
aV_R aV_L aV_F

The leads I, II, aV_L *(aVL also correct)*, and aV_F *(aVF also correct)* are missing in this sequence.

NOTE: *See 27–21, Roman Numerals, for numbers used with* limb leads.

27–9 FRACTIONS

See also 27–5, Decimal Fractions.

✓ **DO** use figures to express numbers referred to as numbers.

multiples of 10   divide by 8   multiply by 4/7

✓ **DO** spell out and hyphenate fractions standing alone.

He smoked a half-pack of cigarettes a day.
He smoked one-half pack of cigarettes a day.
Paresis is noted in four-fifths of the left leg.

✓ **DO** use figures to write mixed numbers *(whole numbers with a fraction)*. Use case fractions (e.g., ¼) when available on your word processing program.

1 ½   7 ⅝   6 ¾   ½
The patient moved to this community 2 ½ years ago.
(mixed number)

✓ **DO** use figures when the fraction is used as a compound modifier.

There was a ¾-inch difference between the two bones.

NOTE: *Common fractions are not used with the metric system or with the percent (%) sign. Decimals are used with the metric system to describe parts of whole numbers.*

Incorrect:
¾%
Correct:
0.75%

27–10 INCLUSIVE (CONTINUED) NUMBERS

✓ DO   use the hyphen to take the place of the word *to* or *through* to indicate ranges.

Take 100 mg Tylenol 1-2 at bedtime.
The L2-3 disk was involved.
30-35 mEq
Rounds were made in Wards 1-4.
practicing there from 1990-1999
checked the records from the 400-450 series
She has a 50-50 chance.
Check V_2-V_6 again.
Cranial nerves II-XII were intact.

🚫 DON'T   use a hyphen when one or both ends of the range contain a plus or a minus sign. *(See also 27–20, Ratios and Ranges.)*

at a −2 to a −3 station

27–11 INDEFINITE EXPRESSIONS

✓ DO   write out numbers that are used for indefinite expressions.

I received thirty-odd applications.
He had diphtheria in his mid-forties.
Hundreds thronged to see my "celebrity" patient.
I had about a thousand reasons for doing that.
Several hundred doctors were expected to attend.
There was a five-fold increase in membership.

Correct:
There were nearly eighteen hundred physicians present at the symposium.
Incorrect:
There were one thousand eight hundred present.

27–12 LARGE NUMBERS

☑ DO   use figures to write numbers larger than ten. Use a comma to punctuate large numbers when there are five or more digits represented. Addresses, year dates, ZIP codes, fax numbers, four-digit numbers, and some ID and technical numbers are traditionally not separated by commas, nor are commas used with decimals or the metric system.

The piece of equipment is valued at $12,300.

Piedmont Hospital Association serves a population of 150,500.

Please send this to Union Annex Box 87543.

All of the ZIP codes changed in our area; please note that the new one is 06431.

☑ DO   express round numbers in the millions and billions in a combination of figures and words.

Do you know that Keane Insurance sold over $3 billion worth of medical insurance last year?

☑ DO   use the exponential form of scientific notation for large scientific numbers greater than 1,000,000. Be sure to write the exponent in superscript.

7^3 (*seven to the power of three*)
2.5×10^7 (*not 25,000,000*)

☑ DO   express large technical numbers in figures and punctuate appropriately.

The culture grew 100,000 colonies of E. coli per cubic centimeter.

The insurance reimbursement was $1240.

NOTE: *Red blood cells are usually counted in millions and white blood cells in thousands.*

Dictated:
rbcs three point two one; wbc seven point seven.
Transcribed:
RBCs 3,210,000; WBCs 7700.

27–13 LISTS

✓ **DO**   use serial figures for listing and enclose them in parentheses when enumerating in text material. Use serial figures followed by a period in a vertical *(displayed)* list.

Plan on admittance: (1) Stat WBC, (2) barium enema, (3) urinalysis, (4) routine chest x-ray.

Rule out: 1. Acute appendicitis.
                2. Ectopic pregnancy.
                3. Endometritis.
                4. Polycystic ovary.

27–14 MONEY

✓ **DO**   use figures to express amounts of money.

She was offered a $62,000 annual salary.

🚫 **DON'T**   use periods and zeros with whole dollar amounts unless two or more amounts are used in the same context in the sentence.

Correct:
My consultation fee was $150.00, but the insurance reimbursement was just $112.37.
Correct:
The initial consultation fee is $150.
Incorrect:
The initial consultation fee is $150.00.

🚫 **DON'T**   use symbols for less than whole dollar amounts.

Correct:
Please give her the 35 cents change.
Incorrect:
Please give her the 35¢ change.
Incorrect:
Please give her the $0.35 change.

✓ **DO**   express round dollar amounts in the millions and billions in a combination of figures and words preceded by the dollar symbol.

Do you know that Keane Insurance sold over $3 billion worth of medical insurance last year?

✔️ **DO** spell out indefinite amounts of money.

I think there was just a few dollars' difference.
He was offered several thousand dollars more to stay.

27–15 NAMES

✔️ **DO** use Roman numerals *(I, II, and so forth)* or ordinals *(2d, 3d, and so forth)* without punctuation after a person's surname, following the individual's preference.

Jon-Pierre Wolffstetter II
William Paul Denny 3d

✔️ **DO** use figures or written-out numbers in the names of business firms as the firms prefer.

Twenty-first Century Research
The 99-cent Emporium

27–16 NEIGHBORING AND RELATED NUMBERS

✔️ **DO** use a figure for one number and spell out the other number when two numbers are used together to modify the same noun. *(Note also the use of the hyphen in the compound modifier.)*

two 1-liter solutions
six 3-bed wards
twenty 4 × 4 sponges

✔️ **DO** use figures to write numbers less than ten when they are related to a large number on the same subject.

There are 3 beds available on the medical wing, 14 on the surgery wing, and 12 on the pediatric floor.

27–17 ORDINAL NUMBERS

✔️ **DO** *spell out* ordinal numbers *(first through ninth)* when used to indicate a time sequence and numbered streets under ten. Use *figures* for ordinals when they are part of a series that includes a higher ordinal *(10 and above),* for street numbers 10 and above, and when the number indicates any other technical term.

Spelled-out numbers
This is her second visit to the clinic.

The patient was discharged to his home on the fifth postoperative day.

The first stage of the disease went by relatively unobserved.

Most spontaneous abortions occur during the first or second week of pregnancy, just after the first menstrual cycle is missed.

Her new office is located at 924 Fifth Avenue, Suite 10.

Figures
The clinic was for children in the 1st through 12th grades.

The 4th, 5th, and 6th ribs were fractured.

The injury was between the 1st and 2nd cervical vertebrae.

Only the 7th (or seventh) cranial nerve was involved.

second-degree burn
the 5th percentile
3rd-degree burn

It occurred sometime between the 14th and 30th weeks of pregnancy.

Change the mailing address from PO Box 254 to 1335 11th Street.

Give the patient an appointment for the 6th of August.

HOWEVER: *Give the patient an appointment for August 6.*

NOTE: *As with all numbers, use a spelled-out ordinal number to begin a sentence or recast the sentence to avoid beginning with a number.*

Twelfth-grade students in the honor programs are simultaneously enrolled in community college classes.

 DON'T space between the number and the *th, d,* or *st.*

DO hyphenate compound ordinals.

the eighty-fifth congress

27–18 PLURALS

✓ **DO**   form the plural of figures by adding *s*.

⊘ **DON'T**   use an apostrophe unless the combination resembles a word.

Be sure that your 2s don't look like z's.
A binary notation is a combination of 1's and 0's.

✓ **DO**   form the plural of written-out numbers just as you form the plural of other words. *(See Chapter 31, Plural Forms.)*

She moved here sometime in the forties.
He refused to do his serial 7s.

27–19 PUNCTUATION WITH NUMBERS
Colon

✓ **DO**   use a colon between numbers to express ratios. The colon takes the place of the word *to*. *(See also 27-20, Ratios and Ranges.)*

The solution was diluted 1:100.
a 3:1 ratio *but* a ratio of 3 to 1

✓ **DO**   use a colon between the hours and minutes indicating the time of day in figures.

The patient expired at 10:30 a.m.

⊘ **DON'T**   use the double zero with an even time of day.

Incorrect:
10:00 a.m.

Comma

✓ **DO**   use a comma between a pair of numbers to facilitate reading the numbers and to avoid confusion.

In 2004, 461 cases were reviewed by the Tumor Board.

✓ **DO**   use a comma to set off a year date that is used to explain a preceding date of the month.

He was born on March 3, 1933, in Reading, Pennsylvania.

✓ **DO**   use commas to group numbers with five or more digits in units of three.

300,000 units   platelets 250,000   wbc 15,000

EXCEPTION: *Numbers used with metric measurements, telephone numbers, social security numbers, insurance and other ID numbers, addresses, credit card numbers, and binary notation (a combination of 0's and 1's).*

🚫 **DON'T** use commas to separate two units of the same dimension.

The infant was 3 days 4 hours old.
She was a gravida 4 para 2 abortus 1 white female.
The surgery was completed in 2 hours 40 minutes.
He was 6 ft 3 in. tall.
(Note the period after in. *in the previous example. This abbreviation is punctuated since it can be misread as the word* in *rather than the abbreviation for* inch.*)*

Hyphen

✓ **DO** use a hyphen to join the isotope number to the radiopharmaceutical brand names.

Glofil-125

🚫 **DON'T** use a hyphen in the generic form

sodium iodide I 131   iothalamate sodium I 125
(Elements are written with superscript, e.g., ^{131}I.*)*

✓ **DO** use a hyphen with words and numbers describing chemical elements

HDL-cholesterol   5-azacytidine
5-FU   17-hydroxycorticosteroids

✓ **DO** use a hyphen with words and numbers describing immunostimulants and interleukins.

interferon alfa-n3   interferon gamma-1b
IL-16   IL-1RA

✓ **DO** use hyphens and close up punctuation in chemical formulas.

9-nitroanthra(1,9,4,10)bis(1)oxathiazone-2,7-bisdioxide

✓ **DO** hyphenate numbers from 21 to 99 when they are written out.

Fifty-five medical transcriptionists attended the meeting last night.

DO   use a hyphen to take the place of the word *to* in numerical ranges.

Take 1-2 at bedtime.
30-35 mEq   a 50-50 chance

 DO   use hyphens in some descriptive classifications of drugs and diseases. *(See also 27-21, Roman Numerals.)*

M-1 to M-7 with M-0 *(zero)* describes nonlymphocytic leukemias.

Roman numbers I-V including IIa and IIb describe hyperlipoproteinemia.

 DON'T   repeat the symbol used in a range.

99-102°F temperature

 DO   use a hyphen and parentheses with telephone numbers.

Call (800) 626-3126 between nine and five.
800-626-3126 *(also correct)*

DO   use a hyphen to join numbers to words in a compound modifier.

6-kg weight   35-mm film
4-mm-thick layer   2-week convalescence

DO   use a hyphen with numbers 21 through 99 when they are written out.

Fifty-five medical transcriptionists attended the meeting last night.

Ninety-nine percent of the time I am confident of the diagnosis.

DO   use a hyphen with spelled-out fractions.

She has spent one-third of her life concerned about the appearance of this scar.

DO   hyphenate the modifier attached to a CPT code in narrative copy.

99255-32
69502-99

DO hyphenate compound modifiers composed of numbers and words.

4-cm long incision
3-month-old infant
5 × 5 × 1-mm glass fragment
35-hour week
4- to 5-year history
.45 caliber weapon
figure-of-8 sutures

 DO use the hyphen to take the place of the word *to* or *through*, to identify numeric and alphabetical ranges. *(See 27-10, Inclusive [Continued] Numbers for further help with numeric ranges.)*

Take 100 mg Tylenol, 1-2 at bedtime

C7-T1 disk
30-35 mEq

Rounds were made in Wards 1-4.
practicing there from 1990-1999
cranial nerves II-XII
Check V2-V6 again.

We eliminated every diagnosis from A-Z.

Note the P-R interval.

 DON'T use a hyphen to express a range when one or both of the numbers contain a minus or plus sign.

at a –2 to a –3 station

NOTE: *Use through to describe ranges of vertebra and spinal nerves.*

The L2 through L5 vertebrae were involved
There was C1 through C6 nerve damage.

 DON'T use commas or hyphens with four-digit numbers, the metric system, street numbers, dates, ZIP codes, and some ID and technical numbers unless they are actually part of the number.

My bill to Medicare was $1250.
Correct:
1000 mL

Incorrect:
1,000 mL

Parentheses

✔️ DO   use parentheses to separate numbers used in text. *(See 27–13, Lists.)*

27–20   RATIOS AND RANGES

✔️ DO   use figures in writing technical ratios and ranges.

The solution was diluted 1:100.

There is a 50-50 chance of recovery.

NOTE: *A ratio expresses the relationship between elements of a proportion. A range is the linking of a sequence of values or numbered items by expressing only the first and last items in the sequence or the difference between the smallest and the largest varieties in a statistical distribution.*

Ratios made up of words are expressed with a slash, a hyphen, or the word *to*.

The odds are ten to one.
the female/male ratio *or* the female-male ratio

Numerical ratios are expressed by using a colon.

The odds are 10:1.
The solution was diluted 1:100,000.
a 3:1 ratio *but* a ratio of 3 to 1

NOTE: *Symbolic ratios are written with a slash.*

The a/b ratio
The word *to* or a hyphen may be used in expressions of range. Avoid using a hyphen when other symbols are used in the range.
We released all the medical records from 1994-2004 to microfilm storage.
There is a waiting period of 3-6 months.
The projected salary increases are $2.75 to $3.00 per hour.
Avoid:
The projected salary increases are $2.75–$3.00 per hour.

🚫 **DON'T** use the hyphen when the range includes a plus or a minus sign.

There was a weight change expected of anywhere from −6.5 kg to +10.5 kg.
The presenting part was at a −2 to a −3 station.

✓ **DO** Use the symbol or abbreviation with each of the figures in the range.

The survival rate was consistent at 20% to 25%.
The fever fluctuated daily between 100° and 103°.

✓ **DO** use a slash in expressing a heart murmur range. *(Other heart sounds may be expressed with subscripts. See 27-24, Subscripts and Superscripts.)*

Dictated:
There was a grade four over six systolic murmur.
Transcribed:
There was a grade 4/6 systolic murmur.

27–21 *ROMAN NUMERALS*

🚫 **DON'T** use a type font that is sans serif *(sans means without; serifs are small lines to finish off tops and bottoms of capital letters)* because the capital letter *I* needed for roman numerals looks like the number one.

✓ **DO** use roman numerals for major divisions in an outline. *(See Figures 25–7 and 25–8.)*

✓ **DO** use roman numerals as part of established nomenclature. They are generally used with nonmathematical or with noncounting listings.

The patient was scheduled for a Verdict-II drug screening panel during his next visit.

The surgeon asked that we prepare Dexon II sutures for the procedure.

The treatment described for this particular lung cancer stage I and II is surgical resection.

The following are examples of some of the many uses of roman numerals in medical documents. Every example cannot be given, but there should be enough here to help you decide if the number is roman or arabic. Because there are some very similar expressions that require arabic figures, they are included to help you to determine proper usage. The arabic examples are in italics.

Expression	Example
anemia	*stage 1-5*
angiotensin	angiotensin I
antithrombin	antithrombin III *or* AT-III
axis	axis I-V
Bethesda system	cervical and vaginal: *group 1-6*
Billroth I	first stage of an operative procedure
block	Mobitz II block (heart block)
blood factors	blood factor I-XII
carcinoma	stage II carcinoma, stage IVB (subdivision)
	FIGO staging ovarian cancer
	cervical carcinoma stage 0 to IVB
	grade 2 cancer cells
	Dukes C2 (colon cancer)
cardiac disease	NYHA cardiac disease I-IV
CIN	*CIN-2* or *CIN grade 2*
class	class II malignancy
	class III intubation
	class III lead poisoning
	class IV diabetes
	Angle's class III malocclusion
	Pap smear cervical cytology class IV
cognitive function scale	level I-VI
collagen	bone collagen type I; human collagen type III
coma	stage I coma
cranial leads (EEG)	lead I reading
cranial nerves (I-XII)	cranial nerves II-XII are intact
decubitus ulcer	stage II decubitus ulcer, left heel
diet	step I diet
disease/disorder	type III von Willebrand disease
	stage I-V and III$_1$ and III$_2$ Hodgkin disease
	mucolipidosis III
	bipolar mood disorder I
	Lynch syndrome II
	type 2 schizophrenic disorder
drugs/agents	CAP-II
	Oxydess II
	Diab II
	agent III for cardiovascular disease

Expression	Example
drug reaction	phase I and II (overdose stage I-IV)
EDSI	connective tissue disorder type I-XI
endometrial	stage IA-IVB
equipment*	Sensolog III pacemaker
	Accu-Chek II instrument
	Accucore II
	Pico-ST II catheter
	Cordguard II
	Crit-Line III
	AeroTech II nebulizer
	Eagle II spirometer
	Mark VII cooling vest
	NeuroLink II
	Guepar II prosthesis
factors	missing factor VII
FIGO staging	ovarian cancer: FIGO stage IIb
fracture	Salter III fracture
	LeFort fracture I
	Neer fracture (I, II, III)
	SER-IV fracture
glycogen storage diseases	types I through XII
grade	grade II hip dysplasia
	reflux esophagitis grade IV
	cognitive scale rating I-VIII
	GVHD2 or *grade 2*
	grade 1 and *2 cancer*
	CIN *grade 2* (cervical cancer)
	grade 4/6 murmur (heart murmur)
Hodgkin disease	stage I-V and III_1 and III_2
human collagen	types I and II
hyperlipo-proteinemia	I through V, including IIa and IIb
hyperprolinemia	I or II (metabolic condition)
immune reaction	type I-IV (in renal disease)
intubation	class III intubation
leukemia	*M-1* to *M-7* and *M-0* (zero)
level	level III lymph node
	cognitive function scale level II
	Clark level III (skin cancer)
limb lead (ECG)	lead II reading (I to III)
lues (I to III)	lues II (secondary syphilis)
lymphoma	I-IV National Cancer Institute

---

*There are countless names for instruments and devices that use roman numerals as part of the trade name.

Expression	Example
MEN	multiple endocrine neoplasia type I, IIa, IIb
neoplasms	stage I-IV (also type I)
oncology staging	I-II to IVA and IVB
phases	*phase 2 clinical trial*
	phase I physiologic jaundice
	phase I and II drug reaction
procedures	Billroth stage I
	Insall/Burstein II
	Belsey Mark IV
	NicCheck-I test
stage	stage II carcinoma; subdivision IVB
	stage I coma
	stage III drug overdose
	stage III endometrial involvement
	stage III cervical carcinoma
	Tanner stage III development
	Rome II criteria
	stage II B Hodgkin disease
	stage III$_2$ Hodgkin disease
	stage III lues
	stage II Billroth
	Reyes syndrome staging III
	stage I-IV neoplasms
	stage III decubitus ulcer
	stage II degenerative fibrosis
	stage 1-5 anemia
step	step I diet
Tanner stage	stage IV sexual maturity
technique	Coffey technique III
test	Hemoccult II test
type	type I hyperlipoproteinemia
	type I neoplasm
	type XI glycogenosis
	type I herpesvirus
	type IIb MEN
	type II lupoid hepatitis
	type VII glycogen storage disease
	type III variant (of a disease)
	type I bone collagen
	type III human collagen
	type IV immune reaction (renal disease)
	type I-XI connective tissue disorder
	type 1 and type 2 diabetes
	type 1 immune-mediated beta-cell diabetes
	type 1 and type 2 aortic dissection
	type 1 and type 1 schizophrenic disorder

27–22   SPACING WITH SYMBOLS AND NUMBERS

✓ **DO**   type the following symbols directly in front of or directly following the number they refer to, with no spacing.

+	=	%	#	$
o	@	&	–	/

✓ **DO**   space on each side of the x that takes the place of the word times or the word by.

3 × 5 card

27–23   SPELLED-OUT NUMERIC TERMS

✓ **DO**   spell out numbers at the beginning of a sentence *(or reword the sentence to avoid beginning with a number.)*

Fourteen patients were studied at the request of the staff, four were studied at the request of their physicians, and eleven were studied as interesting problems for discussion.

NOTE: *When several related numbers are used in a sentence, be consistent; type all numbers in figures or write them all out. Normally, it is easier to type all of them in figures. If the number beginning the sentence is large* (more than two words), *it may be necessary to rewrite the sentence so that the number may be used as a figure within the sentence. However, if you must begin a sentence with a numeric term, you are not bound to write out the other large numbers in the sentence.*

Seventy-one percent responded to the questionnaire; 33% were positive, 21% were negative, and 17% gave a "no opinion" response.

✓ **DO**   remember to spell out an abbreviation or symbol used with a number if the number has to be spelled out for some reason *(see previous example.)*

✓ **DO**   spell out numbers *one* through and including *ten* when they do not refer to technical items and do not appear in the same sentence with larger numbers.

The EEG was run for three minutes with no activity.
but
The EEG was run for 20 minutes with no activity.
also
The EEG was run for 5 ½ minutes with no activity.

The address for our risk management team is One East Wacker Drive, Chicago, IL 60601.

He will have to convalesce for five to six weeks before returning to work.

She had pulmonary tuberculosis three years ago and spent seven months in a sanatorium.

We had seven admissions Saturday and three already this morning.

✓ **DO** spell out numbers that are used for indefinite expressions.

I received thirty-odd applications.
He had diphtheria in his mid-forties.

✓ **DO** spell out fractions when they appear without a whole number or are not used as a compound modifier.

He smoked a half-pack of cigarettes a day.
He smoked one-half pack of cigarettes a day.
but
He smoked 1½ packs of cigarettes a day.

A ½-inch incision was made in the thenar eminence. *(use of modifier)*

There was damage to one-fourth of the distal phalanx. *(no use of modifier)*

NOTE: *With the keyboard, make all fractions by using the whole number, the slash, and the second whole number, with no spacing. Mixed fractions are made with a space between the whole number and the first number of the fraction.*

1/2 inch
1 1/2 inch *(not 1 and 1/2 inch, which the dictator might say)*
1/2-inch incision *(compound modifier)*

✓ **DO** use case fractions when they are available on your word processing menu.

Keyboard fraction:
3/4
Case fraction:
¾

✓ **DO** spell out one number and use a figure for the other when two numbers are used together to modify the same noun.

> two 1-liter solutions
> six 3-bed wards
> 130 two-day admissions

✓ **DO** spell out the even time of day when written with or without *o'clock* and without *a.m.* or *p.m.*

> The staff meeting is scheduled to begin at three.
> He is due at nine this evening.
> Give her an appointment for two o'clock.
> Give her an appointment for 2 o'clock. *(also correct)*

✓ **DO** spell out large round numbers that do *not* refer to technical quantities.

> There were eighteen hundred physicians present at the symposium.
> **Incorrect:**
> He was given six hundred thousand units of penicillin. *(This is a technical number.)*
> **Correct:**
> He was given 600,000 units of penicillin.

27–24 SUBSCRIPTS AND SUPERSCRIPTS

At one time, many numbers were typed in subscript or superscript *(slightly below or above the line)*. With the advent of word processing equipment, this technique has become easier, but it still takes time to leave the routine of keying letters and numbers to create the proper formatting. Numbers are more easily read when typed on the line because most reports are single spaced. Again, some authors may insist on proper formatting, so be alert to this.

> H_2O *(the formula for water)*
> A_2 is greater than P_2 *(the aortic second sound is greater than the pulmonic second sound)*
> The L_4 area was bruised *(reference to the fourth lumbar vertebra)*
> ^{131}I was given *(reference to radioactive iodine)*

You might want to learn this technique. It is shown in the examples, along with numbers typed on the line. An exception to the general rule of avoiding subscripts and superscripts is in the case of numbers given to the power of 10, such as "urine culture grew out 10^5 colonies of E. coli." It is obvious that in this case, to write the superscript on the same line would change the value of the number.

DO use subscript or superscript as appropriate in writing the following values:

Superscripts
Scientific notation: 7^{10} *(seven to the power of ten)*

Place the mass number in the superior position to the left of the symbol.
^{195m}Hg ^{238}U ^{18}F-FDG
krypton: Kr 81 m *or* ^{81m}Kr
xenon: Xe 133 *or* ^{133}Xe
technetium: Tc 99m *or* ^{99m}Tc

NOTE: *The isotope number is keyed on the same line as the rest of the drug name.*

iodohippurate sodium I 131
glucose 14 C *or* glucose ^{14}C

Subscripts
Chemical elements and compounds:
  O_2 (oxygen)
  CO_2 (carbon dioxide)
Vitamin components: B_{12}
Vertebral column: L_{4-5} *(fourth and fifth lumbar)*
Chest leads: V_1-V_6
Heart sounds: A_2, P_2
EEG electrodes: F_3
(See also 27–32, Vitamins.)

NOTE: *All these expressions can be typed on the same line if your equipment is not capable of printing small numbers above or below the line, with the exception of scientific notation.*

V4   L4-5   B12   CO2   O2   14C   A2   F3   U 238

27–25   SUTURE MATERIALS
In the USP system, sutures range in size from the smallest *(11-0)*, which are described with the appropriate number of zeros, to the largest *(7)*, which are described as #1 through #7. In the Brown & Sharp *(B&S)* sizing of stainless steel sutures, the range is from the smallest *(#40)* through the largest *(#20)*.

 DO use figures in writing suture materials.

NOTE: *When the dictator says "three oh" or "triple oh" in referring to suture materials, you type 3-0. For reading ease, use only the number, hyphen and the zero when the number is larger than two, that is, from 3-0 through 11-0.*

Correct
The incision was closed with #6-0 fine silk sutures.
She used 3-0 chromic catgut for suture material
She used #3-0 chromic catgut for suture material.

Please order a box of #1 silk.

Number 6-0 fine silk sutures were used to close the incision.

Incorrect
The incision was closed with #000000 fine silk sutures.
The incision was closed with #60 fine silk sutures.

 DO be consistent throughout the report in describing the suture materials.

 DON'T confuse these markings with the Vicryl sutures or stainless steel sutures when a different gauge designation may be dictated.

The corneoscleral incision was closed with interrupted #70 Vicryl sutures.

A Bunnell 34-gauge pull-out wire was woven through the extensor tendon and tied over a button.

27–26 SYMBOLS AND NUMBERS

 DO use figures and symbols when writing plus or minus with a number.

1 to 2+
pulses were 2+
The presenting part was at a −2 station.
Visual acuity with correction was increased to 20/200 by +8.50 lens.

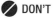 **DON'T** use symbols and hyphens together.

Incorrect:
a 3″-incision
Correct:
a 3-inch incision

 DO use symbols in preference to the spelled-out word when they occur in immediate association with a number and are used to express technical terms.

8 × 3	eight by three
4-5	four to five
#3-0	number three oh
2+	two plus
Vision: 20/20	vision is twenty-twenty
6/d	six per day
diluted 1:10	diluted one to ten
at −2	at minus two
60/40	sixty over forty
grade 4/5	grade four over five
nocturia × 2	nocturia times two
25 mg/h	twenty-five milligrams per hour
limited by 45%	limited by forty-five percent
35 mg%	thirty-five milligrams percent
30°C	thirty degrees Celsius
99°F	ninety-nine degrees Fahrenheit
BP: 100/80	blood pressure is one hundred over eighty
1+ protein	one plus protein
+2.50	plus two point fifty
120/80	one hundred twenty over eighty
Rh−	"are-h" negative
2%	two percent
$10 (*not* $10.00)	ten dollars
#14 Foley	number fourteen Foley
6 in.	six inches
serial # 526-4A	
order No. 3BA-L	
model #13W	

 DON'T assume that you must use the degree symbol (°) in describing temperature if the word *degree* is not dictated.

Temperature: 36 C.
Temperature: 36°C.

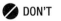 **DON'T** use the percent symbol (%) in nonscientific text.

Incorrect:
Only 25% of those invited were on time.
Correct:
Only a quarter of those invited were on time.
Only twenty-five percent arrived on time.

DON'T use simple fractions with percent.

Incorrect:
45½ percent
45½ %

Correct:
45.5%

 27.27 TIME

☑ DO spell out the *even time of day* when written without *o'clock* or without *a.m.* or *p.m.*

The staff meeting is scheduled to begin at three.
He is due at nine this evening.
Give her an appointment for half-past two.
His plane is due at seven tomorrow night.

☑ DO use the phrases *in the morning, in the afternoon,* and *at night* with *o'clock* and not with *a.m.* or *p.m.* Do not use *o'clock* with *a.m.* or *p.m.* or when both hour and minutes are expressed.

I met her in the emergency room at 3 o'clock in the morning.
Incorrect:
She is expected at 3 o'clock p.m.
She is expected at 3:30 o'clock.
Correct:
She is expected at 3 o'clock.
She is expected at 3:30 p.m.
She is expected at 3:30.

NOTE: *It is also acceptable to write out an even time of day with the expression o'clock.*

Please ask her to come at three o'clock.
Please ask her to come at 3 o'clock.

☑ DO use figures to express the time of day with *a.m.* or *p.m.* and the time of day when both hours and minutes are expressed alone.

Office hours are from 10 a.m. to noon. Your appointment is for 11:30.
He arrived promptly at 2:30.

🚫 DON'T use the colon and double zeros for even periods of time.

Incorrect:
Office hours are from 10:00 a.m. to noon.
Correct:
Office hours are from 10 a.m. to noon.

DON'T   use *a.m.* or *p.m.* with 12. You may use the figure 12 with the word *noon* or *midnight* or use the words alone without the figure 12.

> We close the office at 12 noon. (*or simply* noon)
> My shift is over at midnight.

✓ **DO**   use four figures without a colon when writing the military time of day.

> 0315 *(oh three fifteen; 3:15 a.m.)*
> 1200 *(twelve hundred hours; noon)*
> 1400 *(fourteen hundred hours; 2 p.m.)*
> 1630 *(sixteen thirty; 4:30 p.m.)*
> **Incorrect:**
> Your appointment is set for 16:30.
> Your appointment is set for 1630 p.m.
> **Correct**
> Your appointment is set for 1630.

✓ **DO**   use the expression *o'clock* to refer to points on a circular surface, and use figures with *o'clock.*

> The sclera was incised at about the 3 o'clock area.

> The cyst was in the left breast, just below the nipple, between 4 and 5 o'clock.

> Then 1:2 mL of 1% lidocaine was injected at the 4 o'clock and 8 o'clock positions.

✓ **DO**   write out numbers to express *periods of time* when the number is less than ten; when the number is ten or greater, use the figure.

> She is to return in three months' time.
> The B-R Medical Supply invoice is marked "net 30 days."

27–28   *UNRELATED NUMBERS*

✓ **DO**   follow the rules governing the use of each number when unrelated numbers appear in the same sentence.

> He has three offices and employs 21 medical assistants and 2 transcriptionists.

27–29 *VERTEBRAL COLUMN AND SPINAL NERVES, SPACES, AND DISKS*

✔ DO use figures with capital letters to refer to the vertebral *(spinal)* column and spinal nerves as follows:

C   cervical 1 through 7
T *(or D)*   thoracic *(or dorsal)* 1 through 12
L   lumbar 1 through 5
S   sacral 1 through 5

✔ DO use a hyphen to indicate the intravertebral spaces and intervertebral disks.

C2-3 space   C2-3 disk
C7-T1 space   C7-T1 disk

✔ DO use subscript if preferred; but typing on line is easier to do and easier to read.

He has a herniated disk at C_{4-5}.
He has a herniated disk at C4-5.

There was an injury to the spine between C_7 and T_1.
There was an injury to the spine between C7 and T1.

27–30 *VISUAL ACUITY AND REFRACTIONS*

✔ DO use figures and symbols to express visual acuity.

OD: +3.25+0.75 × 125 = 20/30−1
Vision was corrected to 20/200

NOTE: *Use care in transcribing numbers that make sense. The preceding expression may have sounded like 22/100, which would not make sense. Visual acuity numbers always begin with a 20 (20/20, 20/25, 20/200, 20/500). Therefore, there will not be a 22 hundred, or 22-100 or 22/100 by mistake.*

27–31 *VITAL STATISTICS*

✔ DO use figures in writing vital statistics such as age, weight, height, blood pressure, pulse, respiration, dosage, size, temperature, and so forth.

He is a 16-year-old, well-developed, well-nourished white male. Height: 72 in. Weight: 145 lb. Blood Pressure: 120/80. Pulse: 72. Respirations: 18.

The patient has 20/40 vision in his right eye and 20/100 in his left eye.

27–32   VITAMINS

 DO   write the abbreviation for vitamins by using subscript numbers or numbers on the line, as preferred.

B_1 B1
B_{12} B12
D_3 D3
K_1 K1

27–33   WORDS USED WITH NUMBERS

 DO   use figures *(roman or arabic)* for numbers used in close association with words. *(See also 27–21, Roman Numerals, and 5–15, Numbers with Nouns.)*

#14 Foley catheter
No. 14 Foley catheter
Grass Ten Channel Serial #627-B
Medicare ID 527-40-7201A
grade II systolic murmur
alpha-1 electrophoresis

28

Obstetric Terms

INTRODUCTION

In describing a patient's obstetric history, physicians may dictate abbreviations, brief forms, and/or complete words. For clarification, Table 28–1 (located at the end of the chapter) illustrates basic obstetric abbreviations and terminology.

28–1   ABORT

✓ DO   use the word *abort* or *terminate* to indicate the premature expulsion *(spontaneous or induced)* of products of conception. A pregnancy *(not a fetus or a woman)* may be aborted.

> She elected to abort as soon as possible.
> She elected to terminate the pregnancy as soon as possible. *(preferred)*

28–2   APGAR SCORE

Virginia Apgar, MD, created the Apgar scoring system to tell quickly which infants require treatment right away or transfer to an intensive care nursery. The infant's heart rate, breathing, muscle tone, reflexes, and skin color are rated from a low value of 0 to a normal value of 2. The five values are added to give the total score at one minute and five minutes after birth. Thus, an Apgar score of 9/10 reflects the totals at one minute (9) and at five minutes (10). The maximum score of 10 indicates that these five vital signs are those of a healthy infant.

✔ DO   use Arabic numbers to express the condition of a newborn infant.

He was a male infant weighing 9 pounds 13 ounces, and he had Apgars of 7 at one minute and 9 at five minutes.

🚫 DON'T   write *Apgar* in full caps. It is not an acronym.

28–3 CESAREAN SECTION

🚫 DON'T   use the brief form *C-section* unless it is dictated, and do not use it in the title section of operative reports or discharge summaries.

🚫 DON'T   capitalize the word *cesarean.*

28–4 FUNDAL HEIGHT

✔ DO   express the fundal height (distance from symphysis pubis to dome or top of uterus) in centimeters.

Fundal height is 27 cm.

28–5 GRAVIDA, PARA, ABORTUS

✔ DO   use arabic numbers when describing a patient's obstetric history. Use roman numerals only when preferred by the dictator.

gravida 3 para 2 abortus 1
gravida III para II abortus I

✔ DO   capitalize abbreviations of these terms.

G3 P2 A1

🚫 DON'T   use commas or periods with obstetric abbreviations.

🚫 DON'T   separate gravida, preterm parity, term parity, abortion, and living children sections by commas; spelled-out terms should appear in lowercase.

OB: G3 P1 A1

Case study:
A patient is 14 weeks pregnant *(third pregnancy).* She tells the physician that her 2-year-old daughter was born prematurely *(preterm parity)* at 30 weeks. She has had one miscarriage *(documented as an abortion)* at 9 weeks' gestation.

 DO spell out the terms when one or more of the *gravida, para, abortus* numbers is 0. Lowercase is preferred.

gravida 1 para 0 abortus 3

 DO separate TPAL numbers by hyphens. TPAL numbers are an abbreviation used to describe a patient's obstetric history. *T* indicates *term infants; P, premature infants; A, abortions;* and *L, living children.*

Obstetric history: 3-2-1-3
Optional:
Spell out the terms.
Preferred:
G3 P2 A1 L3
Acceptable alternative:
G3, P2, A1, L3
Obstetric history: 3 term infants, 2 premature infants, 1 abortion, 3 living children.

 DO use arabic numbers and spell out terms describing the obstetric history.

The patient is gravida 2 para 2-0-0-2. *(sentence format)*
OB: Gravida 5 para 4-1-0-5 *(outline format)*

28–6 OBSTETRIC HISTORY FORMAT

 DO make sure that the history and physical examination for a patient, when performed by an Ob-Gyn, includes the following gynecologic information:

Number of pregnancies.
Deliveries.
Complications.
Living children.
Abortions.
Sexual activity.
Menarche *(onset of menses).*
Menstrual flow.
Last menstrual period *(LMP).*
Menopause.
Problems associated with menses.

28–7 PRESENTATIONS

✓ DO   spell out or use abbreviations, depending on which is dictated, when expressing the presentation of the fetus at birth.

ALA *or* LAA *(for acromion left anterior).*
OP *or* occiput posterior *or* occipitoposterior.
Mentoanterior.
Mentoposterior.
Breech vertex.
Sacroanterior.
Sacroposterior.
Occipitoanterior.

28–8 STATION

✓ DO   use plus or minus and arabic numbers (–5 to +5) for expressing in centimeters the location of the presenting fetal part in the birth canal. This location will be below *(minus values)* or above *(plus values)* an imaginary plane *(station 0)* through the ischial spine.

The presenting part was at a –2 to a –3 station, and the amniotic fluid had become brownish green, suggesting some degree of fetal distress.

◆ TABLE 28-1

CURRENT OBSTETRIC TERMINOLOGY AND ABBREVIATIONS

Abbreviation	Term	Definition
G	gravida	Number of pregnancies
T	term parity	Number of deliveries at term (38-42 weeks of gestation)
P	preterm parity	Number of preterm deliveries (prior to 37 weeks' gestation)
A or Ab	abortions	Termination of pregnancy prior to viability (24 weeks' gestation); may be spontaneous (miscarriage), therapeutic, or induced
L	living children	Number of living children at the present time
P	para	Number of births of viable offspring
G0	nulligravida	No pregnancies
nullip or para 0	nullipara	No deliveries of viable offspring
P1	primigravida	One pregnancy
para 2	secundigravida	Two pregnancies
	bipara	Two offspring at one time
para 2, 3, 4	multipara	Two or more pregnancies with viable offspring
P or para 1	primipara	One pregnancy with viable fetus
para 4	quadripara	Four pregnancies with viable offspring
para 3	tripara	Three pregnancies with viable offspring
para 1	primipara	Initial pregnancy with viable offspring
unipara	primipara	Initial pregnancy with viable offspring

Parentheses

INTRODUCTION

Parentheses, commas, and dashes are all used to set off incidental or nonessential elements in text. References and instructions are often enclosed in parentheses. Parentheses are used to add needed information without harming sentence rhythm. Your choice will be determined either by the author of the material or by the relationship between the material to be set apart and the rest of the sentence. In general, commas are used to slightly set apart closely related material; parentheses are used when commas have already been used within the nonessential element or the material itself is neither grammatically nor logically essential to the main thought. The dash is a more forceful and abrupt division and draws attention to a statement; parentheses de-emphasize. Enclosed material can range from a single punctuation mark (!) to several sentences.

29–1 BRACKETS

 DO use brackets to enclose additional, nonessential material within material already enclosed in parentheses.

We will be tested on the technical material in Chapter 6 (pages 31-52 [Figures 6–1 and 6–2]).

DO   use brackets to add material within a quote for clarification. The brackets indicate that the added material was not written by the author of the quote.

His phone message was "add Ringer's [lactate] to the current protocol."
He said emphatically, "The diagnosis is Lou Gehrig disease [amyotrophic lateral sclerosis]."

NOTE: *The person being quoted did not say amyotrophic lateral sclerosis; it was added by the writer of the sentence.*

29–2 ENUMERATIONS

 DO   use parentheses around figures or letters in enumerated items run in with narrative text.

It is my impression that she has (1) progressive dysmenorrhea, (2) uterine leiomyoma, and (3) weakness of the right inguinal ring.

I did not hire her for the position because (a) she lacked enthusiasm, (b) her spoken grammar lacked polish, and (c) her typing speed was fairly low (45 wpm).

NOTE: *You may also use figures or letters followed by a period rather than enclosed in parentheses in enumerations except in narrative text material.*

1. Sterile field.
2. Suture materials.
3. 4 × 4 sponges.

29–3 EXPLANATIONS OR COMMENTS

 DO   use parentheses to enclose material that is an explanation, definition, identification, translation, or comment.

Because of his condition (emphysema) and age (88), he is a poor risk for anesthesia at this time.

The patient thought that she had inhaled some sort of ornamental dust (gold, silver, bronze) while working in her flower shop.

The administrative medical assistant (receptionist, secretary, bookkeeper, insurance clerk, file clerk) requires the same length of training as the clinical medical assistant.

He says he is a "doctor" (PhD) and prefers to use that title.

NOTE: *A complete sentence enclosed within parentheses does not require a capital letter to open it or a period to close it.*

Her temperature peaked at 106.5 degrees (we were relieved when this occurred) and the seizures subsided.

✓ DO use brackets for comments or explanations within quoted material or material enclosed in parentheses. *(See 29–1, Brackets.)*

29–4 IDENTIFICATION

✓ DO use parentheses to enclose an abbreviation after the first completely spelled-out use of a term.

All newborns are routinely tested for phenylketonuria (PKU). As a result, the incidence of PKU as the cause of infant . . .

✓ DO use parentheses to enclose the brand name of a drug after the proprietary name has been used in the text.

I would like to start him out on a nonsteroidal, anti-inflammatory agent such as ibuprofen (Motrin) or indomethacin (Indocin).

29–5 LEGAL DOCUMENTS

✓ DO in preparation of medicolegal documents, place parentheses around numerals after a spelled-out figure.

The patient will not be permitted to return to his full usual and customary duties for a period of thirty-five (35) working days.

29–6 NONESSENTIAL ELEMENTS

✓ DO use parentheses to set off words or phrases that are clearly nonessential to the sentence.

According to the pathology report (see enclosed), there is no evidence of active pulmonary tuberculosis at this time.

29–7 PUNCTUATION AND CAPITALIZATION

✓ **DO**   generally place punctuation marks outside the material enclosed in parentheses.

✓ **DO**   use punctuation inside the parentheses when it is required for definition within the material itself. *(See 29–2 through 29–6 for examples.)*

 DON'T   capitalize the beginning of a sentence when it occurs in parentheses *within* a sentence.

> We are leaving for the workshop in Phoenix early tomorrow (who got me into this?), and we should be back by Friday evening.

> We are leaving for the workshop in Phoenix early tomorrow, and we should be back by Friday evening. (Who got me into this?)

> Her temperature peaked at 106.5 degrees (we were relieved when this occurred), and the seizures subsided.

 DON'T   place a comma in front of a parenthesis.

✓ **DO**   use a comma after a closing parenthesis if the sentence requires a comma.

> After the last holiday (Thanksgiving), we had a very low census.

✓ **DO**   use dashes with parentheses when two or more overlapping parenthetical elements are used to interrupt the same sentence.

> The debate concerning the approval of lay visitors to the Tumor Board Conference became heated–we had to recess several times (once for 40 minutes)–and we finally adjourned with no definitive policy established.

29–8 REFERENCES

✓ **DO**   use parentheses to enclose a reference notation.

> A complete list of all the rules in this section is given on the first page of the chapter (see page 32).

Dr. Norman F. Billups is best known to medical transcriptionists as the author of the *American Drug Index* (J. B. Lippincott).

Grubman S, Oleske J: "HIV Infection in infants, children, and adolescents." *AIDS and Other Manifestations of HIV Infection*, 3rd ed. Wormser GP (Ed). Lippincott-Raven, New York (In press).

29–9   SCIENTIFIC USE

✓ DO   use parentheses to enclose certain mathematical elements, formulas, certain chemical and molecular components that must be grouped, immunoglobulin notations, and genetic notations concerning chromosomes.

Immunoglobulin notation: IgG(Pr)

Unknown sequences of amino acids in polypeptides: (Asp, His, Pro)

Biochemical conventions: $(CH_3)_2ChCh_2Ch(NH_2)COOH$

Symbolization for structurally altered chromosomes: 46,XX,t(4;13)(p21;q32)

29–10   SPACING

⊘ DON'T   space after the left *(opening)* parenthesis or before the right *(closing)* parenthesis.

29–11   TELEPHONE NUMBERS

✓ DO   use parentheses to separate the area code from the seven-digit phone number.

(800) 555-1212
Also acceptable:
800-555-1212

Period and Decimal Point

INTRODUCTION

The period is a mark of terminal punctuation. Some physicians from foreign countries dictate *full stop* when indicating the end of a sentence. Other authors may say *period* or rely on voice inflection to indicate the end of a sentence.

30–1 ABBREVIATIONS

✓ DO   use a period with some abbreviations as follows:

Single capitalized words and single letter abbreviations with one space typed after the period:

Mr.   Jr.   Dr.   Inc.   Co.   Ltd.
Chas.   Geo.   Joseph P. Myers
Mr. John A. Jeffreys Jr. was the guest speaker.

The name of the genus when it is abbreviated and used with the species name:

E. coli   M. tuberculosis   E. histolytica

Lowercase Latin abbreviations with no spaces between the period and the next letter, one space after the period:

a.m.   p.m.   e.g.   t.i.d.   p.r.n.

 DON'T use a period with the following lowercase abbreviations:

Units of measurement:
wpm   mph   ft   oz   sq in.   ml   mL   cm

EXCEPTION: *Don't use in for inch; it is better to spell it out or to punctuate it* (in.)

Certification, registration, academic degrees, religious orders, and licensure abbreviations:

CMA	CMT	RN	RRA	ART	LVN
LPN	PhD	SJ	DDS	MFCC	FACCP

NOTE: *Some individuals prefer that academic degrees be expressed with punctuation. It is not incorrect to do this.*

M.D.   Ph.D.   D.D.S.

Acronyms and metric abbreviations:
CARE   HOPE   AIDS   mg   mL   L   cm

Most abbreviations typed in full capital letters:

UCL	APKU	BUN	CMC	COPD	D&C
T&A	KSON	CBS	SOAP	PERRLA	

Abbreviations written in a combination of uppercase and lowercase letters

Rx	Dx	ACh	Ba	Hb	IgG
Rh	pH	Pap	mEq	mOsm	

Brief forms/short forms
polys appy   prep   eval   strep

Two-letter state abbreviations
AZ   NY   DC   TX   MO

NOTE: *The trend is toward elimination of the use of periods from some single letter abbreviations such as following the middle initials in names and the abbreviations for genus names.*

30–2   FRACTIONS

✓ DO   use a period *(decimal point)* to separate a decimal fraction from whole numbers, with no spacing before or after the period.

> **Correct:**
> His temperature on admission was 99.9°F.
> The new surgical instrument cost $64.85.
> The fee for the exam was $85.
> **Incorrect:**
> The fee for the exam was $85.00.

✓ DO   use a zero and a decimal point when the quantity is less than one.

> Epinephrine dose: 0.3 ml.

> **EXCEPTION:** *He used a .22-caliber rifle.*

✓ DO   use a decimal point fraction in expressions of specific gravity. *(These values use four digits.)*

> The urine specific gravity was 1.003.

✓ DO   use a decimal point fraction to express pH values, which indicate hydrogen ion concentration. If there is no fraction component, use a zero.

> The patient's stomach contents had a pH of 5.2.
> The midpoint between acidity and alkalinity is 7.0.

30–3   INDIRECT QUESTION

✓ DO   use a period at the end of a request for action that is phrased out of politeness as a question. This usage places greater emphasis on the requested action.

> Would you kindly fill out and return the Medicare form.

> Will you please send a copy of the operative report to Dr. Franks.

30–4   OUTLINE FIGURES AND NUMBERS

✓ DO   use a period after a number or letter in alphanumeric outlines or lists and space twice after it. If you desire closure, use a period and double-space after each word or group of words in your outline.

Diagnoses
1. Bilateral external canal exostoses.
2. Deafness, left ear, unknown etiology.

Resume preparation
1. Accurate.
2. Grammatically correct.
3. Attractively arranged on the page.

I. ....
   A. ....
   B. ....
      1. ....
      2. ....

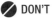 **DON'T** use periods with lists run in with narrative text. The numbers are enclosed in parentheses.

The job description should include (1) stat duties, (2) daily responsibilities, (3) weekly duties, and (4) periodic reports.

30–5 QUOTATIONS

 DO place a period inside quotation marks when the quotation closes the sentence.

The patient related that she spoke with her hands "like an Italian."

30–6 REFERENCES

 DO use a period to close a bibliographic reference.

Book:
Clark, James L. and Lyn R. Clark. *HOW 10: A Handbook for Office Professionals*. 10th ed. Mason, Ohio: South-Western Publishing, 2004.
Web site:
http://www.wedi.org/snip/
public/articles/200211012.0final.pdf.

30–7 SENTENCE

 DO use a period followed by a single or a double space at the end of a declarative sentence, an imperative sentence, a group of words that express a complete thought, an indirect question, and a footnote.

Declarative:
His chest was clear to percussion and auscultation.
Imperative:
You must be seen by a surgeon at once.
A group of words expressing a complete thought:
Diagnosis: Myocardial infarction.
An indirect question:
Will you please send a copy of the operative report to
Dr. Franks.

🚫 **DON'T** put another period at the end of a sentence that is closed
with an abbreviation that requires a period.

Send this to J. P. Chase and Company Inc.

✓ **DO** use ellipses *(three periods, called suspension points, with a
space before and after each period)* to show missing words
in text or to indicate a hesitation. Ellipses can be used to
show a pause for dramatic effect or to interrupt the main
thought.

I don't know how I get myself in to these messes . . .
maybe you can help me out?

✓ **DO** use four periods to show missing words at the end of
sentence. *(There is no space before the first period.)*

If we don't get more help in the ED soon. . . .

Plural Forms

INTRODUCTION

A reference list of common plural forms is in Appendix I, p. 593.

31–1 ABBREVIATIONS

✓ DO   use an apostrophe to form the plural of lowercase
abbreviations.

dsg's *(dressings)* jt's *(joints)*
wbc's *(white blood cells)*

🚫 **DON'T** use an apostrophe with other plural abbreviations unless the abbreviation could easily be misread.

EKGs BMRs TMs DTRs

EXCEPTION: *You used four I's in the first paragraph.*

NOTE: *For abbreviations of units of measure, singular and plural forms are the same. (See 31–21.)*

31–2 BRIEF FORMS

✅ **DO** add an *s* to a brief or short form to make it plural.

bands	segs	monos
lymphs	polys	exams

31–3 COLLECTIVE NOUNS

✅ **DO** treat a unit of measure as a singular collective noun.

Only 20% of the fluid *is* scheduled to be used.
Forty milliequivalents of KCl *was* given.

31–4 COMPOUND WORDS
See also Chapter 3, Apostrophe, and 8–9, Plural Formation of Compounds, in Chapter 8.

✅ **DO** add the appropriate plural ending to compound nouns written as one word.

birthdays	forefeet
bookshelves	spokesmen
eyelashes	teaspoonfuls
fingerbreadths	

✅ **DO** add the appropriate plural ending to the word that is the essential noun in compound nouns written with hyphens or spaces. Compounds are made plural on the main word when there is one. When there is not a main word, the plural is formed at the end.

hangers-on	mothers-in-law
go-betweens	followups
chiefs of staff	surgeons general
sisters-in-law	culs-de-sac

✔ DO   pluralize the final element of a compound when the first element of a compound noun is a possessive.

       traveler's checks   physicians' rotations

✔ DO   add *s* to form the plural of a compound noun that ends in *ful*.

       cupfuls   handfuls   teaspoonfuls

31–5   *ENGLISH WORDS*

✔ DO   form the plural by adding *s* to the singular word.

Singular	Plural
myelogram	myelograms
disease	diseases
bronchoscope	bronchoscopes

✔ DO   form the plural by adding *es* to nouns that end in *s, x, ch, sh,* or *z.*

Singular	Plural
stress	stresses
helix	helixes
fax	faxes
crutch	crutches
patch	patches
mass	masses
sinus	sinuses
virus	viruses

EXCEPTION: Os *has two meanings and becomes* ora *for mouths or* ossa *for bones.*

       os   ora
       os   ossa

✔ DO   form the plural of a noun that ends in *y* preceded by a consonant by changing the *y* to *i* and adding *es.*

Singular	Plural
mammoplasty	mammoplasties
artery	arteries
ovary	ovaries
therapy	therapies

☑ **DO** form the plural of a noun that ends in *o* preceded by a consonant by adding *es* to the singular.

Singular	Plural
veto	vetoes
potato	potatoes
tomato	tomatoes
zero	zeroes

NOTE: *In regard to this rule, many words are pluralized by simply adding an s to the singular.*

albino	albinos
ego	egos
placebo	placebos
embryo	embryos

EXCEPTIONS

comedo	comedones
lentigo	lentigines
ambo	ambones

☑ **DO** form the plural of most nouns that end in *f* or *fe* by changing the *f* or *fe* to *ves*.

Singular	Plural
scarf	scarves
life	lives
calf	calves
knife	knives

☑ **DO** form the plural of a noun that ends in *y* preceded by a vowel by adding *s* to the singular word.

Singular	Plural
attorney	attorneys
boy	boys
gurney	gurneys
ray	rays

NOTE: *There are only a few of these nouns.*

31–6 EPONYMS

See 31–18, Possessive Nouns, and Chapter 14, Eponyms.

31–7 EXCEPTIONS: IRREGULAR PLURAL ENDINGS

The following are irregular plural forms in addition to those found in some of the lists following general rules:

Singular	Plural
arteritis	arteritides
arthritis	arthritides
calix	calices
calyx	calyces
caput	capita
comedo	comedones
cornu	cornua
epididymis	epididymides
epiglottis	epiglottides
femur	femora
index	indexes
index	indices *(numeric expressions)*
iris	irides
os	ora *(mouths)*
os	ossa *(bones)*
pancreas	pancreata
paries	parietes
plexus	plexuses
pons	pontes
pus	pura
syllabus	syllabuses *or* syllabi
vas	vasa

31–8 FRENCH ENDINGS

✔ **DO** generally form the plural of words that end in *eau* and *eu* by adding an *x*.

Singular	Plural
milieu	milieux
rouleau	rouleaux
bandeau	bandeaux
beau	beaux
faux pas	faux pas *(no change)*

EXCEPTIONS

chapeau	chapeaus
chateau	chateaus
adieu	adieus
tableau	tableaus

Unusual French plural formations *(both words made plural)*

fait accompli	faits accomplis
chargé d'affairs	chargés d'affaires
nouveau riche	nouveaux riches

31–9 GENUS

 DO use the plural form of the organism when stating several organisms of the same type. Genus names are not changed. Only names for the individual organisms are pluralized. If there is no plural form, add plural nouns such as *organisms* or *members* to indicate plural usage.

Singular	Plural
streptococcus	streptococci
gonococcus	gonococci
salmonella	salmonellas
pneumococcus	pneumococci
members of the genus Pseudomonas	
Trichomonas organisms	

31–10 GREEK ENDINGS

 DO form the plural of words that end in *on* by dropping the *on* and adding an *a*.

Singular	Plural
criterion	criteria
enteron	entera
zygion	zygia

31–11 GREEK AND LATIN ENDINGS

 DO form the plural of words that end in *itis* by dropping the *s* and adding *des*.

Singular	Plural
arthritis	arthritides
meningitis	meningitides

 DO form the plural of words that end in *is* by changing *is* to *es*.

Singular	Plural
metastasis	metastases
diagnosis	diagnoses

31–12 ITALIAN ENDINGS

 DO form the plural of words that end in *o* by changing the *o* to an *i*.

Singular	Plural
virtuoso	virtuosi
graffito	graffiti

31–13 LATIN ENDINGS

 DO form the plural of words that end in *um* by changing the *um* to *a* (*pronounced* ah).

Singular	Plural
labium	labia
datum	data
medium	media
diverticulum	diverticula

NOTE: The word *diverticula* is often incorrectly dictated to sound like *diverticuli*.

 DO add an *e* to words that end in *a* (*variably pronounced* i, e, *or* a—*dictionaries do not agree on pronunciation*) to form the plural.

Singular	Plural
bursa	bursae
vertebra	vertebrae

 DO form the plural of words that end in *us* by changing the *us* to *i* (*pronounced* eye).

Singular	Plural
alveolus	alveoli
meniscus	menisci
coccus	cocci

 DO form the plural of additional words that end in *us* by dropping the *us* and adding *era* or *ora*.

Singular	Plural
corpus	corpora
genus	genera
glomus	glomera
latus	latera
tempus	tempora
ulcus	ulcera

Singular	Plural
viscus	viscera
vulnus	vulnera

EXCEPTIONS

plexus	plexuses
abortus	abortus
meatus	meatus
genius	geniuses

 DO   form the plural of words that end in *is* by changing the *is* to *es* (*pronounced* ez *or* es).

Singular	Plural
anastomosis	anastomoses
urinalysis	urinalyses

 DO   use an English plural if it has become an accepted form.

Singular	Plural
appendix	appendixes
enema	enemas
equilibrium	equilibriums
femur	femurs
formula	formulas
forum	forums
hernia	hernias
myoma	myomas
syllabus	syllabuses

 DON'T   use Latin plurals if the English equivalent has become an accepted form. Thus, *formulas* is preferred over *formulae*.

 DO   form the plural of words that end in *ax* or *ix* by changing the *x* to *c* and adding *es*.

Singular	Plural
thorax	thoraces
calyx *or* calix	calyces *or* calices

 DO   form the plural of words that end in *ex* or *ix* by changing the *ex* or *ix* to *ices*.

Singular	Plural
appendix	appendices
apex	apices

✅ **DO**   change words that end in *en* by changing the *en* to *ina.*

Singular	Plural
foramen	foramina
lumen	lumina

✅ **DO**   form the plural of words that end in *ma* by changing the *ma* to *mata.* With this ending, it is also permissible to add an *s* to the singular.

Singular	Plural
carcinoma	carcinomata
	carcinomas
leiomyoma	leiomyomata
	leiomyomas

✅ **DO**   form the plural of words that end in *nx* by changing the *x* to *g* and adding *es.*

Singular	Plural
phalanx	phalanges
larynx	larynges

✅ **DO**   change words that end in *on* by changing the *on* to *a.*

Singular	Plural
spermatozoon	spermatozoa

31–14   LETTERS AND ABBREVIATIONS

✅ **DO**   use an apostrophe to form the plural of the capital letters *A, I, O, M, U* and all lowercase single letters. *(See 3–1, Abbreviations and Plural Forms of Numbers and Letters.)*

> When you make an entry in the chart, be careful that your 2s don't look like z's.
> Spell that with three r's.
> You used four I's in the first paragraph.

✅ **DO**   use an apostrophe to form the plural of lowercase abbreviations.

> There were elevated wbc's.

🚫 **DON'T**   use the apostrophe to form the plural of numbers or capital letter abbreviations.

> The TMs were intact.
> There were no 4 × 4s left in the box.

DO   use an apostrophe to form the plural of symbols.

+'s   −'s

31–15 NAMES

DON'T   assume that family names can be made plural by simply adding *s*. If a proper noun, including family names, ends in *s*, *sh*, *ch*, *x*, or *z*, the plural is formed by adding *es*.

Singular	**Plural**
Jones	the Joneses
Bush	the Bushes
Rodriguez	the Rodriguezes
Rex	the Rexes
Wood	the Woods
Woods	the Woodses

See also 3–8, Plural Possessive Nouns, in Chapter 3.

31–16 NUMBERS

 DO   form the plural of figures by adding *s*, but don't use an apostrophe.

1990s
Be sure that your 2s don't look like z's.

 DO   form the plural of written-out numbers just as you form the plural of other words. *(See Chapter 27, Numbers.)*

She moved here sometime in the forties.
See also 3–8, Plural Possessive Nouns, in Chapter 3.

31–17 PARENTHETICAL EXPRESSIONS

 DO   use a singular verb when a singular noun is accompanied parenthetically by its plural form or plural ending.

Incorrect:
Foreign body(s) are not definitely excluded.
Correct:
Foreign body (bodies) is not definitely excluded.
Correct:
Foreign object(s) is not definitely excluded.

31–18 POSSESSIVE NOUNS

✓ DO   add an apostrophe plus *s* to plural forms of nouns to show possession. *(See 3–8, Plural Possessive Nouns, and 32–5, Plural Possessive Nouns.)*

women's studies
children's ward
mice's tracks

✓ DO   use an apostrophe after the *s* in plural nouns that end in *s*.

the typists' responsibility *(more than one typist)*
the Joneses' medical records *(more than one Jones)*
the heroes' methods
the berries' ripeness
the employees' records

31–19 POSSESSIVE PRONOUNS

See 3–9, Pronouns; 3–10, Singular Possessive Nouns; and 32–6, Pronouns.

31–20 SINGULAR OR PLURAL WORDS
Medical Words Commonly Used in the Plural

Some medical terms are commonly used in the plural in all dictation. Because we have two eyes and two ears, physicians commonly dictate the following:

Conjunctivae are clear.
Tympanic membranes are intact.

Because heart sounds are multiple, doctors commonly dictate the word *bruits,* which is the plural form of *bruit.*

The use of the word determines whether it is singular or plural.

There is no bruit heard.
There are no bruits heard.

Some words referring to subjective symptoms are treated as plural.

bends	chills	cramps	hiccups

Singular or Plural Words

Some words can be singular or plural in use.

biceps	triceps	data	facies	caries
series	none (*means* not one *or* not any)			

Words Always Plural

Some words are always plural in use.

adnexa	clothes	confetti	feces	forceps
fauces	genitalia	menses	pubes	scabies
scissors	tongs	tweezers	zucchini	

Words Always Singular

Some words are always singular in use.

ascites	herpes	lues	news	facies
mumps	measles			

Special Plural Forms

 DO consult reference books for those words that change form in the plural.

Singular	Plural
child	children
woman	women
mouse	mice
goose	geese
foot	feet
tooth	teeth

 DON'T assume that a noun ending in *ics* is plural. Many such nouns take singular or plural verbs.

ethics   mathematics   physics   politics

Medical ethics governs the behavior of all employees who work in health care.

Economics *(a course of study)* is a degree requirement for all business majors.

The economics *(economic aspects)* of the free trade zone are very appealing to many organizations.

31–21 UNITS OF MEASUREMENT

 DO use the singular when typing abbreviated units of measurement *(feet, grams, inches, milligrams, pounds, and so forth.)*

7 ft	3 mg	10 g
5 in.	0.3 in.	11 lb

NOTE: *If you interposed of an between 0.3 and inch, you would not say 0.3 of an inches. This "test" works with any measurement and any decimal part thereof. If the number is one plus a fraction, the sentence should read, "One and one-half inches is the length of the little finger." Note that the verb must be singular.*

DO add an *s* to units of measure that are spelled out.

ten centimeters   five milligrams

32

Possessives

32–1   COMPOUND NOUNS

A compound noun consists of two or more distinct words that may be written as one word with a hyphen or hyphens.

 DO   add an apostrophe plus *s* *('s)* to the last element of the possessive compound.

> my brother-in-law's surgery
> my sisters-in-law's book *(two sisters, one book)*
> my sisters-in-law's books *(two sisters, more than one book)*

32–2   EPONYMS

Many eponyms *(adjectives derived from proper nouns)* are used in medical writing. Most of these are not written as possessives. However, some authors prefer the possessive style and wish to have it expressed. You will often find both styles in reference books. When used to describe parts of the anatomy, diseases, signs, or syndromes, eponyms *may* show possession. Follow the guidelines and consult your reference books. If you hear the possessive dictated, use it *(and use it correctly)*. If it is not dictated, do not use it

 DO   use an apostrophe when the possessive is dictated in the following

> **Signs and tests:**
> Bell's phenomenon *or* Bell phenomenon

Hoffmann's reflex *or* Hoffmann reflex
Babinski's phenomenon *or* Babinski phenomenon
Ayer's test *or* Ayer test
Anatomy:
Bartholin's glands *or* Bartholin glands
Beale's ganglion *or* Beale ganglion
Mauthner's membrane *or* Mauthner membrane

EXCEPTIONS *(always use possessive):*

Ringer's lactate
Taber's Cyclopedic Medical Dictionary

Diseases and syndromes:
Fallot's tetralogy *or* Fallot tetralogy
Tietze's syndrome *or* Tietze syndrome
Hirschsprung's disease *or* Hirschsprung disease

 DO use the possessive when the eponym closes the sentence.

The infant shows early signs of Reye's. *(syndrome is understood)*

 DON'T use the apostrophe if the word following begins with the sound of *s*, *z*, or *c*.

Hicks sign   Golgi zones   Langerhans cells

 DON'T show possession for eponyms that describe surgical instruments, are compounds, or represent the names of places or patients.

Surgical instruments:
Mayo scissors
Richard retractors
Foley catheter
Liston-Stille forceps
Names of places or patients:
Christmas factor
Lyme disease
Chicago disease
Compounds:
Stein-Leventhal syndrome
Adams-Stokes disease
Leser-Trélat sign
Bass-Watkins test
Gruber-Widal reaction

EXCEPTION: *The following is not a compound.*

Blackberg and Wanger's test *or* Blackberg and Wanger test

NOTE: *Be careful to check the correct spelling of the name. Is it* Water's view *or* Waters' view? (The second choice is correct.)

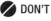 **DON'T**   use the apostrophe with an eponym if it is preceded by an article.

a Pfannenstiel incision
the Babinski sign
the Horner syndrome

 DO   *when writing for publication,* substitute the specific descriptive term for a disease for the equivalent eponymic term. Further, if the author prefers the eponym, *avoid* using the possessive form. Different rules apply when writing for publication.

Preferred:
alopecia parvimaculata syndrome
Second choice:
Dreuw syndrome
Avoid:
Dreuw's syndrome
Preferred:
pancreatic exocrine insufficiency syndrome
Second choice:
Clarke-Hadfield syndrome

32–3   GERUND USE

 DO   show possession when a noun modifies a gerund *(a verb form ending in* ing *used as a noun).*

Dr. Verbaron did not approve the tape's leaving his office.

The safety committee members realized the meeting's being delayed was unavoidable.

 DO   use a possessive pronoun with a gerund.

Correct:
Dr. Wong appreciated your admitting the patient after hours.
Incorrect:
Dr. Wong appreciated you admitting the patient after hours.

32–4   JOINT POSSESSION

 DO   show possession with the last noun when two or more nouns share possession.

Clark and Clark's new reference book is in.
My sisters-in-law's cruise was a success.
Dr. Franklin and Dr. Meadow's patient was just admitted.
Dr. Pate and Dr. Frank's office *(one office)*
Dr. Thomas's associate's diagnosis

 DON'T   use this rule when possession is not shared.

Dr. Franklin's and Dr. Meadow's patients were just admitted.

Dr. Pate's and Dr. Frank's offices *(two offices)*

32–5   PLURAL POSSESSIVE NOUNS

 DO   add an apostrophe plus *s ('s)* to the plural forms of nouns to show possession.

Singular	**Plural**
woman's watch	women's watches
child's toy	children's toys
man's shoe	men's shoes

 DO   use an apostrophe after the *s* in plural nouns that end in *s* to show possession.

the typists' responsibility *(more than one typist)*
the Joneses' medical records *(more than one Jones)*
the heroes' methods
the berries' ripeness
the employees' records

 DON'T   use an apostrophe to show possession of institutions or organizations unless they elect to do so.

Veterans Administration Hospital *(and certainly* not *Veteran's Hospital!)*
Childrens Hospital
St. Josephs Infirmary
Boys Club

✓ **DO**   follow the same rules for forming the possessive of plural abbreviations as for words

It was all the MDs' decision.

🚫 **DON'T**   use an apostrophe with plural nouns that are more descriptive than possessive.

awards banquet
tumor boards conference

32–6 PRONOUNS

✓ **DO**   form the possessive of indefinite pronouns such as *everyone, nobody, someone, anyone,* and *anybody* just as you would with possessive nouns.

It is nobody's fault.
That is anyone's guess.
It is somebody else's responsibility.

🚫 **DON'T**   use an apostrophe with personal pronouns such as *its, hers, yours, his, theirs, ours, whose,* and *yours.*

Incorrect:
The next appointment is her's.
Incorrect:
The dog injured it's foot.
Correct:
The dog injured its foot.
Incorrect:
You're lab coat is soiled.
Correct:
Your lab coat is soiled.

NOTE: *Notice the following contractions, however.*

It's time for your next appointment.
Who's going to clean the operatory?

COMMENT: *One of the most common usage errors concerns the confusion between* its *and* it's. *Both forms are correct when used in the proper context, but writers often make an improper choice. This error is easy to avoid. If you have ever made this error, take the following precaution: Whenever using the word* it's, *always translate it immediately to* it is *and see if it fits. If it does not, remove the apostrophe. When you use the word* its, *do not try to translate it into anything; it is not a contraction.*

Have you ever made an error in it's use? *(What's wrong
here? Read the preceding paragraph again; remove the
apostrophe.)*

32–7 SINGULAR POSSESSIVE NOUNS

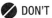 DO   use an apostrophe plus *s (*'s*)* with a singular noun not ending
in *s* to show possession

the typist's responsibility *(one typist)*
Bob's doctor
Dr. Mitch's office

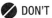 DO   add an apostrophe plus *s (*'s*)* to singular nouns ending in *s* or
an *s* sound when these words have a single syllable.

Mr. Jones's medical record
James Rose's appointment

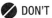 DO   use an apostrophe only (no s) to show possession of singular
nouns that end in *s* or in a strong *s* sound and are more than
one syllable.

the waitress' table
for appearance' sake
Mr. Gomez' surgery

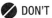 DO   use an apostrophe only after the *s* in two-syllable singular
proper nouns ending in *s*.

Frances' report
Mr. Walters' point of view
Dr. Harris' office

 DON'T   break up a proper noun that ends in an *s* by placing the
apostrophe in front of the *s*.

Concerning Mr. Walters
Incorrect:
Mr. Walter's point of view
Correct:
Mr. Walters' point of view

32–8 TIME, DISTANCE, VALUE, AND SOURCE

 DO   use an apostrophe to show possession of time, distance,
value, and source.

return in a month's time

at 10 weeks' gestation
get your money's worth
too much exposure to the sun's rays
two days' convalescence

🚫 **DON'T** show possession of inanimate things.

the roof of the car *rather than* the car's roof
the color of the bruise *rather than* the bruise's color
the cover of the book *rather than* the book's cover

32–9 UNDERSTOOD NOUNS

✓ **DO** follow the same rules for showing possession when the noun is understood.

That stethoscope is Dr. Green's. *(stethoscope)*
He bought that at William's. *(store)*
I consulted Dorland's. *(dictionary)*
That is where he earned his master's. *(degree)*
I believe this copy is yours. *(your copy)*

33

Progress Notes or Chart Notes

INTRODUCTION

Chart notes *(also called progress notes)* are the formal or informal notes taken by the physician when he or she meets with or examines a patient in the office, hospital, clinic, acute care center, or emergency department. These notes are a part of the patient's permanent medical record and are a vital key to patients' care. Although medical records are used mainly to assist the physician with care of the patient, they can be reviewed by attorneys, other physicians, insurance companies, or the court. It is essential that they be neat, accurate, and complete.

Accurate means that they are transcribed as dictated, and *complete* requires that they be dated and signed or initialed by the author.

For a chart to be admissible as evidence in court, the party dictating or writing entries should be able to attest that the entries were true and correct at the time they were written. The best indication of that is the physician's signature or initials at the end of each typed note. The hospital will insist that the physician sign all dictated material and all entries he or she makes on the patient's record; failure to do so could result in a loss of hospital staff privileges.

✓	DO	transcribe chart notes as dictated. They must be dated and signed or initialed by the author and end with your initials.

33–1   ABBREVIATIONS

See Chapter 1, Abbreviations and Symbols.

✓	DO	type standard abbreviations and symbols freely into office chart notes. Hospital chart notes should reflect only those abbreviations approved by the facility.
⊘	DON'T	use an abbreviation if there is a chance of misinterpretation.
✓	DO	type contractions when dictated if the employer approves. Some physicians prefer that contractions be spelled out.
⊘	DON'T	abbreviate drug names.
⊘	DON'T	abbreviate a diagnosis.

33–2   ABSTRACTING FROM CHART NOTES

✓	DO	abstract information carefully and be extremely accurate when obtaining information from a patient's medical record to complete an insurance claim, letter, or report. Do *not* guess at abbreviations on the chart. Be sure you have a release of medical information form signed by the patient, and give only the information requested (see Chapter 18, HIPAA Guidelines).

33–3   ALLERGIES

 DO key the name of a drug in all capital letters, bold print, or underlined when reporting drug allergies in a *chart note* or in a patient's *history.*

Allergies: Patient is allergic to PHENOBARBITAL and CODEINE.
Allergies: The patient reports a sensitivity to **SULFA**.

33–4   CONTINUATION PAGES

✓ DO type the patient's name on the top of page 2 and on every subsequent page of chart notes.

NOTE: *There is no reason why you cannot continue the notes to the back of the chart paper, and some offices do this to prevent the medical record from becoming bulky. Other physicians prefer to use one side of the chart paper only. The second and all subsequent pages of the progress notes are headed up with the patient's name.*

 DO type the word *continued* at the bottom of the beginning page and head up the following page with the date of the chart entry and the word *continued* as well as the patient's name.

33–5   CONTRACTIONS

✓ DO type contractions when dictated if the employer approves. Some authors prefer that contractions be spelled out.

33–6   CORRECTIONS

Errors that are made while the entry is being keyed are corrected just as you would correct any other material. Errors found subsequently, after the dictation has been signed or entered into the record, are corrected in longhand by following proper procedures.

✓ DO draw a line through the error, being careful not to obliterate the error; make the correct notation either above or below the error, wherever there is room; and date and initial the entry.

 DON'T write over the error, do not erase the error, do not try to "fix" the error, and do not attempt to blot it out with heavy applications of ink or self-adhesive typing strips. *(See Figure 33–1 at the end of the chapter for an example of a chart note that has an entry corrected.)*

33–7 DATES

✓ DO   spell out, abbreviate, or type dates in figures. A date stamp may also be used.

2-4-XX
02/04/XX
Feb. 4, 20XX
February 4, 20XX

33–8 DIAGNOSIS (DX) OR IMPRESSION (IMP)

🚫 DON'T   type an abbreviated diagnosis when dictated, as it is preferred that diagnoses be spelled out in full. Some employers allow diagnoses to be abbreviated when dictated, but an abbreviation can be misinterpreted.

33–9 EMERGENCY DEPARTMENT NOTES

When patients are initially seen in the emergency department, the triage nurse determines the sequence in which patients will see a physician. Laboratory, x-rays, and simple tests may be ordered at this time by the triage nurse. At this point, the level of care is determined.

A nurse or technician initially assesses the patient and handwrites notes or inputs data via computer. When the physician sees the patient, he or she will usually handwrite a brief initial impression and orders to be carried out *(i.e., medications, laboratory tests, x-rays, and treatment)*. At this point, dictation may begin. The author will indicate whether the dictation is STAT *(to be transcribed immediately)*. This dictation may be done with a handheld recorder and the completed tape placed directly on the chart. Dictation for patients requiring admission or transfer is delivered directly to the transcriptionist.

After the release of the patient, the physician will write *(or dictate)* a formal diagnosis and update, append, or complete the dictation. These notes are generally brief, and format may vary with the author. Some authors ask for bold headings for each section, whereas others may prefer the condensed story format. Some emergency departments or urgent care centers place the transcribing station within the facility or in a nearby area so the author can have immediate access to the chart note. If the patient is admitted to the hospital for treatment or observation, this initial note or dictation will accompany the patient. *(See Figure 33–2 at the end of the chapter for an example of a SOAP format in an emergency department record.)*

33–10 FLAGGING QUERIES

See discussion in Chapter 11, Editing.

33–11 FORMAT HEADINGS

☑ DO   verify that all headings include the proper date and the patient's complete name. Usually a brief description for the reason for the physician's contact with the patient immediately follows. This part is the *chief complaint* or *subjective* part of the record.

☑ DO   make headings easy to read and specific so data can be located immediately.

☑ DO   insert outline headings for all but very brief entries.

☑ DO   key outline headings in all capital letters.

☑ DO   use bold with subtopics found *within* text when necessary to help them stand out.

⊘ DON'T   overuse double spacing, all capital letters, and underlining.

☑ DO   select a style that has a purpose: new topic, an alert, emphasis, outline, need for white space.

NOTE: *Format headings can be as varied as the authors of the records in private offices. Hospitals and clinics usually have an established format and a macro into which the data is easily inserted. The headings commonly used are as follows:*

SOAP Format

S **(Subjective):** The information in this section represents the patient's point of view and explains why the patient is seeking care. The main problem requiring care is also referred to as the *chief complaint.* This section relates what the patient tells the physician about the problem.

O **(Objective):** The information in this section describes what the physician finds on examination, x-ray film, or laboratory work: the clinical evidence.

A **(Assessment):** This part covers the examiner's evaluation of what may be wrong on the basis of the subjective and objective information. The assessment is also called the *diagnosis* or *interpretation.*

P **(Plan):** This section outlines the physician's recommendations for further evaluation and treatment: laboratory tests, surgery, medications, referral to another practitioner, other treatment procedures, management, and so forth.

DO   write out the outline or abbreviate it.

Subjective: Epigastric pain. Improved with diet. Plan
               previously described.
Objective: Abdomen: Benign.
Assessment: Epigastric discomfort improved; obesity.
Plan: Cont 1200 ADA diet RTC 3 m for F/U or
               sooner p.r.n.

NOTE: *Abbreviated format uses less space and is easily understood.*

S: Epigastric pain. Improved with diet. Plan
      previously described.
O: Abdomen: Benign.
A: Epigastric discomfort improved; obesity.
P: Cont 1200 ADA diet RTC 3 m for F/U or sooner
      p.r.n.
*(See Figure 33–3 at the end of the chapter for an example of a
chart note done in the SOAP format.)*

HX, PX, DX, RX Method

HX: Epigastric pain. Improved with diet. Plan
       previously described.
PX: Abdomen: Benign.
DX: Epigastric discomfort improved; obesity.
RX: Cont 1200 ADA diet RTC 3 m for F/U or sooner
       p.r.n.
*(See Figure 33–4 at the end of the chapter for an example of
the HX, PX, DX, RX method of charting.)*

Single Paragraph, No Outline Format

Pt complains of epigastric pain. Improved with diet. Plan
previously described. The abdomen is benign. Her
epigastric discomfort improved.
Diagnosis: Obesity.
Pt is to cont 1200 ADA diet RTC 3 m for F/U or sooner
p.r.n.

POMR (Problem-Oriented Medical Record) Format

The problem-oriented format is a problem list with corresponding
numbered progress notes, including the following:

- *Data base: The chief complaint, the history of this
  complaint, a review of the body systems, physical
  examination, and laboratory work.*
- *Problem list: A numbered list of every problem that the
  patient has that requires further investigation.*
- *Treatment plan: Numbered list to correspond with each
  item on the problem list.*

- Notes: Numbered progress notes to correspond with each
  item on the problem list.

Additional headings that may be used include the following:

- PH (past history) or PMH (past medical history)
- Hx (history) or HPI (history of present illness)
- CC (chief complaints, signs, or symptoms)
- DRUGS
- ALLERGIES (allergies to drugs and foods should be in
  all capital letters and underlined)
- PX or PE (physical examination)
- VS (vital signs—blood pressure, pulse, respirations,
  temperature)
- HEENT
- LAB, X-RAYS, ECG
- CHEST
- IMP or DX (impression or diagnosis)
- PLAN, RX, or TX (treatment, advice, recommendation)

33–12 FORMAT STYLES

✓ **DO**   use abbreviations and symbols freely, as dictated, but be sure
that the abbreviations are standard. *(Remember that the
records could be viewed by persons outside the office or
hospital.)* Abbreviations save space, and notes should be as
concise as possible.

✓ **DO**   be sure the patient's complete name is entered and spelling
is verified.

✓ **DO**   date every entry with the month, day, and year. These may be
spelled out, abbreviated, or made with a date stamp.

✓ **DO**   single-space and keep the margins narrow *(not less than ½
inch, however).* Double-space between topics or major
headings.

✓ **DO**   condense the note to conserve space. Use phrases rather
than complete sentences and use abbreviations. These
changes do not constitute an alteration of the dictation.

Dictated

Today's date is November 11, 200X, and this is a chart
note on Nancy Marques, a 32-year-old female who came
in today in followup to an upper respiratory tract
infection either viral or secondary to mycoplasma. She is
much better except that she has had a chronic cough now
for about ten days. The ears, nose, and throat are normal,
and the sinus is nontender. The lymph nodes are normal
and the lungs are clear. The diagnosis is postviral cough.

I have given her a prescription for Hycodan five to ten milliliters for up to ten days and then observation. If the cough is still present in two weeks, I will consider steroid trial.

Transcribed:

Nancy Marques

Age: 32

November 11, 200X

HPI: F/Up URI either viral or secondary to mycoplasma. She is much better except for chronic cough × 10 days.

PX: ENT: Normal. Sinus: Nontender. Lymph nodes: Normal. Lungs: Clear.

DX: Postviral cough.

RX: Hycodan 5-10 mL for 10 days and then observation. If cough present in 2 weeks, I will consider steroid trial. _____

Mary Laudenslayer, MD/ntw

✓ DO insert indentations to make topics stand out. Type the main topics in all capital letters. Use bold type when it is helpful or requested by the author.

✓ DO underline and type drug allergies in all capital letters or use bold.

✓ DO initial the entry just as you initial any other document that you type or transcribe. Initials may be placed at the left margin or following the author's name or initials.

✓ DO type a signature line or leave sufficient space for the author's signature or initials.

See Figure 33–3 at the end of the chapter for an example of a chart note illustrating the SOAP format.

See Figure 33–4 at the end of the chapter for an example showing the HX, PX, DX, RX method of charting.

Figure 33–5 at the end of the chapter shows a chart note in the typical mixed format of handwritten and typed entries. Figure 33–6 at the end of the chapter shows a chart note with preprinted illustrations.

33–13 HANDWRITTEN ENTRIES

✓ DO abstract accurately. Any entry that is questionable as to its interpretation should be verified by the physician. Some examples of misinterpretations follow:

NBM can mean *no bowel movement* or *normal bowel movement*, depending on the dictation site.
U (units) can be mistaken for a *zero (0)*. For example, 6 U of insulin can be mistaken for 60 units of insulin.
Units should always be written out in chart notes.
OD can mean *right eye* or medication to be taken *once daily*. The abbreviation *q.d. (once a day)* has been misinterpreted as *q.i.d. (4 times daily)*.
C, MS, and *CF* have more than 10 possible meanings each.

✓ **DO**   verify with the physician any abbreviated drug names. Here are just a few of the many examples of misinterpretations.

CPZ *(Compazine* or *chlorpromazine)*
PBZ *(phenylbutazone, pyribenzamine,* or *phenoxylbenzamine)*
HCT250 *(hydrocortisone)* may be misinterpreted as HCTZ50 *(hydrochlorothiazide).*

33–14   HISTORY AND PHYSICAL

See also Chapter 19, History and Physical Format. Some chart notes can be a formal history and physical, a report to an attorney, a workers' compensation insurance company document, or a consultation report to a referring physician.

✓ **DO**   place an entry in the medical record if the physician dictates a document rather than a formal chart note.

2-7-9X See note to Dr. Normington./mlo *(Generally a note of this brevity is handwritten.)*
(also correct)

Feb. 7, 199x See note to Dr. Normington mlo

33–15   INFORMATION OR DATA SHEET

✓ **DO**   transfer all the appropriate patient information to the initial page of the medical record.

33–16   INSURANCE DOCUMENTATION

✓ **DO**   be aware of the general principles for the complete documentation of medical records to ensure that these notes are written or transcribed into the record, documenting services for which the provider of care expects to be paid.

The following is a general outline of the principles through which payments are made. It is important to observe that these components are documented and to alert your employer when they are not mentioned. To provide documentation of services rendered, you must know what billing codes are used by the facility for the service documented. The nature and amount of physician work and documentation vary by the type of service performed, the place of the service, and the status of the patient (*e.g., new or established*). These general principles are applicable to all types of medical and surgical services in all settings. The billing and diagnostic codes reported on the health insurance claim forms should be supported by the documentation in the record.

1. Each patient encounter should include the following documentation:
   - *date;*
   - *reason for the encounter;*
   - *history, physical examination, prior diagnostic test results;*
   - *diagnosis (assessment, impression);*
   - *plan for care; and*
   - *name of the observer.*
2. Rationale for ordering diagnostic or other services documented or inferred.
3. Health risk factors identified.
4. Progress, response to treatment, changes in treatment, and revision of diagnosis.

33–17 MEDICATION

✓ DO   underline and use bold or all capital letters for drug and food allergies. *(See Fig. 33–5, at the end of the chapter, December 18 entry.)*

✓ DO   spell out all drug names.

✓ DO   make entries for refill prescriptions given via telephone.

33–18 NUMBERS
See Chapter 27, Numbers.

33–19 OFFICE NOTES, ESTABLISHED PATIENT
Although the office notes for patients' initial visits can be lengthy, subsequent or followup notes may be as brief as one line, but the notes will vary according to the patient's complaint and type of visit to the office.

✓ **DO**   check daily about any previous day's house calls, emergency calls, and hospital discharges and admissions so that entries are made.

✓ **DO**   log in instructions to the patient, prescription refills, or telephone calls for advice.

✓ **DO**   make an entry showing another document has been prepared if the author prefers not to make a formal chart entry. *(You may have transcribed this document.)* This entry is inserted where the normal chart entry would have been placed.

> 4-20-XX Please see consultation report to Dr. Normington. brd

33–20   OFFICE NOTES, NEW PATIENT, INITIAL CONTACT

The records of office visits by new patients vary just as physicians and their medical specialties vary. There is no best method.

✓ **DO**   set up the record by following a consistent format.

✓ **DO**   be sure that records are neat, accurate, complete, and timely *(made as soon as possible after the patient is seen)*.

✓ **DO**   follow the guidelines for insurance reimbursement if it is your responsibility to make sure that these components are included. *(See 33–16, Insurance Documentation.)*

✓ **DO**   make an entry showing another document has been prepared if the author prefers not to make a formal chart entry. *(You may have transcribed this document.)* This entry is inserted where the normal chart entry would have been placed.

> 4-20-XX Please see history and physical. brd

33–21   PHYSICAL EXAMINATION (PX OR PE)

See Chapter 19, History and Physical Format, 19–4 for headings.

33–22   POSTOPERATIVE NOTES

Postoperative progress notes not only furnish basic information on the procedure and the patient's immediate condition but also give the next caregivers in line help so they can provide the best possible care and avoid any contingencies or problems.

✓ **DO**   include the following in postoperative notes:

> Name of surgeon and assistant.
> Procedure performed.

Findings.

Postoperative diagnosis.

Blood loss, if any.

Specimen removed, if any.

33–23   PRESSURE-SENSITIVE PAPER

Several companies manufacture pressure-sensitive paper for transcribing medical notes. This paper comes in a variety of forms, including a continuous sheet of paper folded or on a roll. It is placed behind the pin-feed printer where the regular paper is placed or is fed into the laser printer when needed. One simply keys the patient's name, date, and dictation, leaving a space at the end for the author's signature or initials. Each note is typed without removal of paper from the medical record. Then, when the transcript is printed, the entire sheet is cut off and given to the author for signature. The use of this method makes it easier for the physician as well, because individual charts do not have to be opened and signed. This method of transcribing notes is particularly helpful when dictation is sent out of the office and the medical records do not accompany it. After approval, the notes are cut apart with a paper cutter or scissors or separated at the perforations. The backing is peeled off each one, and the note is then placed on the next blank space of the progress sheet so as not to obliterate the information previously entered. *(Figures 33–7 and 33–8 at the end of the chapter illustrate the use of this type of paper.)*

33–24   SIGNATURE LINE

✓ DO   type a signature line or leave adequate space for the author's signature or initials.

33–25   TELEPHONE

✓ DO   make entries in regard to telephone advice.

✓ DO   make entries for prescription refills via telephone.

JUL 2 6 200X   The patient is a white male, age 4, who came in to see me today with a history of yellow discharge in the right ear a fever and a sore throat of two days duration. His oral temperature was 100°. The pharynx was infected, the tonsils inflamed, and there was crusted purulent material seen in the right ear canal. The tympanic membrane was normal.

DIAGNOSIS: Tonsillitis and otitis externa.

Medication: Erythrocin, 400 mg, q4H.

lr   Michael R. Stearn, MD

JUL 2 7 200X   After 24 h of therapy, the pt was afebrile and comfortable. Temperature is 996°. The throat is slightly infected. Secretions in the ear canal were dry and both TMs normal.

lr   Michael R. Stearn, MD

AUG 2 200X   Follow-up exam showed him to be completely asymptomatic and free of unusual physical findings. The drug was stopped at this time.

lr   Michael R. Stearn, MD

OCT 1 9 200X   Stepped on a piece of glass. Cleansed wound. Mother said Norman had tetanus booster just six weeks ago in Boyd Hosp. ER after a dog bite. Pt not to return unless problem develops.

jt   Michael R. Stearn, MD

OCT 3 0 200X   Pt caught right index finger in car door 2 days ago; finger became inflamed, red, swollen yesterday. Today there is seropurulent discharge present; no lymphangitis visible. Distal phalanx is involved.

Advice: Hot compress to right hand t.i.d. To return in 24 hours if no change.

DIAGNOSIS: Cellulitis, right index finger, distal phalanx.

lr   Michael R. Stearn, MD

Figure 33–1   Example of a properly corrected chart note. Note the August 2 entry. (Reprinted with permission from Diehl, Marcy O., *Medical Transcription: Techniques and Procedures*, 5th ed. Philadelphia, Saunders, 2002.)

			EMERGENCY DEPARTMENT RECORD	**CHART REQUEST**				

LOCATION	DATE	TIME REGISTERED	TRIAGE TIME	OUTPT.	INPT.	NAME
202	10-08-0X	2:45 ☐ AM ☒ PM	☐ AM ☐ PM	☐	☐	REILLY, RANDA O

ARRIVED	☐ WALKED	☐ WC	☐ AMB	☐ PARA AMB	☐ OTHER
ACCOMPANIED BY	☐ ALONE	☐ SPOUSE	☐ PARENT	☐ FRIEND	☐ RELATIVE

PATIENT'S ADDRESS	MED. REC. NO.	BIRTHDATE
3228 East Main, Century City, XX 12345		11-10-XX

HOME TELEPHONE	WORK TELEPHONE	PRIMARY CARE CLINIC	PERSONAL PHYSICIAN
(800) 654-9863	( )		John Lambert, MD

AGE	SEX	TEMP.	B.P.	PULSE	RESP.	WEIGHT (Peds)	CHIEF COMPLAINT
25	F	98.7	120.70				Head pain, post fall

ALLERGIES	MEDICATIONS
	none

S: This 25 YO pt presents with a HX of falling from a horse into a heavy wooden fence, breaking the fence. Pt complains primarily of head pain, neck pain, right knee pain and some mild coccyx pain. There was a brief loss of consciousness observed by her brother and regaining of consciousness with repetitive questioning. Thereafter she again lost consciousness for a short period of time. Pt has been slow to answer questions and has been noted to have repetitive questions since the accident.

O: Pt in no acute distress. Appears to be stable with C-collar and rigid back board. HEENT: Minimal tears in the occipital area. Pupils: Equal and reactive. EOMs: Full. EARS: TMs without blood. NECK: C-collar in place, with a tenderness over the mid C-spine bony area without obvious swelling or deformity. (C-collar left in place) CHEST: Nontender to compression. Equal breath sounds. CVA: Regular rhythm. ABDOMEN: Soft. Nontender extremities. NM: Moves all fours well. There is mild tenderness on palpitation over the right patella but no instability, no limitation of ROM. Cranial nerves II-VII intact. No meds.

A: Mild concussion.

P: CT of the head after C-spine is clear. Home with head injury instructions. Recheck with private doctor in 1-2 days or return here PRN with any change in mental status.

D: 10-08-0X
T: 10-08-0X
m l o

ER PHYSICIAN	DATE
[signature]	10-08-0X

NS-7672 (9-95)

Figure 33–2 Example of an emergency department chart note illustrating the SOAP format. (Reprinted with permission from Diehl, Marcy O., *Medical Transcription: Techniques and Procedures,* 5th ed. Philadelphia, Saunders, 2002.)

Flanagham, Michael R.   AGE: 82

March 17, 200X

SUBJECTIVE: Pt presented complaining of insomnia, weakness,
                     and shortness of breath. Described Hx of
progressive dyspnea on exertion over a 2-3 year period.

OBJECTIVE: BP: 110. Pulse 120 and regular. Visible neck vein
                     distention at 45 degrees elevation; rales at both
lung bases. Cardiac examination revealed an enlarged heart with
PMI felt at the midclavicular line. Sounds were distant, but a systolic
murmur was described.

        ECG: Sinus tachycardia, left axis deviation, and rt bundle branch
        block.

        ECHO: Enlarged left ventricle and calcified and stenotic aortic
        valve. Left ventricular hypertrophy also demonstrated.

ASSESSMENT: 1. Calcified aortic stenosis.
                     2. Congestive heart failure.

PLAN: 1. Admit to hospital.
                     2. Treat with sodium restriction, digitalis, diuretic.

                                    Joseph D. Becquer, MD
mlo

Figure 33–3   Example of a chart note illustrating the SOAP format. (Reprinted
with permission from Diehl, Marcy O., *Medical Transcription: Techniques and Procedures,*
5th ed. Philadelphia, Saunders, 2002.)

Flanaghan, Michael R.   AGE: 82

March 17, 200X

HX	Pt presented complaining of insomnia, weakness, and shortness of breath. Described Hx of progressive dyspnea on exertion over a 2-3 year period.
PX	BP: 110. Pulse 120 and regular. Visible neck vein distention at 45 degrees elevation; rales at both lung bases. Cardiac examination revealed an enlarged heart with PMI felt at the midclavicular line. Sounds were distant, but a systolic murmur was described.
ECG	Sinus tachycardia, left axis deviation, and rt bundle branch block.
ECHO	Enlarged left ventricle and calcified and stenotic aortic valve. Left ventricular hypertrophy also demonstrated.
DX	1) Calcified aortic stenosis. 2) Congestive heart failure.
RX	1) Admit to hospital. 2) Treat with sodium restriction, digitalis, diuretic.

Joseph D. Becquer, MD/mlo

Figure 33–4   Example showing the HX, PX, DX, RX method of charting. (Reprinted with permission from Diehl, Marcy O., *Medical Transcription: Techniques and Procedures,* 5th ed. Philadelphia, Saunders, 2002.)

Mary Neidgrinhaus   DOB: 06-11-XX

REF: Yuen Wong, MD
       555-527-8765

<u>12-18-0X</u>
HX: This 4½-year-old girl has been having URIs beginning in October,
           200X. She has had several of these infections since that time and has
           been seen by another otolaryngologist who recommended that she have
           surgery including an adenotonsillectomy and bilateral myringotomies
           with tubes. The mother desired another opinion and the family doctor
           referred her to me.

ALLERGIES: <u>AMPICILLIN and SEPTRA</u>

PX: Well-developed, well-nourished girl in no acute distress.
VS: Pulse: 84/min. Resp: 20/min. Temp: 98.80 axillary.
HEENT: Eyes: PERRLA. EOMs normal. Ears: The rt TM was retracted and slightly
           injected The left TM was retracted but not injected. Both canals were
           negative. Nose: The nasal septum was roughly in the midline. Mucous
           membrane lining somewhat pale and slightly swollen. Throat: Tonsils
           were +3 and very cryptic. Neck: There were tonsillar nodes palpable in
           both anterior cervical triangles.

CHEST: Lungs: Clear to P&A. Heart: Regular rate and rhythm, no murmurs.

IMP: 1. Hypertrophy of tonsils and adenoids.
           2. Bilateral recurrent serous otitis media.

RX: Dimetapp elixir, 4 oz, 1 t q.i.d.

mlo   Gene M Kasten, MD

<u>12-28-0X</u>   Rt ear improved; no change in the left. Mother still does not want surgery.

RX: Actifed syrup, 2 oz, 1/2 t q.i.d.

mlo   Gene M. Kasten, MD

1-3-0X   *Mother telephoned: Actifed "not working." Called in Ceclor, 4 oz
          1 t q.i.d. per Dr. Kasten mlo*

<u>1-14-0X</u>   No improvement in left ear. Rt ear significantly the same as when last
           seen. Mother now approves surgical removal of the tonsils and
           adenoids and bilateral myringotomies with tube insertions.

mlo   Gene M. Kasten, MD

2-5-OX   See Copy of History and Physical dictated for View of the Lakes Memorial.
2-6-0X   *Pt admitted 3:30 p.m. mlo*
2-8-0X   *See letter to Dr. Wong mlo*

Figure 33–5   Example showing the typical mixed format of handwritten and
typed entries. (Reprinted with permission from Diehl, Marcy O., *Medical Transcription:
Techniques and Procedures,* 5th ed. Philadelphia, Saunders, 2002.)

Allergic to PCN

EAR NOSE & THROAT

Kingersley, Margaret O.
Patient's name

Address: 145 West Cuvamaca, Roseland Hills, XX
Tel No. 555-9743   Referred by : Dept. of Rehabilitation

Insurance Rehab   Date: 1-9-XX
Age: 60   Sex: F

CC: This is a 60-year-old pt who was seen in the office on May 15, 200X, on referral from the Department of Rehabilitation.

HX: I obtained a history from the patient that she has been aware of hearing loss in both ears, worse in the left ear, since about 1998. She was first tested in Dr. Victor Goodhill's office at the University Clinic in 1999, and at that time showed a bilateral sensorineural deafness worse in the left ear. Because there was some asymmetry of her hearing, mastoid and middle ear tomograms were performed and these were normal. She also had a ENG, which was also normal.

Beginning in 1999, she was fitted with first, a hearing aid in her left ear, and later one in her right ear, and these are in-the-ear types. She states that she does not find them very satisfactory, in most situations, unless it is very quiet.

The pt does report some tinnitus in both ears, which has been present for a number of years. She is unable to describe this noise.

The pt has no problems with vertigo.

JHJ/ro

Figure 33–6   Example of a chart note showing preprinted illustrations. (Reprinted with permission from Diehl, Marcy O., *Medical Transcription: Techniques and Procedures*, 5th ed. Philadelphia, Saunders, 2002.)

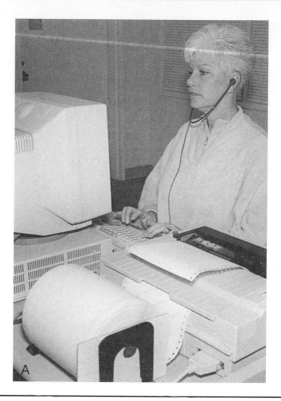

Figure 33–7 *A,* Transcriptionist using PAT Systems pressure-sensitive paper on a roll. *Continued*

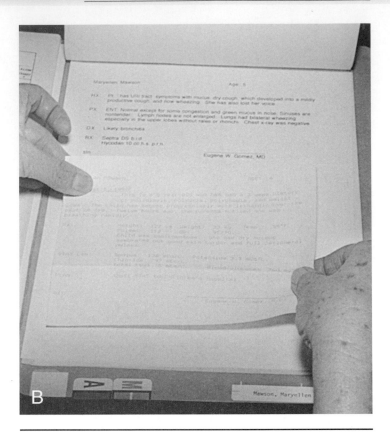

Figure 33–7 Cont'd. *B,* Demonstration of ease of placing the pressure-sensitive paper onto the existing chart note in the medical record. (Paper courtesy of PAT Systems 1-800-543-1911; photograph courtesy of John Dixon, Grossmont College. Reprinted with permission from Diehl, Marcy O., *Medical Transcription: Techniques and Procedures,* 5th ed. Philadelphia, Saunders, 2002.)

Barbara Anne Noonan
7-7-0X

The patient returns today feeling rather poorly. She was admitted to the GrandView Hospital for fluid accumulation which came on rather suddenly last week. Fluid has been removed but the patient is still short of breath. No chest pain and no hemoptysis.

On examination, the patient looks progressively sicker than when first seen. Ankles are quite swollen. Moderately short of breath at rest. P&A of the lungs reveal probable fluid accumulation along the right base. The liver is still prominent and hard.

It would seem advisable that radiation therapy stop at this point. I am not sure what, if any, palliation we have afforded the lady, but I do not think her general situation would permit further radiation to curative doses. This was discussed with her and her husband. It was with some relief as she accepted my recommendation.
LR/do

John W. Issabel
7-7-0X

Patient's weight is up slightly at 124 lb. Requires 4-6 Dilaudid a day, about the same as he has been taking earlier. Pain is a little better. Still localized to soft tissues about 3 cm to the right of the midline at about the level of C7. His wife notices some return of night sweats, though no symptoms of this were noted by the patient and he has not measured his temperature. He is otherwise feeling well.

To exam he looks better than he has looked on previous visits here. There are no palpable nodes. He has tan skin reaction over both ports, more so on the posterior than anterior. Chest is clear to percussion and auscultation. No distinct bone tenderness. No palpable axillary masses or liver masses. No peripheral cyanosis or edema.

PLAN: Chest x-ray with films on the right side, upper chest. Liver function test, CBC. Return here 1 month and to see Dr. Tu on 7-11-0X. I have asked that he keep track of his temperature twice a day in the interim.
LR/do

7-7-0X
Edward Fredrickson

Bilateral femur and hip films show only osteoporosis. Will consider for palliative treatment should reproducible pain persist.
LR/do

Herbert Frenay
7-7-0X

Mr. Frenay returns to be sure that his groin has healed up following significant reaction from irradiation treatments.

On exam, he has no adenopathy in the area. There is some edema. The skin has healed well. There is also distal edema of the lower extremity which is quite significant and I'm sure related to the combination of radiation and surgery. He has seen Dr. Hoffman, and Dr. Hoffman has given him a Jobst stocking for this. He will follow up with Dr. Hoffman and here only on a p.r.n. basis.
LR/do

Figure 33–8 Chart notes on four patients transcribed on pressure-sensitive paper. After the notes are signed by the dictator, they will be cut apart just above each patient's name and placed in the individual charts. (Reprinted with permission from Diehl, Marcy O., *Medical Transcription: Techniques and Procedures,* 5th ed. Philadelphia, Saunders, 2002.)

34

Proofreading and Revisions

INTRODUCTION

Proofread your work carefully on screen while transcribing, at the completion of transcription, and again after printing the document. Accuracy is important in spelling, grammar, figures, word division, and punctuation. Professional quality is demanded in all medical reports. The importance of errors varies, of course. For example, transposed letters in the name of a drug could be very serious, whereas variations in a format and style may be acceptable. Equipment limitations are never an excuse for less than professional quality copy. *(See Figure 34–1 at the end of the chapter for the symbols used in proofreading and their meanings.)*

34–1 ABBREVIATIONS, SYMBOLS, AND NUMBERS

✓ DO   know the technical symbols in your specialty area and use them correctly. Avoid the use of abbreviations in records where they are inappropriate. *(See Chapter 1 for help with abbreviations and Chapter 27 for help with numbers.)*

Incorrect:
Postoperative diagnosis: PID
Correct:
Postoperative diagnosis: Pelvic inflammatory disease
Incorrect:
a 3-cm. incision was carried along the . . .

Correct:
a 3-cm incision was carried along the . . .
Incorrect:
Cultures grew out 10 to the fifth per mL
Correct:
Cultures grew out 10^5/mL

34–2   CAPITALIZATION

✓ DO   know why you are using a capital letter. When in doubt, always take the time to check on a rule or look for the word in a reference book. *(See Chapter 5 for help with capitalization problems.)*

34–3   FLAGGING QUERIES

⊘ DON'T   transcribe material that does not make sense to you. If you cannot understand a word and the author is unavailable, leave a *blank space* in your material, long enough to allow the correct word to be inserted later. Attach a flag sheet to the material. This flagging *(also called carding, tagging, or marking)* can be done by using the repositionable adhesive notes. You can also staple or paper clip your card or flag. The flag should include the patient's name, the page number, the paragraph, and the line with the missing word(s). If you are in a large organization, add your name. It will help the author if you put the missing word(s) in context, that is, include a few words that come before and after it. An example of a flag follows:

Williams, Maribeth #18-74-78.
Under PX, CR.
(page 2, line 8) "_____? respirations present."
Sounds like "chain smokes." Judy, 5-17-XX
(The author will return a note that reads "Cheyne-Stokes respirations present.")
(See Figure 11–1 at the end of Chapter 11 for an example of a flag you might place on a document.)

✓ DO   leave an electronic flag in a situation in which the hard copy is unavailable to you or is printed off-site. The off-site editor will then be alerted to the blank or questionable material and will correct it before final printing. These sites will demonstrate the use of their own electronic flag system.

⊘ DON'T   key in a line (_____) or a series of question marks (???) in the copy. Doing so is inappropriate.

34–4 PROOFREADING

 DO proofread carefully and correct all errors on screen while transcribing.

- *Double-check any vital materials you have transcribed before and after printing the document.*
- *Reread the copy that comes immediately before and after areas where revisions have been made, because computer edits can develop added errors.*
- *Flag the area for the author's attention when there is any doubt about the material.*
- *Check for unintended expansion when you are using a text expander. (Memphis, Tennessee could end up Memphis, Tenderness because your abbreviation for TN expands to cause this problem.)*
- *Be sure no letters, words, or word endings have been dropped.*
- *Be sure no words, phrases, or sentences have been repeated.*
- *Check for consistency of style and overall appearance.*
- *Be sure there are no orphans or widows* (single lines of a paragraph at the bottom or top of a page).
- *Check headers and footers.*
- *Look carefully for another typo near the first one you find; mistakes tend to cluster.*
- *Use the spell-check feature of your word processing software and be alert for homonyms and transposed letters such as* form *and* from.

DO learn where you generally make errors and check these areas again. Read everything in the copy straight through from beginning to end: titles, subtitles, punctuation, capitalization, indented items, and page numbers.

DO use the print preview before printing

DO put your copy aside for a break before checking it. It is also helpful to work on another project and alternate proofreading and production.

DO read your copy aloud to check for punctuation errors.

DO double-check references such as *see the enclosed report.*

DO scrutinize features that come in sets, such as brackets, parentheses, quotation marks, and dashes, to be sure one has not been omitted.

DON'T proofread your own copy whenever possible. Trade transcripts with someone unfamiliar with the material but familiar with the general topic.

✓ **DO** use all electronic shortcuts slowly and with caution, and carefully double-check a final draft after printing out your corrected copy. Often the changes in a document will affect the printout in unexpected ways: the last line appearing alone on the final page; one parenthesis or bracket being printed on the line following; a number being separated from the symbol following it; page numbers being changed inappropriately; long spaces appearing between words or figures; indenting appearing inconsistently; type fonts, italics, underlining, superscript, or boldface printing out inappropriately.

 DON'T rely on grammar software to find all the grammatical errors.

 DON'T rely on electronic spell checkers to alert you to all the possible spelling errors.

34–5   PUNCTUATION

✓ **DO** know why you are using a particular punctuation mark. Remember that leaving out required punctuation is as much an error as putting in an unneeded mark or using the wrong mark. Review the rules from time to time, and refer to the chapters in this book for guidance when you need it.

34–6   ROUGH DRAFT

✓ **DO** double-space rough draft material that is intended for revision or editing and print out a fast, low-quality copy on machines with this feature.

34–7   SPELLING

✓ **DO** consult a dictionary, speller, or word book whenever you have the slightest doubt about your spelling.

 DON'T rely on an electronic spell checker to correct the overall document, but stop as you go along and check any questionable words with a reliable reference.

 DON'T depend on the drug name that the electronic spell checker provides, but check your drug reference for additional information concerning the drug to be sure that you have made the proper selection.

34–8   WORD DIVISION

✓ DO   divide words only at the proper point when you must divide a word. Consult a word book for assistance when you are in doubt about word division. *(See Chapter 20, Hyphen Use and Word Division, for help.)*

Proofing Symbol	Meaning	First Draft	Final Copy
#	insert space	Mr. Jones is here.	Mr. Jones is here.
C	close up space	Too much space here.	Too much space here.
ℓ	delete	There are too many waiting.	There are many waiting.
⋏	insert comma	Dictate the summary but not the formal report.	Dictate the summary but not the formal report.
⋏	insert semicolon	Jean Bradley your patient was seen in the office.	Jean Bradley, your patient, was seen in the office.
⋏	remove one mark; insert another	He agreed to the surgery scheduled it.	He agreed to the surgery; I scheduled it.
ℓ ⋏	insert colon	I wanted to remove the the tumor however, he refused.	I wanted to remove the tumor; however, he refused.
⋏	insert apostrophe	Gentlemen	Gentlemen:
⋎		The patients incision...	The patient's incision...

Figure 34–1 Proofreading marks with explanations. (Reprinted with permission from Diehl, Marcy O., *Medical Transcription: Techniques and Procedures*, 5th ed. Philadelphia, Saunders, 2002.)

Proofing Symbol	Meaning	First Draft	Final Copy
⌄	insert quotes	She had these seizures frequently⊙	She had these "seizures" frequently.
⊙	insert a period	Joaquin R⦵Navarro, MD	Joaquin R. Navarro, MD
=	insert a hyphen	She is well⹀developed, well⹀nourished...	She is well-developed, well-nourished...
⋁	insert a word	The blood pressure⹁was 160/90.	The blood pressure on admission was 160/90.
↻	transpose	A new medication was prescribed and⹁she...	A new medication was prescribed, and she...
→	move copy	She was, however, seen as an outpatient.	She was seen as an outpatient, however.
stet ····	let it alone	He should have cobalt-65 radiation therapy.	He should have cobalt-65 radiation therapy.
≡	caps	College park hospital	College Park Hospital
(one word)	caps	College Park hospital	College Park Hospital

Continued

Proofing Symbol	Meaning	First Draft	Final Copy
lc	lower case	The patient's Mother died of heart disease.	The patient's mother died of heart disease.
circle word	spell out	She was placed in the (ICU.)	She was placed in the intensive care unit.
circle word	spelling error	(Their) was no evidence of	There was no evidence of...
circle word	correct this	③ of the most serious problems we have ...	Three of the most serious problems we have...
circle word	correct this	The patient's temperature was (ninety-nine)	The patient's temperature was 99.
¶	insert paragraph	Her history is well known to you, so I will not repeat it.	Her history is well known to you, so I will not repeat it.
		¶ On physical examination, I found. ...	On physical examination, I...
⌐	move the copy to the right	⌐ On physical examination,	On physical examination,
circle word	spell it out	On (PX,) I ...	On physical examination, I...
⌐	move the copy to the left	On physical examination ⌐ I found a well-developed ...	On physical examination I found a well-developed...

Figure 34–1, Cont'd.

35

Question Mark

35–1 DASHES

✓ **DO** use dashes to set off a parenthetical question within a sentence. Place the question mark before the closing dash.

The pharmaceutical representative from Burroughs Wellcome—do you know her?—has called again for an appointment.

✓ **DO** use a question mark to end an interrogative phrase following a closing dash.

Is the medical convention in Hawaii?—on Maui?

35–2 PARENTHESES

⊘ **DON'T** use a question mark within the closing parenthesis unless the question mark refers to the parenthetical item.

Can you send me a copy of the pathology report (and can you send me two?), or must I request it in on a special form?
The patient's name is Mary Barker (or is it Merry Parker?).

✓ **DO** place a question mark outside the closing parenthesis if the phrase in parentheses is to be incorporated within the sentence, and the entire sentence is a question.

Do you know Barry Smith (or is it Berry Smyth)?

427

Can you order a CBC on Mrs. Warren and have the report by Friday (or better yet, have the lab fax me the results)?

35–3 PUNCTUATION

 DO   use a question mark at the end of a sentence to indicate a direct question.

NOTE: *Leave one or two spaces after a question mark before typing the next sentence.*

When will Mr. Hamlin have the gallbladder surgery?

 DO   use question marks to indicate a series of questions pertaining to the same subject and verb.

NOTE: *Leave only one space after a question mark within a sentence.*

Shall I send the report to Dr. Jones? Dr. Keystone? Dr. Avery?

 DO   use a question mark to show doubt.

The complete blood cell count showed 20,000 (?) white blood cells.

35–4 QUOTATION MARKS

 DO   type a question mark outside a closing quotation mark if the entire sentence is in the form of a question.

Will you answer my question, "What year were you born"?

 DO   type a question mark inside a closing quotation mark if only the quoted material is a question.

The medical report answers my original question, "What is the secondary diagnosis?"

 DO   use the question mark within quotation marks when the quoted material is a question.

"Can you dictate the report on Mr. Bowen right now?" she asked.

35–5 *SPACING*

 DO   use one or two spaces after a question mark at the end of a sentence.

> **NOTE:** *There is no space after a question mark when another mark of punctuation* (closing quotation mark, parenthesis, or dash) *immediately follows.*

36

Quotation Marks

INTRODUCTION

Quotation marks are used to set off words that have been either spoken or written by another person. They may also be used to set off words for some special use.

36–1 CAPITAL LETTERS AND QUOTATIONS

✓ **DO**   use a capital letter at the beginning of the quotation if the quoted material is not an integral part of the sentence itself.

36–2 EXACT WORDS

✓ **DO**   use quotation marks to enclose the *exact* words of a speaker.

> The patient said, "There has been hurting in the pelvis bones."
> The patient said that there had been some pain in the pelvis.
> **Correct:**
> The patient said he's always felt like "something's hung up in there." *(Note where the quotes begin.)*
> **Incorrect:**
> The patient said "he's always felt like something's hung up in there." *(Patient would not say "he's always felt . . .")*
> **Incorrect:**
> The patient said, "she had this identical problem as a child."

Correct:

The patient said that she had this identical problem as a child.

The patient said, "I had this identical problem as a child."

36–3 PUNCTUATION WITH QUOTATION MARKS

✓ DO place periods and commas *inside* the closing quotation mark; semicolons and colons go *outside* the closing quotation mark.

The tenth chapter, "Editing," is the most difficult for me.

The patient related that she spoke with her hands "like an Italian."

✓ DO place a question mark or an exclamation point inside the closing quotation marks when it applies to the material quoted and outside when it applies to the entire sentence.

Dr. Matthews exclaimed, "I must return to the Coronary Care Unit at once"!

Why must patients often report, "I've waited too long to be seen"?

The medical report answers my original question, "What is the secondary diagnosis?"

✓ DO use a colon to introduce quoted material if the introductory material is an independent clause.

Patients often ask me this: "When can I return to work?"

✓ DO use a comma to introduce an informal quotation.

The patient stated, "A roll of paper fell and struck me across the upper back and knocked me to the ground."

⊘ DON'T use a comma when the quoted material is an integral part of the sentence.

Her favorite response is that "we've always done it this way."

36–4 SIC

If a quotation contains a grammatical error, a misspelling, or a thought that is somewhat confusing, the term *sic (thus it is, so, this is the way it was)* is inserted in brackets immediately following the error. *Sic* lets the reader know that an error appeared in the original material.

36–5   SINGLE QUOTATION MARKS

 DO   use single quotation marks to enclose a quote within a quote.

He said emphatically, "I am sure that she asked, 'Where did you put it?'"

36–6   SPECIAL ATTENTION

 DO   use quotation marks to enclose single words or phrases for special attention.

The word "accommodate" is at the top of the list of most frequently misspelled words.

I can see no need for "temper tantrums" in the operating suite.

The German expression "Gemütlichkeit" exactly described the feelings we had during your father's visit.

 DO   use quotation marks to enclose slang, coined, awkward, whimsical, or humorous words that might show ignorance on the part of the writer if it is not known that he or she is aware of them.

See if you can schedule a few "well" patients for a change.

Some of the expressions that startle the novice transcriptionist are "pink puffer" and "blue bloater."

If you have "clergyman's knee," "tailor's seat," "tennis elbow," or "trigger finger," what you really have is a form of bursitis or tendinitis.

 DO   use quotation marks for technical terms or jargon used in nontechnical writing.

She was reminded not to tell the patients to come in "n.p.o. midnight."

 DO   use quotation marks to define a word or expression.

When she says she wants it transcribed "stat," that is "immediately."

36–7 TITLES

 DO place titles of articles, essays, and other brief literary works within quotation marks and capitalize the main words.

His photographic entry "The Country Doctor" won first place in the contest.

 DO place titles of chapters, sections, and other subdivisions of a published work within quotation marks. *(The titles of published books, magazines, and articles are underlined. See 5–21, Titles, Literary, in Chapter 5 for proper capitalization of literary works.)*

Your homework assignment is to read "Capitalization" in <u>Medical Transcription: Techniques and Procedures</u>.

37

Reference Materials and Publications

INTRODUCTION

There are special skills involved in using reference books, and it is important that you develop them before you really need to use them.

✔ DO   select current references appropriate to your transcription responsibilities.

🚫 DON'T   think you need shelves full of reference books.

🚫 DON'T   think you can get by with a "good" medical dictionary along with a drug book and an English dictionary. *(You can't.)*

✔ DO   be open to purchasing *(at a discount)* or accepting older editions of books until you are able to purchase the current edition. Having an older, used edition helps you to decide if the book is appropriate for your needs.

✔ DO   develop research skills before you really need to use them.

✔ DO   review these general guidelines for using reference books.

- *Make an attempt to spell out your target word, write it out, use the sound table in the appendix, if necessary. Don't be concerned about the spelling and spell the word as many ways as you think it could be spelled so you are not mind-locked into something that is nowhere near your appropriate word. Remember silent letters at the beginning of some words make research very difficult.*
- *Write down the words or phrases that accompany the word.*
- *Try to have a sense of the word or phrase that you are looking for.*
- *Determine the type of word you are seeking; is it an abbreviation, verb, noun, a plural form, and so on.*
- *Keep the specialty or body part or body system foremost to use as a clue or guide.*
- *Remember that there are many tables in books listing muscles, bones, arteries, abbreviations, units of measurement, and so on. Choose one of these to be your constant when you need any of these word types.*
- *Be aware that there are lists of words in the appendix of this book to help you in your word search that include*

both English and medical homonyms, unusual terms, brief forms, problem words, Latin phrases, plural forms, French words used in medical documents, abbreviations, and genus and species names.

- *Select a reference.* Read the introduction so you can see how the book is set up if this is your first opportunity to use this reference or if you have forgotten exactly how it is set up. Learn about the main entries and subentries.
- Go to the proper section in the reference you have selected for your search.
- *Verify your final selection with a dictionary when appropriate.* (Generally, the dictionary is the final book of choice when doing research, not the first. The dictionary is the reference you need when you have to verify that you have made the correct selection from a "speller-type" reference book that provides the word for you but not the meaning.)
- *Record the word accurately in your own reference book.* (See Chapter 38, Figure 38–1.)

37–1   ABBREVIATIONS DICTIONARIES, GENERAL

Reverse International Acronyms, Initialisms, and Abbreviations Dictionary, Crowley and Sheppard, Gale Research, Inc., 1993, phone 800-877-4253.

World Guide to Abbreviations, vols. 1-3, Spillner, Gale Research, Inc., 1995, phone 800-877-4253

37–2   ABBREVIATIONS DICTIONARIES, MEDICAL

Common Medical Abbreviations, DeSousa, Delmar Publishers/ITP, 1995, phone 800-347-7707.

Dictionary of Medical Acronyms and Abbreviations, Jablonski, Hanley & Belfus, Inc., 2001, phone 800-962-1892.

Dorland's Medical Abbreviations, Saunders, 1994, phone 800-545-2522.

Lexikon: Dictionary of Health Care Terms, Organizations, and Acronyms for the Era of Reform, O'Leary et al., Joint Commission on Accreditation of Healthcare Organizations, 1997, phone 630-916-5600.

Medical Abbreviations: 12,000 Conveniences at the Expense of Communications and Safety, Davis, Neil M. Davis Association, 2000, phone 215-947-1752.

Medical Abbreviations and Eponyms, Sloane, Saunders, 1997, phone 800-545-2522.

Medical Abbreviation Guide, Campbell, Saunders, 1994, phone 800-545-2522.

Medical Acronyms, Eponyms and Abbreviations, Delong, Practice Management Information Corporation, 2002, phone 800-633-7467.

Melloni's Illustrated Dictionary of Medical Abbreviations, Melloni and Dox, Parthenon Publishing Group, Inc., 1998, phone 800-735-4744.

Mosby's Survival Guide to Medical Abbreviations, Acronyms, Prefixes, Suffixes, Symbols, and the Greek Alphabet, Campbell and Campbell, Mosby, Inc., 1995, phone 800-426-4545.

Stedman's Abbreviations, Acronyms and Symbols, Lippincott Williams & Wilkins, Waverly, Inc., 2003, phone 800-527-5597.

37–3 ANTONYMS, EPONYMS, HOMONYMS, SYNDROMES, AND SYNONYMS

A Dictionary of Medical Eponyms, Firkin and Whitworth, Parthenon Publishing Group, Inc., 2003, phone 800-735-4744.

Dictionary of Medical Syndromes, Magalini, Lippincott Williams & Wilkins, 1996, phone 800-777-2295.

Medical Abbreviations and Eponyms, Sloane, Saunders, 1997, phone 800-545-2522.

Medical Acronyms, Eponyms and Abbreviations, Delong, Practice Management Information Corporation, 2002, phone 800-633-7467.

Stedman's Medical Eponyms, Forbis and Bartolucci, Lippincott Williams & Wilkins, 1998, phone 800-638-3030

37–4 CAREER DEVELOPMENT

Administrative Medical Assisting, Fordney and Follis, Delmar Publishers/ITP, 1998, phone 800-347-7707.

American Association for Medical Transcription Journal, American Association for Medical Transcription (quarterly), phone 209-551-0883 or 800-982-2182.

Analysis: Civil Service Classification of Medical Transcriptionist, American Association for Medical Transcription, 1981, phone 209-551-0883 or 800-982-2182.

Business Start-Up Guide: Medical Transcription Service #1392, Entrepreneur Magazine Media, 1995, phone 800-421-2300.

Career Development for Health Professionals, Haroun, Saunders, 2001, phone 800-545-2522.

HIPAA for MTs 2002, American Association for Medical Transcription, phone 800-982-2182.

The Independent Medical Transcriptionist, Avila-Weil and Glaccum, Rayve Productions Inc., 2002, phone 800-852-4890.

Perspectives on the Medical Transcription Profession, Health Professions Institute (quarterly), phone 209-551-2112.

The Small Business Start-up Kit, Pakroo, Nolo Press, 2000, phone 800-992-6656.

37–5   CERTIFICATION

The AAMT Test Guide, American Association for Medical Transcription, phone 209-551-0883 or 800-982-2182.
Professional Skillbuilding Wizard, Kropko and Francis, M-Tec, Inc., 2001, phone 877-733-4346.

37–6   COMPOSITION

Basic Verbal Skills, Burnham and Lederer, Ongman, 1986.
Edit Yourself—A Manual for Everyone Who Works with Words, Ross-Larson, W.W. Norton & Company, 1995, phone 800-223-2584.
Woe is I, O'Conner, Riverhead Books, 1998.
Words Fail Me, O'Conner, Harvest-Harcourt, 2000.
Words into Type, Warren, Brady Prentice-Hall, 1992, phone 800-223-1360.
The Write Way, Lederer and Downs, Pocket Books, 1995, phone 800-223-2336.

CONFIDENTIALITY

See also Law and Ethics.

37–7   EDITING

Developing Proofreading Skills, Camp, Glencoe/McGraw-Hill, 2002, phone 800-334-7344.
The Elements of Editing: A Modern Guide for Editors and Journalists, Plotnik, Macmillan Publishing Company, 1986, phone 800-223-2336.

37–8   ENGLISH HANDBOOKS (GRAMMAR, PUNCTUATION, AND GENERAL CLERICAL INFORMATION)

The AAMT Book of Style for Medical Transcription, American Association for Medical Transcription, 2002, phone 209-551-0883 or 800-982-2182.
American Medical Association Manual of Style, American Medical Association, Lippincott/Williams & Wilkins, 1998, phone 800-527-5597.
Chicago Manual of Style, University of Chicago Press, 2003, phone 800-621-2736.
Diehl and Fordney's Medical Transcription: Techniques and Procedures (includes software), Diehl, Saunders, 2002, phone 800-545-2522.
The Gregg Reference Manual, Sabin, Glencoe/McGraw-Hill, 2000, phone 800-334-7344.
How to Write and Publish Papers in the Medical Sciences, Huth, Lippincott Williams & Wilkins, 1997, phone 800-527-5597.
Mark My Words: Instruction and Practice in Proofreading, Smith, Editorial Experts Incorporated, 1993, phone 703-683-0683.

Medical English Usage and Abusage, Schwager, Oryx Press, 1990, phone 800-279-6799.

Medical Style and Format, Huth, Lippincott Williams & Wilkins, 1987, phone 800-527-5597.

Medical Transcription: Fundamentals and Practice, Health Professions Institute, Brady Prentice-Hall, 1999, phone 800-638-0220.

The Medical Transcriptionist's Handbook, Blake, Delmar Publishers/ITP, 1993, phone 800-347-7707.

The Merriam-Webster Concise Handbook for Writers, Merriam-Webster, Inc., 1998, phone 800-828-1880.

Saunders Manual of Medical Transcription, Sloane and Fordney, Saunders, 1993, phone 800-545-2522.

Scientific English: A Guide for Scientists and Other Professionals, Day, Oryx Press, 1995, phone 800-279-6799.

Scientific Style and Format: The CBE Manual for Authors, Editors, and Publishers, Council of Biology Editors, Cambridge University Press, 1994, phone 800-872-7423.

Sleeping Dogs Don't Lay, Lederer and Dowis, St. Martin's Press, 1999, www.stmartins.com.

Substance and Style: Instruction and Practice in Copyediting, Revised, Stoughton, Editorial Experts Incorporated, 1996, phone 703-683-0683.

Talking About People: A Guide to Fair and Accurate Language, Maggio, Oryx Press, 1997, phone 800-279-6799.

The Write Way: The Spell˚ Guide to Real-Life Writing, *Society for the Preservation of English Language and Literature, Lederer and Dowis, Pocket Books, 1995, phone 800-223-2336.

37–9   ENGLISH DICTIONARIES

The American Heritage Dictionary of the English Language, Houghton Mifflin Company, 2000, phone 800-225-3362.

Merriam-Webster's Collegiate Dictionary, Merriam-Webster, Inc., 2003, phone 800-828-1880.

Random House Unabridged Dictionary, Random House, Inc., 1997, phone 800-733-3000.

Talking About People: A Guide to Fair and Accurate Language, Maggio, Oryx Press, 1997, phone 800-279-6799.

Webster's Third New International Dictionary, Unabridged, Merriam-Webster, Inc., 1993, phone 800-828-1880.

EPONYMS

See Antonyms, Eponyms, Homonyms, Syndromes, and Synonyms.

37–10   ERGONOMICS

Carpal Tunnel Syndrome: How to Relieve and Prevent Wrist "BURNOUT!" Atensio, HWD Publishing, 1993, phone 800-935-7323.

The Dvorak Keyboard, Cassingham, Kinesis Corporation, 1997, phone 800-454-6374 ext 21.
Preventing Computer Injury: The Hand Book and KeyMoves Software, Brown, Ergonome, 1995, phone 212-222-9600.
Shoulders, Upper Back and Neck: Free Yourself from PAIN! Atensio, HWD Publishing, 1995, phone 800-935-7323.
Zap! How Your Computer Can Hurt You—and What You Can Do About It, Sellers, Peachpit Press, 1994, phone 800-283-9444.

37–11 FOREIGN LANGUAGE

Building a Medical Vocabulary, Leonard, Saunders, 2001, phone 800-545-2522.
Delmar's English-Spanish Pocket Dictionary for Health Professionals, Kelz, Delmar Learning, 1997, phone 800-998-7498.
Medical Spanish: An Instant Translator, Nasr and Cordero, Saunders, 1996, phone 800-545-2522.
Medical Spanish: An Instant Survival Guide, Wilbur and Lister, Butterworth-Heinemann, 1995, phone 800-366-2665.
Medical Spanish in Pediatrics, Nasr and Cordero, W. B. Saunders, 2001, phone 800-545-2522.
Medical Terminology with Human Anatomy (includes Spanish terminology), Rice, Appleton & Lange, 1994, phone 800-423-1359.
Saunders International Medical Word Book, Saunders, 1991, phone 800-545-2522.
Say It in Spanish: A Guide for Health Care Professionals, Joyce, Saunders, 2000, phone 800-545-2522.
Spanish-English Handbook for Medical Professionals, Perez-Sabido, Practice Management Information Corporation, 1994, phone 800-633-7467.
Spanish-English, English-Spanish Medical Dictionary, McElroy and Grabb, Lippincott Williams & Wilkins, 1996, phone 800-638-3030

GRAMMAR

See English Handbooks.

37–12 HIPAA GUIDELINES

HIPAA Compliance Alert, DecisionHealth (monthly), phone 877-602-3835.
HIPAA for MTs 2002, American Association for Medical Transcription, phone 800-982-2182.
HIPAA Guidelines Policy and Procedure Manual, hcPro, 2002, phone 800-639-8511.

37–13 HUMOR AND GAMES

The Best of Medical Humor, Bennett, Hanley & Belfus, Inc., 2000, phone 215-546-7293.

Dictation PRN, Keller, American Association for Medical Transcription, 1992, phone 209-551-0883.

The eMpTy Laugh Book, Pitman (Ed.), American Association for Medical Transcription, 1981, phone 800-982-2182.

Fritz Spiegl's Sick Notes: An Alphabetical Browsing-Book of Derivatives, Abbreviations, Mnemonics and Slang for the Amusement and Edification of Medics, Nurses, Patients, and Hypochondriacs, Spiegl, Parthenon Publishing Group, Inc., 1996, phone 800-735-4744.

Medical Knowledge for Fun, Worcester, Parthenon Publishing Group, Inc., 1995, phone 800-735-4744.

Medical Wit and Wisdom, Brallier, Running Press Publishers, 1993, phone 800-345-5359.

Medicate Me, Marshall, Health Professions Institute, 1987, phone 209-551-2112.

Medicate Me Again, Marshall, Health Professions Institute, 1994, phone 209-551-2112.

[sic] Humor, American Association for Medical Transcription, 1995, phone 209-551-0883.

IMAGING
See Specialty References, Radiology/Imaging.

37–14 INSURANCE AND CODING

Insurance Handbook for the Medical Office, 8th edition, Fordney, Saunders, 2004, phone 800-545-2522.

Step by Step Medical Coding, 5th edition, Buck, Saunders, 2004, phone 800-545-2522.

37–15 INTERNET

Health and Medicine on the Internet, Practice Management Information Corporation, 2002, phone 800-633-7467.

Medical Information on the Internet, Kiley, Saunders, 2002, phone 800-545-2522.

37–16 LAW AND ETHICS

AAMT Code of Ethics, American Association for Medical Transcription, 1995, phone 209-551-0883.

AAMT Guidelines on Confidentiality, Privacy, and Security of Patient Care Documentation Through the Process of Medical Dictation and Transcription, American Association for Medical Transcription, 1996, phone 209-551-0883.

Ethics and Jurisprudence, Ehrlich, The Colwell Company, 1983, phone 800-637-1140.

Guidelines for Establishing Information Security Policies, CPRI Workgroup, Computer-Based Patient Record Institute, 1995, phone 301 657-5918

The Health Care Workers' Primer on Professionalism, Makely, Prentice Hall, 2000, phone 800-445-6991.

Health Information Management, Huffman, American Health Information Management Association, 1997, phone 800-335-5535.

HIPAA Compliance Alert, DecisionHealth (monthly), phone 877-602-3835.

HIPAA Guidelines Policy and Procedure Manual, hcPro, 2002, phone 800-639 8511.

In Confidence, American Health Information Management Association (bimonthly newsletter), phone 800-335-5535.

Law and Ethics for Health Occupations, Judson and Blesie, Glencoe/McGraw-Hill, 1994, phone 800-334-7344.

Law, Liability and Ethics for Medical Office Professionals, Flight, Delmar Publishers/ITP, 1998, phone 800-347-7707.

Legal and Ethical Issues in Health Occupations, Aiken, Saunders, 2002, phone 800-545-2522.

Medical Law and Ethics, Lipman, Brady Prentice-Hall, 2002, phone 800-223-1360.

Medicolegal Forms with Legal Analysis, American Medical Association, 1997, phone 800-621-8335.

Standard Guide for the Training of Persons Who Have Access to Health Information: E1988, American Society for Testing and Materials, phone 610-832-9500.

37–17 LAW DICTIONARIES AND GLOSSARIES

Black's Law Dictionary, Black, West Publishing Company, Electronic edition (3.5 or 5.25 diskettes), 1993, phone 800-328-9352 or 800-328-9424.

The Concise Dictionary of Medical-Legal Terms: A General Guide to Interpretation and Usage, Bailey, CRC Press, Inc. 1998, phone 800-272-7737.

Dictionary of Medical-Legal Terms, Bailey, Parthenon Publishing Group, Inc., 1997, phone 800-735-4744.

Medicolegal Glossary, Scott, Medical Economics, 1989, phone 800-633-7467 or 800-232-7379 or 800-432-4570.

Merriam-Webster's Law Dictionary, Merriam-Webster, Inc., 1996, phone 800-828-1880.

37–18 MEDICAL DICTIONARIES

Churchill's Medical Dictionary, Churchill Livingstone, 1989, phone 800-553-5426.

Current Medical Terminology, Pyle, Health Professions Institute, 2003, phone 209-551-2112.

Current MedTalk: A Dictionary of Medical Terms, Slang and Jargon, Segen, Appleton & Lange, 1995, phone 800-423-1359.

Dictionary of Eye Terminology, Cassin and Solomon, Triad Publishing Company, 2001, phone 352-373-5800.

Dictionary of Medical Acronyms and Abbreviations, Jablonski, Hanley & Belfus, Inc., 2001, phone 800-962-1892.

A Dictionary of Medical and Surgical Syndromes, Gibson and Potparic, Parthenon Publishing Group, 1991, phone 800-735-4744.

Dictionary of Medical Eponyms, Firkin and Whitworth, Parthenon Publishing Group, Inc., 2003, phone 800-735-4744.

Dictionary of Medical Syndromes, Magalini et al., Lippincott Raven Publishers, 1996, phone 800-777-2295.

Dictionary of Medical-Legal Terms, Bailey, Parthenon Publishing Group, Inc., 1997, phone 800-735-4744.

Dictionary of Modern Medicine, Segen, Parthenon Publishing Group, Inc., 1992, phone 800-735-4744.

Dorland's Illustrated Medical Dictionary, 28th ed., Saunders, 2003, phone 800-545-2522.

Dorland's Pocket Medical Dictionary, Saunders, 2001, phone 800-545-2522.

Glossary of Biotechnology Terms, Fleschar and Nill, Technomic Publishing Company, Inc., 2002, phone 800-233-9936.

Glossary of Healthcare Terms, American Health Information Management Association, 1994, phone 800-335-5535.

The HarperCollins Illustrated Medical Dictionary, Dox et al., HarperCollins Publishers, Inc., 1993, phone 800-242-7737.

Health Care Defined: A Glossary of Current Terms, Goldfarb, Lippincott Williams & Wilkins, 1997, phone 800-527-5597.

Heinemann Dental Dictionary (British), Fairpo and Fairpo, Butterworth-Heinemann, 1997, phone 800-366-2665.

Illustrated Dictionary of Obstetrics and Gynecology, Dox, Parthenon Publishing Group, Inc., 1997, phone 800-735-4744.

The Inverted Medical Dictionary, Stanaszek et al., Technomic Publishing Company, Inc., 1991, phone 800-233-9936.

Lexikon: Dictionary of Health Care Terms, Organizations, and Acronyms for the Era of Reform, Joint Commission on Accreditation of Healthcare Organizations, 1998, phone 630-916-5600.

Medical Dictionary of the English and German Language, Unseld, CRC Press, Inc., 1988, phone 800-272-7737.

Melloni's Illustrated Dictionary of the Musculoskeletal System, Melloni and Dox, Parthenon Publishing Group, Inc., 1998, phone 800-735-4744.

Melloni's Illustrated Medical Dictionary, Dox and Melloni, Parthenon Publishing Group, Inc., 2001, phone 800-735-4744.

Merriam-Webster's Medical Desk Dictionary, Merriam-Webster, Inc., 1996, phone 800-828-1880.

Merriam-Webster's Medical Dictionary, Merriam-Webster, Inc., 1998, phone 800-828-1880.

Mosby's Emergency Dictionary, Garcia, Mosby, Inc., 1998, phone 800-426-4545.

Mosby's Medical, Nursing, and Allied Health Dictionary, Mosby, Inc., 2002, phone 800-426-4545.

Mosby's Pocket Dictionary of Medicine, Nursing, and Allied Health, Mosby, Inc., 1994, phone 800-426-4545.

Physician's Rx Shorthand, Jablonski, Hanley & Belfus, Inc., 1996, phone 800-962-1892.

Stedman's Concise Medical Dictionary for the Health Professions, Lippincott Williams & Wilkins, 1997, phone 800-527-5597.

Stedman's Medical Dictionary, Lippincott Williams & Wilkins, Waverly, Inc., 2000, phone 800-527-5597.

Szycher's Dictionary of Biomedical Materials and Medical Devices, Szycher, Technomic Publishing Company, Inc., 1992, phone 800-233-9936.

Taber's Cyclopedic Medical Dictionary, F. A. Davis Company, 2001, phone 800-523-4049.

37–19 MEDICAL RECORDS

Annual Book of ASTM Standards, Healthcare Informatics: Computerized Systems, ASTM International, phone 610-832-9500.

ASTM Standards: Emergency Medical Care; Confidentiality, Privacy, Access and Data Security Principles; Content and Structure of the Electronic Health Record; Management of the Confidentiality and Security of Dictation, Transcription and Transcribed Health Records; Identification and Establishment of a Quality Assurance Program for Medical Transcription, ASTM International, phone 610-832-9500.

Electronic Health Records: Changing the Vision, Murphy et al., Saunders, 1999, phone 800-545-2522.

Comprehensive Accreditation Manual for Hospitals: The Official Handbook, Joint Commission on Accreditation of Healthcare Organizations, 2003, phone 630-916-5600.

Health Information: Management of a Strategic Resource, Abdelhak et al., Saunders, 1996, phone 800-545-2522.

Information Management: The Compliance Guide to the JCAHO Standards, hcPro, 2000, phone 877-727-1728.

Journal of the American Medical Informatics Association, Hanley & Belfus, Inc. (bimonthly), phone 800-962-1892.

Physician Documentation for Reimbursement, Kotoski, Aspen Publishers, Inc., 1994, phone 800-638-8437.

37–20   MEDICAL TERMINOLOGY

Building a Medical Vocabulary (includes software), Leonard, Saunders, 2001, phone 800-545-2522.

Concise Introduction to Medical Terminology, Lillis, Appleton & Lange, 1996, phone 800-423-1359.

Davies' Medical Terminology: A Guide to Current Usage (British), Loveday, Butterworth-Heinemann, 1991, phone 800-366-2665.

The Elements of Medical Terminology, Applegate and Overton, Delmar Publishers/ITP, 1995, phone 800-347-7707.

Exploring Medical Language: A Student-Directed Approach, LaFleur-Brooks and Starr, Mosby, Inc., 2002, phone 800-426-4545.

The Language of Medicine, Chabner, Saunders, 2001, phone 800-545-2522.

The Latest Word, Grow, Saunders (bimonthly), phone 800-545-2522.

Learning Medical Terminology: A Work Text, Austrin and Austrin, Mosby, Inc., 1999, phone 800-426-4545.

Medical Language: A Programmed Body Systems Approach, Layman, Delmar Publishers/ITP, 1998, phone 800-347-7707.

Medical Terminology: An Illustrated Guide, Cohen, Lippincott Raven Publishers, 1994, phone 800-777-2295.

Medical Terminology: The Language of Health Care, Willis, Lippincott Williams & Wilkins, 1996, phone 800-527-5597.

Medical Terminology: A Programmed Text, Smith et al., Delmar Publishers, 1999, phone 800-347-7707.

Medical Terminology: A Self-Learning Text, Birmingham, Mosby, Inc., 1999, phone 800-426-4545.

Medical Terminology: A Short Course, Chabner, Saunders, 2003, phone 800-545-2522.

Medical Terminology: A Systems Approach, Gylys and Wedding, F. A. Davis Company, 1999, phone 800-523-4049.

Medical Terminology for Health Professionals, Ehrlich, Delmar Publishers, Inc., 2001, phone 800-347-7707.

Medical Terminology in Action, Wistreich, William C. Brown/McGraw-Hill Book Company, 1994, phone 800-338-5578.

Medical Terminology Made Easy, Dennerll, Delmar Publishers/ITP, 2003, phone 800-347-7707.

Medical Terminology Simplified: A Programmed Learning Approach by Body Systems, Gylys, F. A. Davis Company, 1999, phone 800-523-4049.

Medical Terminology with Human Anatomy, Rice, Appleton & Lange, 1999, phone 800-423-1359.

Medword: The Basic Roots of Medical Vocabulary, Cassellman et al., Parthenon Publishing Group, Inc., 1997, phone 800-735-4744.

Quick and Easy Medical Terminology, Leonard, Saunders, 2000, phone 800-545-2522.

Quick Medical Terminology: Self-Teaching Guide, Smith et al., John Wiley & Sons, Inc., 1999, phone 800-225-5945.

Stedman's Word Watcher, Lippincott Williams & Wilkins, (3 times a year), phone 800-527-5597.

Terminology for Allied Health Professionals, Sormunen and Moisio, Delmar Publishers/ITP, 2003, phone 800-347-7707.

Understanding Medical Terminology, Frenay and Mahoney, WCB/McGraw-Hill, 1998, phone 800-338-3987.

37–21 PERIODICALS

ADVANCE for Health Information Professionals, Merion Publications, Inc. (biweekly), phone 800-355-5627.

AMWA Journal, American Medical Writers Association (quarterly), phone 301-493-0003.

Briefings on Joint Commission on Accreditation of Healthcare Organizations, Opus Communications (monthly), phone 800-650-6787.

CPRI-Mail, Computer-Based Patient Record Institute (bimonthly), phone 847-706-6746.

Drug Newsletter, Facts and Comparisons (monthly), phone 800-223-0554.

The Editorial Eye, Editorial Experts Incorporated (monthly), phone 703-683-0683.

FAX-STAT, Facts and Comparisons (weekly), phone 800-223-0554.

For the Record, Great Valley Publishing (biweekly), phone 800-278-4400.

Healthcare Informatics, McGraw-Hill Healthcare Publications (monthly), phone 800-525-5003.

In Confidence, American Health Information Management Association (bimonthly), phone 800-335-5535.

JAAMT (Journal of the American Association for Medical Transcription), American Association for Medical Transcription (bimonthly), phone 209-551-0883.

JAMIA (Journal of the American Medical Informatics Association), Hanley & Belfus, Inc. (bimonthly), phone 800-962-1892.

Journal of AHIMA, American Health Information Management Association (monthly), phone 800-335-5535.

The Latest Word, Grow (Ed.), Saunders (bimonthly), phone 800-545-2522.

MD Computing, Springer-Verlag (bimonthly), phone 800-777-4643.

Medical Records Briefing, Medical Records Briefing (monthly), phone 800-650-6787.

Monthly Prescribing Reference, Prescribing Reference, Inc. (monthly), phone 800-436-9269.

MT Monthly, Computer Systems Management (monthly), phone 800-951-5559.

Perspectives on the Medical Transcription Profession, Health Professions Institute (quarterly), phone 209-551-2112.

PMA (Professional Medical Assistant), American Association of Medical Assistants (bimonthly), phone 800-228-2262.

Stedman's Word Watcher, Lippincott Williams & Wilkins, (3 times a year), phone 800-527-5597.

Toward an Electronic Patient Record, Medical Records Institute (monthly), phone 627-964-3923.

37–22 PHARMACEUTICAL REFERENCES

American Drug Index, Billups, Facts and Comparisons (annually), phone 800-223-0554.

Compendium of Pharmaceuticals and Specialties, Canadian Pharmaceutical Association, 2001, phone 613-523-7877.

Drugs Facts and Comparisons, Facts and Comparisons (loose-leaf edition updated monthly; bound edition updated yearly), phone 800-223-0554.

Essentials of Pharmacology for Health Occupations, Woodrow, Delmar Publishers/ITP, 2002, phone 800-347-7707.

Instant Drug Index, Aloisi, Blackwell Science, Inc. (annually), phone 800-215-1000.

Monthly Prescribing Reference, Prescribing Reference, Inc. (monthly), phone 800-436-9269.

Physician's Rx Shorthand, Jablonski, Hanley & Belfus, Inc., 1996, phone 800-962-1892.

Physicians' Desk Reference, Medical Economics Company (annually), phone 800-633-7467 or 800-232-7379 or 800-432-4570.

Physicians' Desk Reference for Nonprescription Drugs, Medical Economics Company (annually), phone 800-232-7379 or 800-633-7467 or 800-432-4570.

Physicians' Desk Reference for Ophthalmology, Medical Economics Company (annually), phone 800-232-7379, or 800-633-7467 or 800-432-4570.

Quick Look Drug Book, Lippincott Williams & Wilkins, (annually), phone 800-527-5597.

The Review of Natural Products (monographs), Facts and Comparisons (monthly), phone 800-223-0554.

Saunders Pharmaceutical Word Book, Drake and Drake, Saunders (annually), phone 800-545-2522.
Understanding Pharmacology, Turley, Brady Prentice-Hall, 2002, phone 800-223-1360 or 800-374-1200.

37–23 REFERENCES FOR THE HANDICAPPED
Associations

American Association for Medical Transcription, Visually-Impaired MT Committee, c/o Frances Holland, 635 West Grade, Apt. 306, Chicago, IL 60613.

American Foundation for the Blind, 15 West 16th Street, New York, NY 10011 (annual catalog of publications).

American Printing House for the Blind, PO Box 6085, Louisville, KY 40206 (large-print books, books on tape, books put into braille).

Clearinghouse-Depository for the Handicapped Student, State Department of Education, 721 Capitol Mall, Sacramento, CA 95814 (for information on large-print books, books on tape, and books put into braille).

Sensory Aids Foundation, 399 Sherman Avenue, Palo Alto, CA 94306 (quarterly journal, research sensory aids, job opportunities, information on latest equipment).

Publications and Tapes

AAMA Guided Study Course: Anatomy, Terminology, and Physiology (cassettes), American Association of Medical Assistants, Inc., 20 North Wacker Drive, Chicago, IL, 60606.

Audio Tapes for Building a Medical Vocabulary, Leonard, Saunders, Independence Square West, Philadelphia, PA 19105-3399.

Audio Cassettes for Medical Terminology, Smith and Davis, John Wiley & Sons, 330 West State Street, Media, PA 19063.

Basic Medical Terminology (audio cassettes), Fisher, Bobbs-Merrill Educational Publishing Company, 4300 West 62nd Street, Indianapolis, IN 46268.

Current Medical Terminology (braille), Pyle, contact Mrs. Gerri Beeson, Volunteer Services Director, Oklahoma Library for the Blind and Physically Handicapped, 1108 N. E. 36th Street, Oklahoma City, OK 73111.

Dynamic Job Interviewing for Women (braille), Russell, Federally Employed Women, PO Box 251, Port Hueneme, CA 93041.

The Language of Medicine (audio tapes), Chabner, Saunders, Independence Square West, Philadelphia, PA, 19105-3399.

Mastering Medical Terminology (braille), Gross, Braille Institute, 1150 East Fourth Street, Long Beach, CA 90802.

Medical Transcription: Techniques and Procedures (cassette), Diehl, Recording for the Blind, Inc., 5022 Hollywood Boulevard, Los Angeles, CA 90027.

Patient's Guide to Vision Rehabilitation for the Partially Sighted, Hollander, Sight Improvement Center, Inc., 25 West 43rd Street, New York, NY 10036.

Personal Computers and the Disabled, McWilliams, Doubleday, New York, 1984.

Personal Computers and Special Needs, Bowe, Sybex, Inc., 2021 Challenger Drive, No. 100, Alameda, CA, 94501.

Raised Dot Computing Newsletter (monthly), 310 South 7th Street, Lewisburg, PA 17837.

37–24   SELF-EMPLOYMENT AND FREELANCING

Business Start-Up Guide: Medical Transcription Service (#1392), Entrepreneur Magazine Group, 1995, phone 800-421-2300.

Getting Business to Come to You, Edwards and Edwards, Putnam Publishing Group, 1991, phone 800-847-5515.

Health-Service Business on Your Home-Based PC, Benzel, McGraw-Hill, 1993, phone 800-525-5003.

Hiring Independent Contractors: The Employer's Legal Guide, Fishman, Nolo Press, 1996, phone 800-992-6656.

The Independent Medical Transcriptionist: A Comprehensive Guide for the Health Language Specialist, Avila-Weil and Glaccum, Rayve Productions, Inc., 2003, phone 800-852-4890.

Making Money with Your Computer at Home, Edwards and Edwards, Putnam Publishing Group, 1993, phone 800-847-5515.

The Medical Transcriptionist: Independent Contractor or Employee? Shulman and Etter, American Association for Medical Transcription, 1993, phone 209-551-0883 or 800-982-2182.

Secrets of Self-Employment, Edwards and Edwards, Putnam Publishing Group, 1996, phone 800-847-5515.

Working as a Medical Transcriptionist at Home (articles from MT Monthly), Computer Systems Management, 1995, phone 800-951-5559.

Working from Home, Edwards and Edwards, Putnam Publishing Group, 1994, phone 800-847-5515.

You Can Type for Doctors at Home, de Menezes, Claremont Press, 1993, phone 510-829-2512.

37–25   SPECIALTY REFERENCES
Alternative Medicine

Dictionary of Alternative Medicine, Segen, McGraw-Hill Medical Division, 2001, phone 800-262-4729.

Dorland's Complementary and Alternative Word Book for Medical Transcriptionists, Saunders, 2003, phone 800-545-2522.

Fundamentals of Complementary and Alternative Medicine, Micozzi, Saunders, 2001, phone 800-545-2522

International Dictionary of Homeopathy, Swayne, Saunders, 2000, phone 800-545-2522.

Mosby's Complementary and Alternative Medicine: A Research-Based Approach, Freeman and Lawlis, Mosby, 2001, phone 800-545-2522.

Stedman's Alternative Medicine Words, Lippincott Williams & Wilkins, 2000, phone 800-638-3030.

Anesthesia

See Surgery/Anesthesia.

Bacteriology

See Pathology/Laboratory Medicine/Bacteriology.

Cardiology/Pulmonology

See also Neonatology/Pediatrics/Genetics.

Cardiology Words and Phrases (includes cardiac imaging, cardiac surgery, cardiothoracic, cardiovascular, pediatric cardiology, pulmonary), Health Professions Institute, 1995, phone 209-551-2112.

Cardiopulmonary Anatomy and Physiology, Matthews, Lippincott Raven Publishers, 1996, phone 800-777-2295.

Dorland's Cardiology Speller, Saunders, 2001, phone 800-545-2522.

Nomenclature and Criteria for Diagnosis of Diseases of the Heart and Great Vessels, Criteria Committee of the New York Heart Association, Lippincott Raven Publishers, 1994, phone 800-777-2295.

Stedman's Cardiology and Pulmonary Words (includes respiratory), Littrell and Stedman, Lippincott Williams & Wilkins, 2002, phone 800-527-5597.

Chiropractic

See Orthopedics.

Dentistry/Otolaryngology

Dorland's Dentistry Speller, Saunders, 2003, phone 800-545-2522.

Heinemann Dental Dictionary (British), Fairpo and Fairpo, Butterworth-Heinemann, 1997, phone 800-366-3665.

Jablonski's Dictionary of Dentistry, Jablonski, Krieger Publishing Company, 1992, phone 407-727-7270.

Stedman's Plastic Surgery, ENT and Dentistry Words, Lippincott Williams & Wilkins, 2003, phone 800-527-5597.

Dermatology

Dorland's Dermatology Word Book for Medical Transcriptionists, Saunders, 2003, phone 800-545-2522.

An Illustrated Dictionary of Dermatologic Syndromes, Mallory and Leal-Khouri, Parthenon Publishing Group, Inc., 1994, phone 800-735-4744.

Stedman's Dermatology and Immunology Words, Lippincott Williams & Wilkins, 2003, phone 800-527-5597.

Gastroenterology

Dorland's Gastroenterology Speller, Saunders, 2002, phone 800-545-2522.

Gastrointestinal Words and Phrases: A Quick Reference Guide, Health Professions Institute, 2001, phone 209-551-2112.

Stedman's GI and GU Words (includes nephrology), Lippincott Williams & Wilkins, 2002, phone 800-527-5597.

General Medicine

Churchill Livingstone's Medical Word Guide, Churchill Livingstone, 1991, phone 800-553-5426.

Current Medical Terminology, Pyle, Health Professions Institute, 2003, phone 209-551-2112.

Dorland's Medical Speller, Drake, Saunders, 2002, phone 800-545-2522.

H&P: A Nonphysician's Guide to the Medical History and Physical Examination, Dirckx, Health Professions Institute, 2001, phone 209-551-2112.

Internal Medicine Words, Danna, Rayve Productions Inc., 1997, phone 800-852-4890.

Medical Phrase Index, Lorenzini, Practice Management Information Corporation, 2000, phone 800-633-7467.

The Medical Word Book, Drake and Sloane, Saunders, 2002, phone 800-545-2522.

The Merck Manual of Diagnosis and Therapy of Diseases, Merck Publishing Group, 2003, phone 800-863-7333.

Stedman's Medical Speller, Lippincott Williams & Wilkins, 2001, phone 800-527-5597.

Stedman's Medical and Surgical Equipment Words, Lippincott Williams & Wilkins, 1996, phone 800-527-5597.

Taber's Medical Word Book with Pronunciations, F. A. Davis Company, 1990, phone 800-523-4049.

Genetics

See Neonatology/Pediatrics/Genetics.

Geriatrics/Gerontology

Key Words in Sociocultural Gerontology, Acchenbaum et al., Springer Publishing Company, 1996, phone 212-431-4370.

The Merck Manual of Geriatrics, Merck Publishing Group, 2000, phone 800-523-4049.

Stedman's Internal Medicine and Geriatric Words, Lippincott Williams & Wilkins, 2002, phone 800-527-5597.

Infectious Disease/Immunology

See also Oncology/Hematology.

AIDS Related Terminology, McIntyre and Cartwright, 1484 Old Forest Road, Pickering, Ontario, Canada, L1V 1N9.

A Dictionary of Infections and Infectious Diseases, Potparic, Parthenon Publishing Group, Inc., 1995, phone 800-735-4744.

Stedman's Dermatology and Immunology Words (includes allergy, infectious disease, rheumatology), Lippincott Williams & Wilkins, 2002, phone 800-527-5597.

Stedman's Organism and Infectious Disease Words, Lippincott Williams & Wilkins, 2002, phone 800-527-5597.

Stedman's Radiology and Oncology Words (includes hematology, HIV-AIDS), Lippincott Williams & Wilkins, 2003, phone 800-527-5597.

Neonatology/Pediatrics/Genetics

Cardiology Words and Phrases (includes cardiac imaging, cardiac surgery, cardiothoracic, cardiovascular, pediatric cardiology, pulmonary), Health Professions Institute, 1995, phone 209-551-2112.

A Dictionary of Congenital Malformations and Disorders, Potparic and Gibson, Parthenon Publishing Group, Inc., 1995, phone 800-735-4744.

Dorland's Pediatric Word Book for Medical Transcription, Saunders, 2003, phone 800-545-2522.

Neonatology Word Book, Tank and Gilliam, American Association for Medical Transcription, 1991, phone 209-551-0883 or 800-982-2182.

Stedman's OB-GYN Words (includes genetics, neonatology, pediatrics), Lippincott Williams & Wilkins, 2001, phone 800-527-5597.

Neurology/Neurosurgery

See also Orthopedics.

Orthopedic/Neurology Words and Phrases (includes chiropractic, neurosurgery, podiatry, rehabilitation), Health Professions Institute, 2000, phone 209-551-2112.

Stedman's Neurology/Neurosurgery Words, Lippincott Williams & Wilkins, 2003, phone 800-527-5597.

Obstetrics and Gynecology

Illustrated Dictionary of Obstetrics and Gynecology, Dox, Parthenon Publishing Group, Inc., 1997, phone 800-735-4744.

Dorland's Obstetric and Gynecology Word Book for Medical Transcriptionists, Saunders, 2002, phone 800-545-2522.

Obstetric-Gynecologic Terminology with Section on Neonatology and Glossary of Stedman's OB-GYN Words (includes genetics, neonatology, pediatrics), Lippincott Williams & Wilkins, 2001, phone 800-527-5597.

Stedman's OB-GYN and Genetics Words, Lippincott Williams & Wilkins, 2001, phone 800-527-5597.

Surgical Transcription in Obstetrics and Gynecology, Turrentine, Parthenon Publishing Group, Inc., 1994, phone 800-735-4744.

Oncology/Hematology

Dorland's Hematology/Oncology Speller, Saunders, 1993, phone 800-545-2522.

Handbook for Staging of Cancer: From the Manual for Staging Cancer, Beahrs, Lippincott Raven Publishers, 1995, phone 800-777-2295.

The Oncology Word Book, Littrell, F. A. Davis Company, 1993, phone 800-523-4049.

Stedman's Radiology and Oncology Words (includes hematology, HIV-AIDS), Lippincott Williams & Wilkins, 2003, phone 800-527-5597.

Ophthalmology/Optometry

Dictionary of Eye Terminology, Cassin and Solomon, Triad Publishing Company, 2001, phone 352-373-5800.

Dictionary of Optometry, Millodot, Butterworth-Heinemann, 2002, phone 800-366-2665.

Ophthalmic Drug Facts, Facts and Comparisons, 2003, phone 800-223-0554.

Ophthalmic Terminology: Speller and Vocabulary Builder, Stein et al., Mosby, Inc., 1992, phone 800-426-4545.

The Ophthalmology Word Book, Indovina and Lindh, F. A. Davis Company, 1993, phone 800-523-4049.

Physicians' Desk Reference for Ophthalmic Medicine, Medical Economics Company, 2003, phone 800-232-7379 or 800-633-7467 or 800-432-4570.

Saunders Ophthalmology Word Book, Adams, Saunders, 1991, phone 800-545-2522.

Stedman's Ophthalmology Words, Lippincott Williams & Wilkins, 2000, phone 800-527-5597.

Oral and Maxillofacial Surgery

American Society of Oral Surgeons: The Oral and Maxillofacial Surgery Procedural Terminology with Glossary, American Society of Oral Surgeons, 1975, phone 847-678-6200.

Orthopedics

Dorland's Orthopedic Word Book for Medical Transcriptionists, Saunders, 2002, phone 800-545-2522.

A Manual of Orthopaedic Terminology, Blauvelt and Nelson, Mosby, Inc., 1998, phone 800-426-4545.

Melloni's Illustrated Dictionary of the Musculoskeletal System, Melloni and Dox, Parthenon Publishing Group, 1998, phone 800-735-4744.

Musculoskeletal Anatomy, Colborn and Lause, Parthenon Publishing Group, 1993, phone 800-735-4744.

Orthopaedic Dictionary, Hoppenfeld, Lippincott Raven Publishers, 1993, phone 800-777-2295.

Orthopedic/Neurology Words and Phrases (includes chiropractic, neurosurgery, podiatry, rehabilitation), Health Professions Institute, 2000, phone 209-551-2112.

Stedman's Orthopaedic and Rehab Words (includes chiropractic, occupational therapy, physical therapy, podiatry), Lippincott Williams & Wilkins, 2002, phone 800-527-5597.

Otolaryngology

See Dentistry/Otolaryngology.

Pathology/Laboratory Medicine/Bacteriology

Bergey's Bacteriology Words, Lippincott Williams & Wilkins, 1993, phone 800-638-0672.

Diagnostic Procedure Handbook, Golish et al., Lippincott Williams & Wilkins, 1992, phone 800-527-5597.

Dorland's Laboratory/Pathology Word Book for the Medical Transcriptionist, Saunders, 2003, phone 800-545-2522.

Interpretation of Diagnostic Tests: A Handbook Synopsis of Laboratory Medicine, Wallach, Lippincott Raven Publishers, 1986, phone 800-777-2295.

Laboratory and Diagnostic Tests: A Pocket Guide, McMurrow and Malarkey, Saunders, 1998, phone 800-545-2522.

Laboratory Medicine: Essentials of Anatomic and Clinical Pathology, Dirckx, Health Professions Institute, 1995, phone 209-551-2112.

Laboratory Test Handbook, Jacobs et al., Lippincott Williams & Wilkins, 2001, phone 800-527-5597.

Laboratory Tests and Diagnostic Procedures, Chernecky et al., Saunders, 1996, phone 800-545-2522.

Laboratory/Pathology Words and Phrases, Health Professions Institute, 1996, phone 209-551-2112.

A Manual of Laboratory and Diagnostic Tests, Fischbach, Lippincott Raven Publishers, 2003, phone 800-777-2295.

Stedman's Pathology and Lab Medicine Words, Lippincott Williams & Wilkins, 2002, phone 800-527-5597.

A Word Book in Pathology and Laboratory Medicine, Sloane and Dusseau, Saunders, 1995, phone 800-545-2522.

Pediatrics

See Neonatology/Pediatrics/Genetics.

Physical Therapy

See Rehabilitation/Physical Therapy/Occupational Therapy.

Podiatry

See Orthopedics.

Psychiatry/Psychology

American Psychiatric Glossary, Stone, American Psychiatric Press, Inc., 2003, phone 800-368-5777.

Diagnostic and Statistical Manual of Mental Disorders (DSM-IV), American Psychiatric Association, 1994, phone 800-368-5777.

Dorland's Psychiatry and Psychology Speller, Saunders, 1993, phone 800-545-2522.

Psychiatric Dictionary, Campbell, Oxford University Press, 2002, phone 800-451-7556.

Psychiatric Words and Phrases, D'Onofrio and D'Onofrio, Health Professions Institute, 1997, phone 209-551-2112.

The Psychiatry Word Book with Street Talk Terms, Forbis, F. A. Davis Company, 1993, phone 800-523-4049.

Stedman's Psychiatry Words, Lippincott Williams & Wilkins, 2002, phone 800-638-0672.

Pulmonology

See Cardiology/Pulmonology.

Radiology/Imaging

Cardiology Words and Phrases (includes cardiac imaging, cardiac surgery, cardiothoracic, cardiovascular, pediatric cardiology, pulmonary), Health Professions Institute, 1995, phone 209-551-2112.

Diagnostic Procedures Handbook, Mishod, Lippincott Williams & Wilkins, 2001, phone 800-638-0672.

Dorland's Radiology/Oncology Word Book for Medical Transcriptionists, Saunders, 2001, phone 800-545-2522.

Glossary of MR Terms, American College of Radiology, 1995, phone 800-227-7762.

Radiology/Imaging Words and Phrases, Health Professions Institute, 1997, phone 209-551-2112.

Stedman's Radiology and Oncology Words (includes hematology, HIV-AIDS), Lippincott Williams & Wilkins, 2003, phone 800-527-5597.

A Word Book in Radiology with Anatomic Plates and Tables, Sloane, Saunders, 1988, phone 800-545-2522.

Rehabilitation/Physical Therapy/Occupational Therapy

Key Words in Physical Rehabilitation, Cammack and Eisenberg, Springer Publishing Company, 1996, phone 212-431-4370.

Orthopedic/Neurology Words and Phrases (includes chiropractic, neurosurgery, podiatry, rehabilitation), Health Professions Institute, 2000, phone 209-551-2112.

Rehabilitation Specialist's Handbook, Wolf et al., F. A. Davis Company, 1998, phone 800-523-4049.

Stedman's Orthopaedic and Rehab Words (includes chiropractic, occupational therapy, physical therapy, podiatry), Lippincott Williams & Wilkins, 2002, phone 800-527-5597.

Sports Medicine

See Orthopedics.

Surgery/Anesthesia

Diagnostic Procedures Handbook, Mishod, Lippincott Williams & Wilkins, 2001, phone 800-257-5597.

Dorland's Medical Equipment Word Book for Medical Transcriptionists, Saunders, 2003, phone 800-545-2522.

Encyclopedia of Anesthesia Practice, Yentis et al., Butterworth-Heinemann, 1996, phone 800-366-2665.

General Surgery/GI Words and Phrases, Health Professions Institute, 2001, phone 209-551-2112.

Illustrated Guide to Instrumentation for the Operating Room: A Photographic Manual, Brooks-Tighe, Mosby, Inc., 1994, phone 800-426-4545.

Instrumentation for the Operating Room, Tighe, Mosby, Inc., 1999, phone 800-545-2522.

Stedman's Medical Equipment Words, Lippincott Williams & Wilkins, 2002, phone 800-527-5597.

Stedman's Surgery Words, Lippincott Williams & Wilkins, 2002, phone 800-527-5597.

Surgical Technology: Principles and Practice, Fuller, Saunders, 1993, phone 800-545-2522.

Surgical Transcription in Obstetrics and Gynecology, Turrentine, Parthenon Publishing Group, 1994, phone 800-735-4744.
The Surgical Word Book, Tessier, Saunders, 2003, phone 800-545-2522.
A Syllabus for the Surgeon's Secretary, Szulec and Szulec, Medical Arts Publishing, 1990, phone 313-886-5160.
Synopsis of Common Surgical Procedures, Bodai, Lippincott Williams & Wilkins, 1993, phone 800-638-0672.

Urology

OB and Genitourinary Words and Phrases, Health Professions Institute, 2002, phone 209-551-2112.
Stedman's GI and GU Words (includes nephrology), Lippincott Williams & Wilkins, 2002, phone 800-527-5597.

37–26 SPELLING BOOKS, ENGLISH

One Word, Two Words, Hyphenated? Gilman, National Court Reporters Association, 1992, phone 800-272-6272.

37–27 SPELLING BOOKS, MEDICAL

NOTE: *See lists under each medical specialty.*

Current Medical Terminology, Pyle, Health Professions Institute, 2003, phone 209-551-2112.
For Your Information, Taylor and Collins, PO Box 1842, Santa Ana, CA 92702, FYI Book Co., 1991.
Medical Phrase Index, Lorenzini, Practice Management Information Corporation, 2001, phone 800-633-7467.
The Medical Word Book, Sloane and Drake, Saunders, 2002, phone 800-545-2522.
Webster's Medical Speller, Merriam-Webster Editorial Staff, Merriam-Webster, Inc., 1995, phone 800-828-1880.

37–28 STANDARDS

See also Law and Ethics.
AAMT Book of Style for Medical Transcriptionists, American Association for Medical Transcription, 2002, phone 800-982-2182.
Annual Book of ASTM Standards, Vol. 14.01: Healthcare Informatics: Computerized Material and Chemical Property Databases, American Society for Testing and Materials, 1997, phone 610-832-9500.
Comprehensive Accreditation Manual for Hospitals: The Official Handbook, Joint Commission on Accreditation of Healthcare Organizations, 2003, phone 630-916-5600.
HIPAA Compliance Alert, DecisionHealth (monthly), phone 877-602-3835.

HIPAA for MTs 2002, American Association for Medical Transcription, phone 800-982-2182.

HIPAA Guidelines Policy and Procedure Manual, hcPro, 2002, phone 800-639-8511.

In Confidence, American Health Information Management Association (bimonthly newsletter), phone 800-335-5535.

Information Management: The Compliance Guide to the Joint Commission on Accreditation of Healthcare Organizations Standards, Cofer et al., Opus Communications, 2000, phone 800-650-6787.

Law and Ethics for Health Occupations, Judson and Blesie, Glencoe/McGraw-Hill Book, 1994, phone 800-334-7344.

Law, Liability and Ethics for Medical Office Professionals, Flight, Delmar Publishers/ITP, 1998, phone 800-347-7707.

Legal and Ethical Issues in Health Occupations, Aiken, Saunders, 2002, phone 800-545-2522.

Medical Law and Ethics, Lipman, Brady Prentice-Hall, 2002, phone 800-223-1360.

Medicolegal Forms with Legal Analysis, American Medical Association, 1997, phone 800-621-8335.

Standard Guide for the Training of Persons Who Have Access to Health Information: E1988, American Society for Testing and Materials, phone 610-832-9500.

Standard Guide for Electronic Authentication of Health Care Information: E1762-95, ASTM Subcommittee E31.20, American Society for Testing and Materials, 1995, phone 610-832-9500.

Standard Guide for View of Emergency Medical Care in the Computerized Patient Record: E1744-95, ASTM Subcommittee E31.12, American Society for Testing and Materials, 1998, phone 610-832-9500.

SYNONYMS

See Antonyms, Eponyms, Homonyms, Syndromes, and Synonyms.

37–29 TEACHING MEDICAL TRANSCRIPTION

Advanced Medical Transcription: A Modular Approach, Destafano and Federman, Saunders, 2003, phone 800-545-2522.

Delmar's Medical Transcription Handbook, Blake, Delmar Learning, 1998, phone 800-998-7498.

Diehl and Fordney's Medical Transcription: Techniques and Procedures, 5th edition, Diehl, Saunders, 2002, phone 800-545-2522.

Essentials of Medical Transcription: A Modular Approach, Destafano and Federman, Saunders, 2003, phone 800-545-2522.

Exploring Transcription Practice Modules in General Medicine (1995), *General Surgery* (1996), *Skillbuilding in Medicine/Surgery* (2003), *Skillbuilding in Radiology* (2003), *Skillbuilding with Accents* (2003), American Association for Medical Transcription, phone 800-982-2182.

How to Become a Medical Transcriptionist, Morton, Medical Language Development, 1998, phone 609-924-2403.

Instructor's Manual for Diehl and Fordney's Medical Transcription: Techniques and Procedures, 5th edition, Diehl, Saunders, 2002, phone 800-545-2522.

Medical Transcription: Fundamentals and Practice, HPI, Prentice Hall Health, 1999, phone 800-445-6991.

Medical Transcription: Instructor's Guide, Ettinger and Ettinger, EMC Paradigm Publishing, 1997, phone 800-535-6865.

Medical Transcription Career Handbook, Drake, Prentice-Hall Health, 2002 phone 800-445-6991.

Medical Transcription Guide Do's and Don'ts, Diehl, Saunders, 2005, phone 800-545-2522.

Medical Transcription Text, Ettinger and Ettinger, EMC Paradigm Publishing, 1997, phone 800-535-6865.

The Medical Transcription Workbook, Health Professions Institute, 1999, phone 209-551-2112.

The Model Curriculum for Medical Transcription, American Association for Medical Transcription, 1988, phone 209-551-0883.

The SUM Program: Beginning, Advanced, Surgery, Cardiology, Gastroenterology, Orthopedics, Pathology, Radiology, Health Professions Institute, 2003, phone 209-551-2112.

The Teachers Manual, Campbell and Drake, Health Professions Institute, 1998, phone 209-551-2112.

37–30 WEB SITES

Medical Information on the Internet, Kiley, Elsevier Science, 2003, phone 215-238-7869.

About.com (pharmaceutical): http://www.pharmacology.about.com/health/pharmacology

American Association of Medical Assistants: www.aama-ntl.org

American Association for Medical Transcription: http://www.aamt.org/aamt

American Health Information Management Association: www.ahima.org

American Medical Association: www.ama-assn.org

American Medical Informatics Association: www.amia.org

Association for At-Home MTs: www.mtdaily.com/aahmt.html

ASTM International: www.astm.org

Big Dog Grammar: http://aliscot.com/bigdog/index/htm

The Blue Book of Grammar and Punctuation:
www.grammarbook.com
Doctor's Guide to the Internet: www.docguide.com
Gilbert Medical Transcription Service:
http://gmts.com/resources.html
Guide to Grammar and Writing:
http://www.ccc.commnet.edu/grammar
Health Professions Institute: http://www.hpisum.com
Medical Online Glossaries and Resources:
www.interfold.com/translator/medsites.htm
MedPlanet (medical products): www.medplant.com
Medword (links to services and schools):
www.medword.com/mtlist.html
Mary Morken, Web Monitor, a Networking Center: MT
Daily I: http://angelfire.com/mt and MT Daily II:
http://angelfire.com/mt2/next.html
Medical Transcription Industrial Alliance:
http://www.wwma.com/a2/mtia/
The Online English Grammar:
www.edunet.com/english/grammar
Praxis.md: http://praxis.md

37–31 WORD DIVISION

The Medical and Health Sciences Word Book, Hafer,
Houghton Mifflin Company, 1992, phone 800-225-3362
or 671-351-3500.
Medical Word Finder, Willeford, Brady Prentice-Hall, 1983,
phone 800-223-1360.
*Ten Thousand Medical Words, Spelled and Divided for Quick
Reference,* Byers, McGraw-Hill Book Company, 1972,
phone 800-722-4726.
Twenty Thousand Words, Zoubek, Glencoe/McGraw-Hill
Book Company, 1996, phone 800-334-7344.
Webster's Medical Speller, Merriam-Webster Editorial Staff,
Merriam-Webster, Inc., 1995, phone 800-828-1880.
The Word Book III, American Heritage Dictionary Editors,
Houghton Mifflin Company, 1990, phone 800-225-3362
or 671-351-5000.

37–32 WRITING, SCIENTIFIC AND TECHNICAL

Clear Technical Writing, Brogan, McGraw-Hill Book
Company, 1973, phone 800-722-4726.
Technical Communication: A Practical Guide, Dagher, Brady
Prentice-Hall, 1978, phone 800-223-1360.
Words Into Type, Warren, Brady Prentice-Hall, 1992, phone
800-223-1360.

38

Rules to Transcribe By

38–1   CONTINUING EDUCATION

✓ DO   keep learning.

⊘ DON'T   pass up an opportunity to acquire a new reference book.

✓ DO   network with other medical transcriptionist professionals.

✓ DO   become certified in this profession.

✓ DO   attend meetings, symposia, and conferences to keep abreast of new techniques, laws, materials, equipment, and so on.

38–2   CYBERSPACE

✓ DO   check the professional associations' Web sites for new information.

⊘ DON'T   believe everything you read on the Internet. It provides a wealth of information, but it is unregulated.

38–3   DICTATOR/AUTHOR/EMPLOYER

DO   carry out the wishes of your employer even if they conflict with methods you view as correct.

38–4   ETHICS, ETIQUETTE, AND LEGAL RESPONSIBILITIES (see also Chapter 18, p. 185, HIPAA Guidelines)

DO   educate yourself to conduct your business by the highest standard for patient privacy.

DO   take care that all patient identification information is secure at all times.

DO   complete work on a timely basis so as not to compromise patient care.

DO   avoid using the patient's name in other than the heading and/or footing of a document.

DO   be aware that you are a vital part of the continuity of care in the health care environment.

DO   use diligence to prevent a critical error.

DO   flag any questionable or unclear dictation.

DO   conduct yourself as a professional at all times.

DO   be courteous and dependable.

DO   be a team player.

DO   associate with positive people.

DO   assist others graciously when asked. *(You never know when you might be the one who needs help.)*

DON'T   laugh at anyone else's mistakes.

DON'T   transcribe inflammatory remarks. Bring them to the attention of your supervisor.

DON'T   criticize your employer.

38–5   GRAMMAR AND PUNCTUATION

DO   learn to punctuate properly and check your work carefully.

✔ **DO**   be aware of and on the lookout for homonyms.

🚫 **DON'T**   use a punctuation mark without a reason. When in doubt, leave it out.

38–6   GROOMING

✔ **DO**   dress in a well-groomed manner, attractively and appropriately.

38–7   PERSONALITY

✔ **DO**   be flexible and keep a learning attitude.

✔ **DO**   maintain a sense of humor; learn to laugh at yourself.

🚫 **DON'T**   take yourself too seriously.

🚫 **DON'T**   get discouraged; everyone has a bad day every once in awhile.

🚫 **DON'T**   act like you know everything.

🚫 **DON'T**   point out others' mistakes.

✔ **DO**   try to make your coworkers and employer look good.

✔ **DO**   be prepared to be wrong some of the time.

38–8   PROOFREADING AND EDITING

✔ **DO**   proofread carefully.

🚫 **DON'T**   guess.

✔ **DO**   edit to correct grammatical errors.

✔ **DO**   flag and verify all unknown words.

✔ **DO**   leave a blank and a flag when you don't know or can't hear a word.

✔ **DO**   view your document before printing it.

38–9   RESPONSIBILITY

✔ **DO**   produce the best work of which you are capable.

DO feel a sense of responsibility for the accuracy of the medical record.

DO know and abide by the HIPAA regulations governing your work. *(See Chapter 18, HIPAA Guidelines.)*

38–10 SPELLING

DO use the spell checker before printing.

DON'T depend on the spell checker.

DO make a rule for yourself to check every unfamiliar term with a dictionary.

DO remember that reference books may be in seeming conflict with each other, but there may be more than one way to do something correctly.

DON'T assume that the most prestigious of reference books cannot include an error.

DON'T assume anything—verify everything.

38–11 TRANSCRIPTION TECHNIQUES

DO keep a transcriptionist's notebook and use it faithfully. *(See Figure 38–1 at the end of the chapter).*

DO remember that everything you transcribe is for one person: the patient.

DO be careful about abbreviations. *(See Chapter 1, Abbreviations and Symbols, and the Appendix.)*

DO spell out most brief forms.

DO use the metric system properly. *(See Chapter 26, Metric System.)*

DON'T sacrifice quality for quantity.

DO ask questions.

DO remember that practice makes perfect.

DON'T use a method simply because "we've always done it this way."

✓ DO   be consistent, complete, and correct.

✓ DO   complete documents in a timely manner.

✓ DO   use diligence to prevent a critical error.

✓ DO   learn how to do research quickly and effectively. *(See Chapter 37, Reference Materials and Publications.)*

✓ DO   trust that you can and will be very good at this profession.

---

m-<u>AMSA</u>

<u>M</u>anschot implant

<u>M</u>antoux

<u>maxilla</u> (s)
<u>maxillae</u> (p)

medication-resistant

<u>M</u>ellaril-<u>S</u>

milieu (mee-Loo)

<u>M</u>ill-house murmur

mucous (a)
mucus (n)

Figure 38–1   Page M from an alphabetical pocket-sized transcriptionist's notebook showing the capital letters underlined for emphasis and the following entries: an unusual abbreviation for a drug name, an eponym for a device, an eponym for a test, a singular-plural guide, a hyphenated adjective, a compound brand name for a drug, a French term with pronouncing help, an unusual eponym, and an adjective-noun guide, respectively.

39

Semicolon

INTRODUCTION

Think of a semicolon as stronger than a comma but weaker than a period. There are just four rules for using a semicolon, but when you need to use it, no other mark will suffice.

39–1 INDEPENDENT CLAUSE WITH NO CONJUNCTION

✓ DO use a semicolon to separate two or more closely related independent clauses when no conjunction is used.

You have requested our cooperation; we have complied.

The nose is remarkable for loud congestive breathing; there is no discharge visible.

NOTE: *Usually, you can also use a period and make two sentences. However, because of the nature of the two independent clauses, the break with the period disrupts the link between the two.*

The nose is remarkable for loud congestive breathing. There is no discharge visible.

OPTION: *You can use a comma to separate two independent clauses when the sentences are very brief and closely related.*

She was in today for followup exam, she was doing well.

39–2 INDEPENDENT CLAUSE HEAVILY PUNCTUATED

☑ DO   use a semicolon to separate independent clauses if either one or both of them have been punctuated with two or more commas.

Around the first of July, he developed pain in his chest, which he ignored for several days; and, finally, he saw me, at the request of his family doctor, on July 16.

39–3 SERIES WITH PUNCTUATION

☑ DO   use a semicolon for clarity between a series of phrases or clauses if any item in the series has internal commas.

Among those present at the Utilization Committee Meeting were Dr. Frank Byron, chief-of-staff; Mrs. Joan Armath, administrator; Ms. Nancy Speeth, medical records technician; and Mr. Ralph Johnson, director of nurses.

Medications: He will continue his 1800-calorie ADA diet and usual medicines, which include estradiol 2 mg/d, for 25 of 30 days; flurazepam HCl 30 mg at bedtime; hydrocodone bitartrate 5 mg; and ibuprofen 600 mg q.i.d.

39–4 WITH QUOTATION MARKS AND PARENTHESES

☑ DO   place the semicolon outside quotation marks and parentheses.

39–5 WITH TRANSITIONAL EXPRESSIONS

☑ DO   use a semicolon *before* a transitional expression when it is used to join two independent clauses. *(These are also called conjunctive adverbs and parenthetical expressions.)*

She will be followed by Dr. Abbott; therefore, a copy of her records needs to be forwarded to his office.

☑ DO   use a comma *after* the expression when the expression is composed of two or more syllables.

I attempted a labor induction with Pitocin, and contractions occurred; however, the patient did not develop an effective labor pattern, and I discharged her after eight hours.

NOTE: *Some of the most common conjunctive adverbs used as transitional expressions are* accordingly, also, anyhow, besides, consequently, on the contrary, furthermore, however, indeed, likewise, moreover, nevertheless, otherwise, similarly, still, then, therefore, *and* thus.

40

Slang Expressions and Unusual Medical Terms

INTRODUCTION

Sometimes an author will dictate an unusual expression that may puzzle you, and you may try to find it in a medical or English reference book. Chances are you will not find the expression and will type the phrase the way you heard it and/or flag it for the physician to double-check. *(See also Chapter 11, Editing.)*

✓ **DO**   check with your supervisor before transcribing or editing questionable slang.

> The patient was stupid, a crock (hypochondriac), and boorish.

✓ **DO**   contact the dictator and diplomatically and tactfully question his or her use of the slang or unprofessional expression before it becomes a permanent part of the patient's medical record.

40–1   ACRONYMS

✓ **DO**   spell out acronyms in most medical reports.

Dictated:
The patient was CABGed.
Transcribed:
The patient had a coronary artery bypass graft.
Correct:
Caloric testing produced COWS. (COWS *refers to the Hallpike caloric stimulation response that stands for* cold to the opposite, warm to the same.)

See 1–24, When Not to Abbreviate, in Chapter 1 for rules on when abbreviations and acronyms are inappropriate.

40–2 BRIEF FORMS

See the list in the Appendix of Brief Forms, Short Forms, and Medical Slang. Items shown without an asterisk may be used as is unless they might be misread or misinterpreted in the medical report or chart note. See also Chapter 4, Brief Forms, Short Forms, and Medical Slang.

40–3 FLAGGING QUERIES

DO   flag, tag, or mark a slang expression if you cannot translate the slang term in full, and leave a blank. Attach a note to the transcript with a brief description of where the blank is located. *(See Figure 11–1 at the end of Chapter 11.)*

40–4 PUNCTUATION

 DO   use quotation marks to enclose slang, coined, awkward, whimsical, or humorous words that might show ignorance on the part of the writer if it is not known that he or she is aware of them.

See if you can schedule a few "well" patients for a change.

If you have "clergyman's knee," "tailor's seat," "tennis elbow," or "trigger finger," what you really have is a form of bursitis or tendinitis.

40–5 SLANG TERMS

Some of the unusual terms commonly dictated in medical reports are listed in the Appendix to help you through puzzling dictation. These dictated words and phrases are usually typed as shown.

 DO   translate slang terms in full when dictated.

Appy should be typed as *appendectomy.*
Cathed should be typed as *catheterized.*
Dex should be typed as *dexamethasone.*
H. flu should be typed as *H. influenzae* or *Haemophilus influenzae.*
Lab may be typed as *laboratory* or *lab.*
Lytes should be typed as *electrolytes.*

 DO   edit slang words and phrases.

Incorrect:
She arrived in the ED with a hot appy.

Correct:
She arrived in the ED with acute appendicitis.
Incorrect:
Mrs. Becker's temp was 102°.
Correct:
Mrs. Becker's temperature was 102°.
Incorrect:
At the end of surgery, I introduced an intracath.
Correct:
At the end of surgery, I introduced an intravenous catheter.

41

Slash

INTRODUCTION

The *slash* is also called the *diagonal, bar, virgule, slant,* or *solidus.* The slash is typed with no space on either side. We generally mean the forward slash (/) when discussing the use of the slash.

41–1   BACKWARD SLASH (\)

 DO   use the backward slash as indicated in certain computer commands. It is generally not used in everyday keyboarding.

c: \format a:
a: \JONES\CASES\

41–2   FRACTIONS

 DO   use the slash to write fractions.

2/3   1 1/2

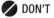 **DON'T**   mix case fractions and those made by typing each number.

Incorrect:
They measured out at ¼, 1/3, ½
Correct:
They measured out at 1/4, 1/3, 1/2.

41–3   SEPARATING CERTAIN TECHNICAL TERMS

 DO   use the slash in writing certain technical terms. The slash sometimes substitutes for the words *per, to,* or *over.*

She has 20/20 vision. *(separates the indicators of visual acuity)*

His blood pressure is 120/80. *(120 over 80)*

Grade 2/4 systolic murmur *(takes the place of the word over)*

The dosage is 50 mg/d. *(milligrams per day)*

Please note the A/B ratio. *(A to B)*

DON'T   use the slash in place of *per* with words.

Incorrect:
He has been smoking three packs of cigarettes/day.
Correct:
He has been smoking three packs of cigarettes per day.
Correct:
Turn it a centimeter per day.
or
Turn it 1 cm/d.

DO   use the slash or the hyphen to separate the parts of a date when dating documents. Use the date spelled out in full in text material.

4-6-XX *(for dating documents)*
04-06-XX *(for dating documents)*
4/6/XX *(for dating documents)*
April 6, 200X *(for dating text material)*

DON'T   use the slash to express a ratio. *(See 27–20, Ratios and Ranges, in Chapter 27.)*

Incorrect:
Serum was diluted 1/200,000.
Correct:
Serum was diluted 1:200,000.
Incorrect:
A 1/2 dilute solution was used.
Correct:
A 1:2 dilute solution was used.

✓ DO use the slash in making the abbreviation for the expression *in care of* in an address.

Ms. Margot Hunter
c/o J. B. Marsh
2387 First Street
La Mesa, CA 92041

41-4 WEB SITE

✓ DO use two slashes to separate the Web site command from the Web site address.

http://www.gccd.cc.ca.us

✓ DO use the slash to separate the file name path from the Web site address.

www.gccd.cc.ca.us/grossmont

41-5 WORD CHOICE

✓ DO use the slash to offer word choice.

and/or   he/she   his/her
plus/minus   +/–
Mr./Mrs./Miss/Ms.

42 ■ Sound Variations of Syllables *see Appendix J*

Spacing with Punctuation Marks

42–1 *NO SPACE*

Following a period within an abbreviation
Following a period used as a decimal point
Between quotation marks and the quoted material
Before or after a hyphen
Before or after a slash
Before or after a dash *(two hyphens)*
Between parentheses and the enclosed material
Between any word and the punctuation following it
Between the number and the colon used to indicate a dilute solution or ratio
On either side of the colon when expressing the time of day
Before an apostrophe
Before or after a comma used within numbers
Before or after an ampersand in abbreviations *(e.g., l&w)*
On either side of the colon when expressing ratios
After the closing parenthesis if another mark of punctuation follows.

Correct	**Incorrect**
25 mg%	25 mg %
98.8°	98.8 °
98.8°F	98.8° F

42–2 *ONE SPACE*

Between words
After a comma
After a semicolon
After a period following an initial
After the closing parenthesis
Between numbers and the abbreviation following

On each side of the x in an expression of dimension
(*e.g.,* 2 ×2)
q.4 h. *not* q.4h.
15 mg *not* 15mg
125 lb *not* 125lb

42–3 TWO SPACES

After a period, question mark, or exclamation point at the
end of a sentence *(optional)*
After a quotation mark at the end of a sentence *(optional)*
After a colon *(optional)* except when used with the time of
day or when expressing a dilute solution

NOTE: *Widespread use of computers and word processors has led
to a common practice of leaving only one space after a colon and
when closing a sentence, that is, after a period, question mark,
and exclamation mark. Do what is comfortable for you.*

43

Spelling

INTRODUCTION

Most word processing computer programs include an ability to spell-check individual words and entire documents as well as allow the user to add words to an electronic dictionary. The user may search for a word on screen while working in a document. However, errors may occur when a spell-check provides a noun when an adjective is needed. The spell-checker only alerts the user to misspelled words; users must refer to dictionaries or drug books to ensure that the proper word is selected and makes sense.

 DO   verify the spelling of a word in an English or medical dictionary when you have any doubt about the accuracy of the spelling.

 DON'T   accept the spelling of a word given by the author or anyone else unless you know the spelling is correct or have checked it in a reference source.

DO   use the medical spelling of a word when there is a difference between spellings given by the medical dictionary and the English dictionary. *(See also 43–16, Words Spelled in More Than One Way, for examples.)*

> **Dorland's:**
> distention *(use this one)*
> **Webster's:**
> distension or distention

43–1   ANATOMIC WORDS

 DO   type out English and Latin names of anatomic parts as dictated.

abductor hallucis muscle   basalis vein
femoralis nerve   infraorbitalis artery

43–2   BRITISH WORDS

When submitting a manuscript to a British journal, these rules may come in handy for reference, since words in the manuscript must conform to British rules. In addition, all names of drugs mentioned in the manuscript must also be listed according to the drug name as known in Great Britain.

 DO   spell the suffix *ize* as *ise* when pronounced *eyes*.

American	British
rationalize	rationalise
rationalization	rationalisation

 DO   use the preferred spelling for the suffix *er* as *re*.

American	British
theater	theatre
meter	metre
center	centre
liter	litre
fiber	fibre

 DO   use the preferred spelling for the suffix *or* as *our*.

American	British
color	colour
humor	humour
labor	labour
honor	honour
vigor	vigour

✓ DO   use the preferred spelling for the suffix *lyze* as *lyse*.

American	British
analyze	analyse

✓ DO   include an internal *e* when words are derived from stems ending in a silent *e* and adding *able* or *ment*.

American	British
likable	likeable
judgment	judgement

EXCEPTION: *Lovable* (British spelling)

✓ DO   watch doubling or nondoubling of consonants.

American	British
fulfill	fulfil
skillful	skilful

✓ DO   watch variances in spelling that differ in phonetic sounds.

American	British
jail	gaol
curb	kerb
mold	mould

✓ DO   use British digraphs *ae* and *oe* for medical terms.

American	British
anesthesia	anaesthesia
orthopedic	orthopaedic
hematology	haematology
esophagus	oesophagus
rectocele	rectocoele

✓ DO   note that the spelling of some British technical words without digraph elements differs from the American spelling.

American	British
aluminum	aluminium

✓ DO   spell titles and proper names when mentioned in text or tables or cited in references by retaining their original spelling.

Haemophilus influenzae (American and British spelling)

✅ DO   consult *Butterworth's Medical Dictionary, Chambers 20th Century Dictionary,* or *International Dictionary of Medicine and Biology* for British spelling.

43–3   COMPOUND WORDS
See Chapter 8, Compounds.

43–4   DIACRITICAL MARKS

✅ DO   add an *e* if your word processor or computer software cannot place an *umlaut* (¨) over *a, o,* or *u.*

Pötzsch   Poetzsch

 DON'T   add an accent mark to most English words taken from French, Spanish, or other foreign languages.

apropos	boutonniere	cabana
cafe	coupe	facade
matinee	melee	puree
role	smorgasbord	
soiree	vicuna	

✅ DO   key the following foreign words with their accents (`) (´) (˜):

à la carte	passé
à la mode	pâté
attaché	père
cause célèbre	piéce de résistance
chargé d'affaires	pied-à-terre
mañana	touché
outré	vis-à-vis

✅ DO   key these French phrases with a circumflex (^):

bête noire	raison d'être
maître d'hôtel	table d'hôte
pâté	tête-à-tête

43–5   DRUG NAMES
See Chapter 10, Drugs and Drug References.

43–6   ELECTRONIC SPELL CHECKING

✓ DO   use your word processing computer program to spell-check individual words and entire documents. *(You can add words to an electronic dictionary and search for a word on screen while working in a document.)*

NOTE: *Errors may occur when a spell-check provides a noun when an adjective is needed. The spell-checker only alerts the user to misspelled words; users must refer to dictionaries or drug books to ensure that the proper word is selected and makes sense.*

43–7   EPONYMS
See Chapter 14, Eponyms.

43–8   FRENCH MEDICAL WORDS

✓ DO   take special care in spelling French medical words because different sounds are given to the letters. *(See also Rule 43–4, Diacritical Marks, and Appendix D for a list of French medical words.)*

43–9   HOMONYMS

✓ DO   look up the meaning of English and medical homonyms to end confusion and help you decide how to spell them. Homonyms sound the same but have different meanings. *(See also Appendix F, Homonyms and Sound-alike Words.)*

mucus, mucous	vesicle, vesical
too, to, two	site, cite, sight
raise, raze	principal, principle

43–10   NOUNS TO VERBS

✓ DO   use an English rule to spell a verb that the dictator has created from a noun or trade name.

Bovie *(trade name)*	bovied *(verb)*
Hyfrecator *(trade name)*	hyfrecated *(verb)*
pedicle *(noun)*	pedicleized *(verb)*

NOTE: *A coined expression may not be acceptable, as shown in the following example.*

Correct:
Mrs. Davis was given diuretics.
Incorrect:
Mrs. Davis was diuresed.

NOTE: *Some physicians have coined verbs from acronyms. These should usually be spelled out in full regardless of the dictation.*

Dictated:
The patient was admitted with severe precordial pain and cardiac arrhythmias and was romied. *(R = rule, O = out, M = myocardial, I = infarction)*
Corrected version:
The patient was admitted with severe precordial pain and cardiac arrhythmias. Treatment plan is to rule out a myocardial infarct.
Dictated:
The patient was CABG'd. *(C = coronary, A = artery, B = bypass, G = graft)*
Corrected version:
The patient had a coronary artery bypass graft.
Dictated:
Blood had proetzed into the sinus cavity. *(from Proetz method of injecting fluid by pressure into a cavity)*
Corrected version
Blood had forcefully hemorrhaged into the sinus cavity.

NOTE: *The medical transcriptionist has the responsibility to edit dictation so that it is accurate, complete, clear, and consistent.* (See Chapter 11, Editing.)

43–11   ONE WORD, TWO WORDS, OR HYPHENATED
See also Chapter 20, Hyphen Use and Word Division, or obtain one of the following books: *Look It Up: A Deskbook of American Spelling and Style* by Rudolf Flesch, Harper & Row, Publishers, New York, New York, 1977; *One Word, Two Words, Hyphenated?* by Mary Louise Gilman, National Shorthand Reporters Association, Vienna, Virginia, 1998.

See Appendix F, Homonyms and Sound-alike Words, for words commonly encountered.

43–12   PLURALS
See Chapter 31, Plural Forms, and Appendix I, Plural Forms.

43–13   REFERENCES FOR SPELLING WORDS
See Chapter 37, Reference Materials and Publications.

43–14   SILENT CONSONANTS

✓ DO   See Appendix J, Sound Variations of Syllables, to learn spelling possibilities for silent consonants so that a word can be located in the medical dictionary. Examples of words with silent consonants include:

Spelling at beginning of word	Phonetic Sound	Example
pn	n	pneumonia *(nu-MO-ne-ah)*
ps	s	psychiatric *(si″ke-AT-rik)*
ps	s	psoriatic *(sor-e-AT-ik)*
pn	n	pneumal *(new′mall)*
pt	t	ptosis *(TO-sis)*
pt	t	ptarmus *(TAR-mis)*
ct	t	ctetology *(te-TOL-o-je)*
cn	n	cnemis *(NE-mis)*
gn	n	gnathalgia *(nath-AL-je-ah)*
mn	n	mnemonic *(ne-MON-ik)*
kn	n	knuckle *(NUK-l)*
eu	you	euphoria *(u-FOR-e-ah)*

NOTE: *Notice the silent g in phlegm* (flem) *and the silent h in hemorrhoid* (HEM-o-roid).

43–15   SLANG AND UNUSUAL MEDICAL TERMS
See Chapter 40, Slang Expressions and Unusual Medical Terms.

43–16   WORDS SPELLED IN MORE THAN ONE WAY

✓ DO   type words spelled in more than one way according to the preferred style of your employer. If there is no preference, use the most popular and current spelling of the medical term. The first column depicts the most common spelling; the second column gives optional acceptable spelling.

Preferred	Alternative
aneurysm	aneurism
curet	curette
disk	disc
dysfunction	disfunction
fontanel	fontanelle
leukocyte	leucocyte
venipuncture	venepuncture

44

Symbols

INTRODUCTION

Symbols are just another form of abbreviation. Most standard symbols can be accessed when using word processing computer software.

Symbols can be inserted by using commands involving the keypad numbers, the keyboard numbers, or the pull-down menu. Most figures you want to use are illustrated in this chapter. The procedure varies, depending on your system. You might press *Alt* plus the number on the number pad, not the keyboard. The character does not appear until the Alt key is released. Some programs use a combination of pressing option + shift + some letter-number combinations on the keyboard. You will learn which method is provided by your software. Here are some examples of a program that uses the Alt + keypad method. *(You may have to turn off your number lock.)*

Alt + 248 = °
Alt + 171 = $\frac{1}{2}$
Alt + 172 = $\frac{1}{4}$
Alt + 251 = ✓
Alt + 254 = •

Here are examples of another system

option + shift + 8 = °
option + v = ✓
option + 8 = •

(See also 1–22, Symbols with Abbreviations, in Chapter 1.)

✓ DO   know the technical symbols in your specialty area. Avoid the use of abbreviations in records where they are inappropriate. See Chapter 1 for help with abbreviations and Chapter 27 for help with numbers.

44–1 ABBREVIATIONS, SYMBOLS, AND NUMBERS

✓ DO   spell out the symbol term when it is used alone, not in association with a number.

What is the degree of difference between the two? *(not* °*)*

🚫 DON'T   use a period after a symbol unless the symbol is at the end of a sentence.

DO use symbols only when they occur in immediate association with a number or another abbreviation.

8 × 3	eight by three
4-5	four to five
#3-0	number three oh
2+	two plus
Vision: 20/20	vision is twenty-twenty
6/d	six per day
diluted 1:10	diluted one to ten *(a ratio)*
at −2	at minus two
60/40	sixty over forty
grade 4/5	grade four over five
nocturia × 2	nocturia times two
T&A	tonsillectomy and adenoidectomy
25 mg/h	twenty-five milligrams per hour
limited by 45%	limited by forty-five percent
35 mg%	thirty-five milligrams percent
30°C	thirty degrees Celsius
99°F	ninety-nine degrees Fahrenheit
BP: 100/80	blood pressure is one hundred over eighty
rSR′	RSR prime
× 3 days	times three days
3.5 cm	three point five centimeters
0.5 cm	point five centimeters
47% segs	forty-seven percent segs
O Rh−	O Rh negative
A Rh+	A Rh positive
#1 French	number one French

 DO use figures when numbers are used *directly* with symbols, words, or abbreviations.

1+ protein	one plus protein
2%	two percent
75 ml/kg/24h	seventy-five milliliters per kilogram per twenty-four hours
the BUN is 45 mg%	the "bee you en" is forty-five milligrams percent
99°F	ninety-nine degrees Fahrenheit
$10 *(not* $10.00)	ten dollars
63 cents *(not* 63¢ or $.63)	sixty-three cents
#14 Foley *or* No. 14 Foley	number fourteen Foley

44–2 AMPERSAND (&) SYMBOL

The *ampersand* (&) means *and*. It is used to save space while keying in data when symbols are commonly used, such as in bills, tables, charts, and technical material. The ampersand is not generally used in the body of letters and reports. It may be used in business names in which the ampersand is part of the incorporated or trade name.

AT&T (no space between symbol)
Bausch & Lomb (space before and after symbol)

✅ DO   use the ampersand (&) symbol in phrases containing abbreviations separated by *and*. There is no space before or after the ampersand.

I&D   D&C   L&W

🚫 DON'T   use the ampersand symbol in operative titles or diagnoses.

Incorrect:
Operation: D&C
Correct:
Operation: Dilatation and curettage

44–3 APOSTROPHE (') SYMBOL
See Chapter 3, Apostrophe.

44–4 ARROW (→) SYMBOL

✅ DO   use an arrow when illustrating from-to in a table.

44–5 AT (@) SYMBOL

✅ DO   use the at (@) symbol in informal business communications.

Order 24 syringes @ $1.50 each. *(a memo)*

✅ DO   use the @ symbol as part of an email address introducing the Internet domain.

wbsinfo@wbsaunders.com

44–6 CARDIOLOGIC SYMBOLS AND ABBREVIATIONS

✅ DO   use cardiologic symbols and abbreviations to express electrocardiographic results.

The P waves are slightly prominent in V_1 to V_3. *(or V_1-V_3 or V1-V3)*
(Subscript is found under Font in the Format pull-down menu.)

It is not clear whether it contains a U wave.
The QRS complexes are normal, as are the ST segments.
There are T wave inversions in I, aVL, and V1-4 and
+/− T in V5.

NOTE: *Please remember to use a lowercase r and an apostrophe when typing rSR' (pronounced RSR prime). See also 3-7, Miscellaneous Apostrophe Use, in Chapter 3.*

44–7   CENT (¢) SYMBOL
See also 27–14, Money, in Chapter 27.

⊘ **DON'T**   use symbols for less than whole dollar amounts.

Correct:
Please give her the 35 cents change.
Incorrect:
Please give her the 35¢ change.
Please give her the $0.35 change.

44–8   CHARTING SYMBOLS
There are many handwritten symbols that may be entered into the patient's chart but these would be written out when dictated.

*	birth
c̄, c, w/	with
s̄, s, w/o	without
c̄c, c̄/c	with correction (eyeglasses)
s̄c, s̄/c	without correction (eyeglasses)
+	positive
−	negative
ō	negative
Ⓛ	left
Ⓡ	right
Rx	recipe, take
℥	ounce
♂	dram
	male
♀	female
μ	micron
±	negative or positive; indefinite
>	greater than
<	less than

44–9   CHEMICAL SYMBOLS

✓ **DO**   use arabic numerals with chemical symbols. They may be keyed on the same line or as superscripts or subscripts.

I 131 *or* iodine 131 *or* ^{131}I

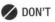 **DON'T**   use periods or hyphens within chemical symbols or compounds.

$$CO_2 \quad K \quad Na \quad O_2 \quad H_2O$$

44–10   COLON (:) SYMBOL
See Chapter 6, The Colon.

44–11   COMMA (,) SYMBOL
See Chapter 7, The Comma.

44–12   DASH (–) SYMBOL
See Chapter 9, Dash.

44–13   DEGREE (°) SYMBOL

☑ **DO**   use the degree symbol in expressing temperature, angles, and imaging studies.

Irrigated with 250 mL of 4° solution.
Rotations of the lumbar motion segments varied between −1.8° and 5.7°.
Adduction between thumb and first finger was limited to 20°.

 DON'T   use the degree (°) symbol if is not accompanied by a number.

Correct:
Temperature: 36°C.
Temperature: 36°
Incorrect:
I noted a small ° of difference.

44–14   DIACRITICAL (˙˙′ ^ ˜) MARKS

☑ **DO**   underscore or use italics for foreign expressions that are not considered part of the English language.

☑ **DO**   use quotation marks to set off translations of foreign expressions.

☑ **DO**   use diacritical marks on proper names.

Ramón Valenzuela
Esmé Manasson
Abbé flap

✓ DO use diacritical marks on some, but not all, foreign words. Check your reference books to be sure.

à la carte   cause célèbre
à la mode   Mönckeberg's arteriosclerosis
bête noire   vis-à-vis
Büngner's band

44–15   DOLLAR ($) SYMBOL
See also 27–14, Money, in Chapter 27.

✓ DO use the dollar symbol and figures to express amounts of money.

Correct:
The patient's outstanding balance is $250.
Incorrect:
The patient's outstanding balance is $250.00. *(Do not use period and zeros when expressing whole dollar amounts.)*

44–16   EQUAL (=) SYMBOL

✓ DO use an equal symbol for indicating digital sums.

$24 + 50 = 74$

44–17   EXCLAMATION (!) POINT
See Chapter 15, Exclamation Mark.

44–18   FEET (') SYMBOL
See also Chapter 26, Metric System.

✓ DO use the ' symbol for foot and the " symbol for inches if desired in tables.

Subject A is 5' 7" tall, B is 5' 10" tall, and C is 5' 9" tall.

The patient is 5 ft 7 in. tall. *(Notice that the abbreviation for inch is punctuated.)*

✓ DO spell out *feet* and *inches* in most medical documents.

The patient is 5 feet 7 inches tall.

44–19   GREATER THAN (>) AND LESS THAN (<) SYMBOLS
The greater than and less than symbols are generally not typed into medical documents but are often used in tables and in published

research articles. They are often handwritten by the author along with other nonkeyboard symbols. *(See 44-8, Charting Symbols.)*

>4 cm   p < 0.05 considered significant

44–20   GREEK LETTERS

✅ **DO**   use symbols for Greek letters if your equipment provides them. Otherwise, type out the English translation of the letter.

α *(alpha)*   β *(beta)*   ω *(omega)*
π *(pi)*   λ *(lambda)*

44–21   HYPHEN (-) AND WORD DIVISION

See Chapter 20, Hyphen Use and Word Division.

44–22   INCHES SYMBOL OR DITTO (") MARKS

✅ **DO**   use the " symbol for inches if desired in tables.

Subject A is 5′ 7″ tall, B is 5′ 10″ tall, and C is 5′ 9″ tall.

The patient is 5 ft 7 in. tall. *(Notice that the abbreviation for inch is punctuated.)*

44–23   MINUS (–) OR PLUS (+) SYMBOLS

✅ **DO**   use a minus symbol for indicating loss or absence.

✅ **DO**   use plus (+) and minus (–) symbols to designate the strength of a response or reaction, as well as for expressing the Rhesus blood factor as Rh positive (*Rh*+) or Rh negative (*Rh*–).

O Rh positive *or* O Rh+
blood type O Rh– or O Rh negative
knee jerks 3+ or knee jerks + + +

✅ **DO**   use a plus/minus (±) symbol in tables and test results.

operative time (n) $7.3 ± 1.3$

NOTE: *When the phrase plus or minus is dictated, it may be typed as ± or +/–.*

✅ **DO**   use a superscript plus symbol with some ion symbols.

intracellular Ca^{2+} *(calcium ion)*

44–24 NUMBER (#) SYMBOL

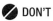 **DO** use the number symbol with an arabic number for sizes of instruments or sutures. The symbol is preferred but may be replaced by the abbreviation *No*. When the word *number* is not dictated, you may choose whether to use the symbol # or the abbreviation *No*.

A #22 French Malecot Silastic suprapubic tube was placed in the anterior bladder dome.

The skin was closed by using #4-0 Prolene interrupted vertical mattress sutures.

 DON'T use the number symbol to indicate pounds (#) after a numeral.

Correct:
She weighed 110 pounds.
She weighed 110 lb.
Incorrect:
She weighed 110#.

 DO use a symbol rather than the spelled-out word when it occurs in immediate association with a number. (*See 27–26, Symbols and Numbers, in Chapter 27*.)

Dictated:
A number three oh chromic catgut suture material was used.
Transcribed:
A #3-0 chromic catgut suture material was used.

DO use the zero (0) and not the capital O for designating the suture size.

44–25 PARENTHESES ( )
See Chapter 29, Parentheses.

44–26 PERCENT (%) SYMBOL

DO use the percent symbol or spell out the word *percent* when a number accompanies the word. There is no space between the number and the percent symbol.

75%   1.2%   0.20% *(preferred)*
5 percent
What is the percentage of difference between the two? *(not %)*

DON'T   use simple fractions with percent.

> **Incorrect:**
> 45 1/2 percent
> 45 1/2%
> **Correct:**
> 45.5%

44–27   PERIOD (.)
See Chapter 30, Period and Decimal Point.

44–28   PLURALS

✓ **DO**   use an apostrophe to form the plurals of symbols by adding **'s** to the singular.

> %'s   &'s $'s   +'s

44–29   PLUS (+) SYMBOL
See 44–23, Minus (–) or Plus (+) Symbols.

44–30   POUND (#) SYMBOL
See 44–24, Number (#) Symbol.

44–31   PROOFREADING SYMBOLS
See Figure 34–1.

44–32   QUESTION (?) MARK
See Chapter 35, Question Mark.

✓ **DO**   use a question mark at the end of a direct question.

> Did he return after three months for a reexamination?

✓ **DO**   use a question mark to express doubt within a sentence.

> Dr. Fritz Coleman graduated from the University of Notre Dame in 1998 (?).

44–33   QUOTATION (" ") MARKS
See Chapter 36, Quotation Marks.

44–34   REFERENCE BOOKS FOR SYMBOLS
See 37–1, Abbreviations Dictionaries, General, and 37–2, Abbreviations Dictionaries, Medical, in Chapter 37.

44–35   ROMAN NUMERALS
See also 27–21, Roman Numerals, in Chapter 27.

DO use roman numerals for major divisions in an outline *(see Fig. 25–8)*.

ROMAN NUMERAL TABLE

Figure	Roman Numeral	Figure	Roman Numeral
1	I	40	XL
2	II	50	L
3	III	60	LX
4	IV	70	LXX
5	V	80	LXXX
6	VI	90	XC
7	VII	100	C
8	VIII	200	CC
9	IX	300	CCC
10	X	400	CD
11	XI	500	D
12	XII	600	DC
13	XIII	700	DCC
14	XIV	800	DCCC
15	XV	900	CM
16	XVI	1000	M
17	XVII	1500	MD
18	XVIII	1900	MCM
19	XIX	2000	MM
20	XX	5000	$\bar{V}$
30	XXX	10,000	$\bar{X}$

NOTE: *A line over a roman numeral multiplies the value by 1000.*

44–36 SEMICOLON (;)
See Chapter 39, Semicolon.

44–37 SLASH, BAR, DIAGONAL, OR SLANT (/) LINE
See Chapter 41, Slash.

44–38 SPACING WITH SYMBOLS AND NUMBERS
See also 27–22, Spacing with Symbols and Numbers, in Chapter 27.

 DO key the following symbols directly in front of or directly following the number they refer to with no spacing.

```
+    %    #    $    °
@    &    –    /
```

 DO place a space on each side of the *x* that takes the place of the word *times* or the word *by*.

44–39 SYMBOLS WITH ABBREVIATIONS

 DO use the ampersand (&) symbol in phrases containing abbreviations separated by *and*. There is no space before or after the ampersand.

I&D D&C L&W

44–40 SYMBOLS WITH NUMBERS

 DO spell out the symbol abbreviation when it is used alone, not in association with a number.

What is the degree of difference between the two? (*not* °)

 DO use a symbol in preference to the spelled-out word when the symbol occurs in immediate association with a number.

8 × 3	eight by three
4-5	four to five
#3-0	number three oh
2+	two plus
Vision: 20/20	vision is twenty-twenty
6/d	six per day
diluted 1:10	diluted one to ten (*a ratio*)
at −2	at minus two
60/40	sixty over forty
grade 4/5	grade four over five
nocturia × 2	nocturia times two
T&A	tonsillectomy and adenoidectomy
25 mg/hr	twenty-five milligrams per hour
limited by 45%	limited by forty-five percent
35 mg%	thirty-five milligrams percent
30°C	thirty degrees Celsius
99°F	ninety-nine degrees Fahrenheit
BP: 100/80	blood pressure is one hundred over eighty

44–41 TIMES (×) OR MULTIPLICATION SYMBOL

 DO use the symbol *x* for *times* followed by a space and then the arabic number. (*This is the lowercase* x.)

He has had nocturia × 2.

 DO use the symbol *x* for *by* to express dimensions.

The cervical stump measures 2 × 3 × 3 cm.

44–42   UNKNOWN (X, Y, Z) SYMBOLS

 DO   use an *X* to denote the unknown in an abbreviation, sentence, word, or phrase. *Y* and *Z* are also used as symbols for unknown quantities or qualities.

X marks the spot.
x-ray or X-ray *(In German it is X-strahlen.)*

Syndrome X involves a patient who complains of chest pain with exertion, a classic symbol of angina.

Patient Bob X is now converted from HIV to AIDS.

Patients X, Y, and Z had low white blood cell counts after being on the experimental chemotherapeutic drug for one month.

NOTE: *This symbol is also used to delete or obliterate.*

 DO   use an *X* to substitute for a group of letters when using an abbreviation.

Rx *(treatment or prescription)*
DX *or* Dx *(diagnosis)*
HX *or* Hx *(history; sometimes used in outlines)*
TX *or* Tx *(treatment or therapy)*
pedestrian Xing *or* railroad Xing *(crossing)*

45

Time

45–1   EVEN TIME OF DAY

 DO   spell out the even time of the day when written with or without *o'clock* or without *a.m.* or *p.m.*

> The staff meeting is scheduled to begin at three.
> He is due at nine this evening.
> Give her an appointment for two o'clock.
> She was seen as an emergency at a quarter past ten.
> I saw her at half-past two.
> His plane is due at seven tomorrow night.

 DO   use the phrases *in the morning, in the afternoon,* and *at night* with *o'clock* but not with *a.m.* or *p.m.*

DON'T   use *o'clock* with *a.m.* or *p.m.* or when both hour and minutes are expressed.

Correct:
I met her in the emergency room at 3 o'clock in the morning.
She is expected at three o'clock.
She is expected at 3 o'clock.
She is expected at 3 p.m.
She is expected at 3:30.
Incorrect:
She is expected at 3 o'clock p.m.
She is expected at 3:30 o'clock.

NOTE: *It is also acceptable to use figures with the expression o'clock.*

Please ask her to come at three o'clock.
Please ask her to come at 3 o'clock.

45–2   HOURS AND MINUTES USING A.M. AND P.M.

 DO   use figures to express the time of day with *a.m.* or *p.m.* or when both hours and minutes are expressed alone.

Office hours are from 10 a.m. to noon. Your appointment is for 11:30 a.m.
Surgery will begin at 7 in the morning. The surgeon will arrive at 6:30.

 DON'T use the colon and double zeros for even periods of time.

Incorrect:
Office hours are from 10:00 to noon.
Correct:
Office hours are from 10 to noon.

45–3   MIDNIGHT AND NOON

 DON'T use *a.m.* or *p.m.* with 12. You may use the figure 12 with the word *noon* or *midnight* or use the words alone without the figure 12.

We close the office at 12 noon.
My shift is over at midnight.

45–4   MILITARY TIME

 DO   use four figures without a colon when writing the military time of day. The word *hours* may or may not be dictated with the time.

0315 *(oh three fifteen; 3:15 a.m.)*
0900 *(oh nine hundred; 9 a.m.)*
1200 *(twelve hundred hours; noon)*
1400 *(fourteen hundred hours; 2 p.m.)*
1630 *(sixteen thirty; 4:30 p.m.)*
Incorrect:
Surgery began at precisely 16:32.
Surgery began at precisely 1632 p.m.
Correct:
Surgery began at precisely 1632.

He was pronounced at 0947. (*Declared officially dead at 9:47 a.m.*)

NOTE: a.m., p.m., and o'clock are not used with military time.

45–5 PERIODS OF TIME

✓ DO   write out numbers to express *periods of time* when the number is less than ten; when the number is ten or greater, use the figure.

She is to return in three months.
The medical supply invoice is marked "net 30 days."

45–6 POSSESSIVE CASE

✓ DO   use an apostrophe to show possession of time.

return in one month's time
convalescence of three weeks' duration

45–7 SURFACE LOCATIONS RELATED TO THE FACE OF THE CLOCK

Although unrelated to the time of day, the location of lesions, injections, and incision sites on round anatomic surfaces, such as the breast or the eye, are often expressed by referring to the face of a clock.

✓ DO   use the expression *o'clock* to refer to points on a circular surface, and use figures with *o'clock*.

The sclera was incised at about the 3 o'clock area.

The cyst was in the left breast, just below the nipple, between 4 and 5 o'clock.

Then 2 mL of 1% lidocaine was injected at the 4 o'clock and 8 o'clock positions.

46

Underlining and Italics

✓ **DO**   Avoid underlining in documents as a general rule. Italics is preferred for emphasis. Use boldface as an alternative.

46-1 ABBREVIATIONS

✓ **DO**   underscore abbreviations for special emphasis.

In the following report, be sure to type b.i.d. in lowercase letters.

46-2 ARTISTIC WORKS

✓ **DO**   use an underscore when keying titles of books, magazines, pamphlets, long poems, movies, plays, musicals, paintings, and other literary and artistic works. Titles of shorter literary works are placed within quotation marks. *(See Chapter 36, Quotation Marks.)*

Mrs. Lee made it a point to see the painting of the Mona Lisa when visiting the Louvre Museum in Paris, France.

<u>A Chorus Line</u> was the longest running musical on Broadway.

46–3   BIOLOGICAL NAMES

 DO   underscore formal taxonomic names for a genus, species, subspecies, or variety in keying a manuscript for publication. If the genus name is abbreviated, this general rule should be followed.

The urinary infection was caused by <u>Pseudomonas aeruginosa</u>.

NOTE: *The underlining will indicate that the words are to be italicized and will thus appear in publication as follows:*

The urinary infection was caused by *Pseudomonas aeruginosa*

A common organism of uncomplicated urinary infections is *E. coli.*

46–4   DEFINITIONS

 DO   italicize or put in quotes words that are defined or referred to.

The insured is known as a *subscriber* or, in some insurance programs, a *member.*

I noticed that she wrote "p.r.n." in capital letters.

46–5   EMPHASIS

 DO   underscore or put in quotes words or phrases for special emphasis or to place emphasis on a task or command.

Dr. Johnson always mispronounces the word <u>bruit.</u>

Make sure everyone on the team has noted the <u>do not resuscitate</u> order.

 DO   underline the full phrase, including spaces and punctuation, except final punctuation.

A style guide for medical transcriptionists is <u>Medical Transcription Guide: Do's and Don'ts</u>.

NOTE: *A period, comma, colon, or semicolon following an italicized or boldfaced word should be italicized or boldfaced as well.*

ALLERGIES: Codeine.

Other punctuation marks—question marks, quotation marks, exclamation points, and parentheses—follow the typeface of the sentence.

46–6 FOOTNOTES

See also Chapter 23, Manuscripts.

✓ **DO** key an underscore 2 inches long to separate footnotes from the main text. The underscore line should be one line below the last line of text, beginning at the left margin.

1. Kathleen Kropko and Susan Francis, *The Professional Skillbuilding Wizard for Medical Transcription*, M-Tec, Inc., 2002, p. 73.

46–7 FOREIGN EXPRESSIONS

✓ **DO** underscore foreign expressions that are not considered part of the English language. Quote marks are used to set off translations of foreign expressions.

The patient kept repeating tzuris ("trouble") to the EMT crew that brought him in.

In the large intestine, there is a 2 1/2-inch area which forms the cul-de-sac known as the cecum *(no underlining since* cul-de-sac *is part of the English language).*

46–8 ITALIC TYPE FOR PRINTED MATERIAL

✓ **DO** use an underscore in keyed material to indicate italic font in printed material.

Code numbers represent diagnostic and therapeutic procedures on medical billing statements and insurance forms.

✓ **DO** underscore as a unit individual words, titles, phrases, or even whole sentences if they should be grasped as a unit.

✓ **DO** underscore only the individual units, not the series as a whole.

Do you know the meaning of terms like respondeat superior and res ipsa loquitur?

✅ **DO**   use italics for the genus and species names in printed material. Indicate italics with an underscore in the manuscript.

> The article is focused on <u>Borrelia burgdorferi</u> (the agent of Lyme disease).

🚫 **DON'T**   use italics when using genus and species names in general transcription.

46–9   LEGAL CITATIONS

✅ **DO**   underscore legal case names referred to in text. The *v.* may or may not be underscored, depending on the employer's preference.

> <u>Allen</u> v. <u>Levine</u>

46–10   LITERARY WORKS

✅ **DO**   use an underscore when keying titles of published books, magazines, pamphlets, long poems, movies, plays, musicals, paintings, and other literary and artistic works. Place titles of chapters, sections, and other subdivisions of a published work within quotation marks. *(See 36–3, Punctuation with Quotation Marks, in Chapter 36.)*

> According to an article in <u>New Woman</u>, real estate investment is future financial protection for the career woman.

46–11   NAMES OF VEHICLES

✅ **DO**   underscore, type with initial capital letters, or italicize individual names given to vehicles.

> Dr. Barry returned on the cruise ship, the S.S. <u>Royal Viking</u>.
> *or*
> Dr. Barry returned on the cruise ship, the S.S. *Royal Viking*.
> Dr. and Mrs. Wertlake have a Mercedes-Benz named *Otto*.

46–12   PLACEMENT OF UNDERSCORING

✅ **DO**   underscore each word individually only when it is used as an individual word. Generally, underscore each expression as a unit.

> As an expression: <u>Respondeat superior</u> means "Let the master answer."
> As individual words: <u>Res, ipsa,</u> and <u>loquitur</u> are Latin words.

✓ **DO**   underline headings in medical reports if it is the preferred format of your employer. *(See Chapter 24, Medical Reports.)*

46–13   PUNCTUATION

🚫 **DON'T**   underline punctuation marks that follow the underlined material.

🚫 **DON'T**   break the underscore to skip punctuation within the underscored material.

Do you have the book by Mary Louise Gilman entitled <u>One Word, Two Words, Hyphenated?</u> in your library?

Have you read that excellent article in the <u>Star Free Press</u>, "The New Pandemic"?

🚫 **DON'T**   underscore a possessive or plural ending that is added on to an underscored word.

There are too many <u>but</u>s in that paragraph.

The <u>New York Times</u>'s editorial gave the projected population of the United States for the year 2010.

46–14   TITLES OF PUBLISHED WORKS

✓ **DO**   use an underscore when keying titles of published books, computer programs *(software)*, journals, magazines, pamphlets, long poems, movies, plays, musicals, paintings, and other literary and artistic works. Place titles of chapters, sections, and other subdivisions of a published work within quotation marks. *(See 36–3, Punctuation with Quotation Marks, in Chapter 36.)*

Our little patient forgot <u>Clarence Goes Out West and Meets the Purple Horse</u>, the book she was reading while waiting to be seen.

NOTE: *Titles of journals (e.g., J. Inf. Dis.) that appear in reference lists or bibliographies do not have to be underscored.*

Vitae Format and Preparation

INTRODUCTION

The physician's curriculum vitae, or professional profile, is used in the following situations:

- *as evidence of the expertise of a physician who is testifying as an expert witness*
- *to introduce a physician who has been invited as a guest speaker or who is appearing on television*
- *to seek employment in a hospital staff position or apply*

513

for a faculty appointment at a teaching hospital
- *to obtain a research grant from a federal or funding agency*
- *to determine if an institution is complying with state and voluntary agency requirements for physicians who have certain positions in hospitals*
- *to obtain agency accreditation for residency training programs*

A cover letter should accompany a mailed or faxed vitae.
- *Keep the letter to one or two pages.*
- *Print on high-quality bond paper.*
- *Write concisely.*
- *Send it to an individual by name.* (Telephone the organization if you don't have a contact name.)
- *Outline your current work environment.*
- *Highlight strengths.*

47–1 ACADEMIC CREDENTIALS

See 47–7, Education.

47–2 AFFILIATIONS

✓ DO list membership in professional associations, showing category of membership, name of the organization, and date membership began, followed by a hyphen and the word *present* if membership is continuing. Double-space between entries if listing more than one organization.

Member, New York State Medical Society, 200X-present

Fellow, American College of Physicians 200X-present

47–3 BIBLIOGRAPHIES OF PUBLICATIONS AND ABSTRACTS

See 47–20, Publications.

47–4 BOARD CERTIFICATION

✓ DO list the name of the board from which the physician received certification, followed by the year certification was received. Double-space between entries if listing more than one specialty area, beginning each entry on a separate line.

American Board of Orthopaedic Surgery, 200X

47–5 BOARD ELIGIBILITY

✓ DO   insert the name of the board examination for which the physician is eligible to sit.

American Board of Internal Medicine—Infectious Diseases

47–6 CONTINUATION PAGES

✓ DO   begin numbering with the second sheet as page 2 in the upper right corner.

47–7 EDUCATION

✓ DO   list chronologically all medical and academic degrees held by the physician by typing the name of the college or university from which the undergraduate degree was earned and then the name of the school from which the medical degree was earned. Double-space between these two groups of information.

✓ DO   state the name of the college or university followed by the names of the city and state where the school is located.

New York University, New York City, New York, B.S., Biology

✓ DO   list the kind of degree earned and the years of attendance or the year the degree was granted.

NOTE: *A subheading under this category might be* Postdoctoral Study.

George Washington University, School of Medicine, Washington, D.C., MD, 2001

47–8 ELECTRONIC CURRICULUM VITAE

✓ DO   use ASCII files and GIF viewer formats when posting a resume or curriculum vitae to an online computer service. The resume or curriculum vitae may be three or four pages long.

✓ DO   keep the format very simple.

✓ DO   use tabulation or indent features rather than the space bar to indent.

🚫 **DON'T** write in all capital letters, and avoid jargon and acronyms.

✓ **DO** use asterisks to frame words or phrases for emphasis.

✓ **DO** use action words *(nouns)* rather than action verbs. The following are some examples of some action words *(nouns)*:

accomplishment	identification
achievement	improvement
attainment	information
clarification	installation
collaboration	institute
creation	manipulation
design	moderation
determination	organization
development	process
education	program
effect	reconciliation
encouragement	review
examination	summary
exchange	

🚫 **DON'T** use decorative or uncommon typefaces.

🚫 **DON'T** use any underlining and minimize the use of abbreviations.

✓ **DO** compress large files. *(Data compression is a method of encoding data to take up less storage space. This file can be decompressed by the receiver and printed out in full text.)*

✓ **DO** check the rules for posting to a service or forum as these can vary.

✓ **DO** update whenever there is a change.

47–9 FACULTY APPOINTMENTS

✓ **DO** mention the academic rank *(assistant, associate, full professor, lecturer)* and the name of the medical school or college. One line below, type the names of the city and state of the school and the years of appointment. Double-space between entries if there is more than one appointment.

Associate Professor, UCLA School of Medicine
Los Angeles, California, 2001-2004

47–10   FELLOWSHIP

✓ DO give the name of the hospital where fellowship training was completed, followed by the names of the city and state where the institution is located. One line below, type the kind of fellowship training, the word *Fellowship*, and the dates of fellowship training.

> Westlake Community Hospital, Westlake Village, California
> Plastic Surgery Fellowship, 2000-2003

47–11   FORMAT

See Figure 47-1 at the end of the chapter.

✓ DO use 8 ½ × 11-inch white or off-white bond paper and leave 1 ½-inch margins all around.

✓ DO use a high-quality photocopying process *(offset or laser printing)*, and keep the original document in a plastic protector so it is not given away by mistake.

⊘ DON'T include personal information *(hobbies or children's names)* other than the physician's office and/or home address, and telephone number.

> OPTIONAL: *Date of birth, place of birth, marital status.*

⊘ DON'T overuse underlining and capitalization.

✓ DO spell out names of organizations and agencies.

✓ DO spell out titles.

✓ DO proofread the curriculum vitae carefully for spelling and punctuation.

47–12   HEADING

✓ DO center the all-capitalized heading *CURRICULUM VITAE* 1 ½ inches from the top of the first page. The physician's name and degree abbreviations are centered and keyed two line spaces beneath the heading.

> CURRICULUM VITAE
> Mary T. O'Connor, MD

47–13   HONORS

✅ DO   list the name of the award or honor and the agency giving the award. One line below, insert the names of the city and state and the year the award was given. Double-space between each award and honor.

Intern of the Year, New York Masonic Medical Center
New York, New York, 2004

47–14   INTERNSHIP
Internship refers to the first year of postgraduate medical education.

✅ DO   state the names of the hospital and the city and state where the internship was completed. One line below, insert the word *Internship* and, in parentheses, the words *Straight Medicine* or *Rotating*, followed by the dates of internship.

New York Masonic Medical Center, New York, New York
Internship (Straight Medicine), 2003

47–15   LICENSURE

✅ DO   list license numbers for all states, giving the name of the state and the month, and year the license was issued, and the date of expiration.

State of California (018-502897) June 2003

47–16   MILITARY SERVICE

✅ DO   list the military position held by the physician and the branch of service. One line below, type the names of the city and state where he or she was stationed and the years of service.

Major, U. S. Army, Chief of Surgery
Baghdad, Iraq 2002-2004

47–17   PERSONAL DATA

🚫 DON'T   include personal information *(hobbies or children's names)* other than the physician's name, office and/or home address, and telephone number.

OPTIONAL: *Date of birth, place of birth, marital status.*

47–18   POSTDOCTORAL TRAINING
See 47–14, Internship, and 47–22, Residency.

47–19 PROFESSIONAL TRAINING AND EXPERIENCE

✓ DO   state the specialty of medical practice *(see Figure 47–1 at the end of the chapter)* followed by the years of service. One line below, type the names of the city and state where the practice is located. Double-space between entries if the physician has more than one practice. This section should be in chronological order. List the current practice and work back to residency and internship.

47–20 PUBLICATIONS

✓ DO   list three categories *(journals, books and other monographs, and meeting presentations)* on separate sheets of paper in chronological order, according to their dates of publication or presentation. *(For further information see 23–2, Bibliography, in Chapter 23.)*

✓ DO   list the authors' names in the same order as they appear in the publication.

Pellegrino ED, Thomasma DC. The Virtues in Medical Practice. New York: Oxford University Press; 1993.

🚫 DON'T   underline any part of a citation except the genus and species names of microorganisms and Latin words.

Vincent, R. and Derby, K. Quantitative testing for *Escherichia coli.* J. Pathol. 1994;23:234–236.

47–21 RESEARCH PROJECTS

✓ DO   insert the name of the project and the name of the company, hospital, or agency for which the physician is conducting research. Give the status of the research project *(ongoing, completed, or expected completion date)* one line below and the beginning and ending dates of the project. Double-space between entries if there is more than one research project.

Electromagnetophoresis, National Institutes of Health Completed research, 1990-2000

47–22 RESIDENCY

✓ DO   list the name of the hospital where residency training was completed, followed by the names of the city and state where the hospital is located. One line below, insert the name of the specialty followed by the word *Residency* and the dates of residency training.

Cook County Medical Center, Chicago, Illinois
Internal Medicine Residency, 2001-2002

47–23 STAFF APPOINTMENTS

✓ DO state the category of the staff appointment *(senior attending physician, associate attending physician, consulting physician, courtesy physician, and so forth)* followed by the name of the institution. One line below, insert the names of the city and state where the hospital is located followed by the years in which the appointment was held. Double-space between entries if there is more than one appointment.

Senior Attending Physician, Bethesda Naval Hospital
Bethesda, Maryland, 2003-present

47–24 STAFF POSITIONS

✓ DO state the name of the position held and the years served. One line below, type the name of the hospital followed by the names of the city and state where the hospital is located. If the physician served on a committee, list the name of the committee.

NOTE: *Staff appointment is an initial appointment to the hospital staff, and staff position is subsequent to that.*

Chairman, Bioethics Committee, 2003-present
Vista Medical Center, Cleveland, Ohio

47–25 SUBHEADINGS

✓ DO key major subheadings flush with the left margin. Single-space each cluster of data beneath the subheadings. Double-space between the subheadings and the first line of the date. Double- or triple-space between subheads, depending on the available space. Subheadings may be in all capital letters with or without underscoring or in capital and lowercase letters and underscored. *(See Figure 47–1 at the end of the chapter.)*

✓ DO use the following categories:

- *staff appointments*
- *staff positions*
- *faculty appointments*

- *practice experience*
- *teaching experience*
- *research projects*
- *journals*
- *books and other monographs*
- *meeting presentations (optional)*

47–26 *TEACHING EXPERIENCE*

✓ DO   list the name of the teaching program, the name of the
hospital and the names of the city and state where located,
and the years the physician was associated with the
program. If the physician was a lecturer, so indicate.

Pain Control, UCLA School of Medicine, Los Angeles,
California, 2003-2004

CURRICULUM VITAE
Josephine B. Wells, MD

PERSONAL HISTORY

Business Address: 329 West Main Street, Suite 430
Weston, PA 19016

Telephone (805) 890-5399

EDUCATION

1990 New York State University, New York, New York
B.S., Biology

1995 George Washington University, Washington, D.C.
M.D. with Honors

INTERNSHIP

1995-1996 UCLA Medical Center, Los Angeles, California
Internship (Straight Medicine)

RESIDENCY

1996-1997 UCLA Medical Center, Los Angeles, California
Internship Medicine Residency

FELLOWSHIP

1997-1999 Cook County Hospital, Chicago, Illinois
Infectious Disease Fellowship

BOARD CERTIFICATION

1998 American Board of Internal Medicine

BOARD ELIGIBILITY

American Board of Internal Medicine-
Infectious Disease

HONORS

1996 Intern of the Year, UCLA Medical Center
Los Angeles, California

MEDICAL LICENSURE

State of California (G027037) June 1995

Figure 47–1 Example of a curriculum vitae.

Josephine B. Wells Curriculum Vitae (continued)

MEDICAL SPECIALTY

1995-present   Internal Medicine

PROFESSIONAL AFFILIATIONS

1995-present   Fellow, American College of Physicians

1995-present   Member, California Medical Association

STAFF APPOINTMENTS

1998-present   Attending Physician, Westside Medical Center
                Los Angeles, California

1999-present   Associate Attending Physician, Community
                Memorial Hospital
                Los Angeles, California

STAFF POSITIONS

1999-present   Chairperson, Bioethics Committee
                Westside Medical Center, Los Angeles, California

FACULTY APPOINTMENTS

1999-present   Assistant Professor, UCLA Medical School
                Los Angeles, California

TEACHING EXPERIENCE

1995-1999   Guest Lecturer, Rheumatology Course
             UCLA Medical School
             Los Angeles, California

Figure 47–1   Cont'd

48

Working from Home

INTRODUCTION

All of the ideas concerning working from home cannot be given here. This material is just to get you thinking.

✓ DO obtain *The Independent Medical Transcriptionist* by Avila-Weil and Glaccum, 4th edition, from Rayve Productions Inc. (800) 852-4890 before you begin to make your plans to work from home.

✓ DO be patient getting your business up and running and making a profit. Keep your regular job and use your new business as a sideline until you can rely on it for income.

✓ DO consider working at home for a service. Unlike the situation when you are working for yourself, the company usually provides equipment as well as employee benefits, such as health insurance, vacation time, and quality assurance.

48–1 ENVIRONMENT

✓ DO set up a comfortable environment for yourself at home. You will need space not only for your desk and chair but also for storage space for books, supplies, reference materials, and, of course, for your telephone, computer, printer, scanner, fax, shredder, and so on.

DO   have a space where will you will not be disturbed by the family living with you if you cannot have a designated office away from the normal family environment.

DO   maintain regular business hours. *(You may have whatever hours you want, but you need to be sure that you are available for your clients when you say you will be.)*

48–2 EQUIPMENT

DO   get a separate telephone line installed for business calls and fax machine.

DO   make sure clients can reach you. Voice mail and other telephone aids will help you when you have to be away from your business. *(Voice mail picks up calls so that clients never get a busy signal.)*

DO   hire a computer/software expert to help you set up your business equipment correctly.

DON'T   try to get started with a skimpy equipment budget.

DO   make a realistic list of your overhead expenses, including equipment, software, supplies, reference books, advertising and marketing expenses, utilities, and so on.

48–3 HELP

DO   arrange for start-up funds.

DO   have written agreements with clients and vendors.

DO   ask colleagues about contracts they use and their marketing strategy.

DO   find a trustworthy mentor.

DO   work for a while for someone who is established in the business you envision for yourself.

DO   attend seminars on small businesses and marketing.

DO   plan for vacation relief and assistance for overflow work. *(See 48–6, Networking.)*

48–4   LAWS AND REGULATIONS

☑ DO   make your business official.

☑ DO   determine what regulations apply to doing business in your area. Obtain a copy of the laws and regulations of your community. Requirements for business licenses and regulations vary greatly.

☑ DO   clarify any zoning restrictions that may apply to having a home-based business.

☑ DO   make sure that you are aware of the tax laws relative to operating as an independent contractor.

☑ DO   take necessary legal steps to safeguard your business.

☑ DO   register your business name.

☑ DO   consider errors and omissions insurance to cover you against claims that your service harmed someone.

☑ DO   consider using the talents of an attorney and/or tax consultant.

☑ DO   be aware of HIPAA regulations that affect you and your work. *(See Chapter 18, p. 185.)*

48–5   MARKETING

☑ DO   write out your marketing plan.

☑ DO   decide whom you want to serve.

☑ DO   make sure to keep a balance in your client base.

🚫 DON'T   allow any one client to account for more than one-third of your business in order to protect yourself in times of shifting sources of transcription.

☑ DO   prepare flyers, mailings, and brochures describing what services you will provide.

☑ DO   decide what you will charge and find out what people will actually pay for your services. *(You will undoubtedly need help in this area; see 48–6, Networking.)*

🚫 DON'T   sell yourself short.

48–6 NETWORKING

 DON'T neglect the importance of networking with other professionals.

DO join or set up a networking group that meets regularly.

DO join organizations of other professional groups.

DON'T neglect the hobbies and friendships you had before you began your business.

DO attend workshops.

48–7 RECORDS

DO open a business bank account to keep your personal and business affairs separate.

DO begin keeping track of everything that could possibly be considered a business expense. Keep your receipts and checks. Don't overlook dues, mileage, journals, advertising, courier charges, and so on.

DO keep good business records.

48–8 WORK SCHEDULE

DO protect your free time.

DO set a schedule for yourself with fixed starting and stopping points and stick to it.

DO schedule minibreaks.

DON'T let errands and household activities enter into your work schedule.

DON'T let extraneous phone calls from friends or relatives disrupt your work schedule.

DON'T interrupt yourself.

DO pay attention to detail.

DO make sure your family understands and respects your work schedule.

49

ZIP Codes

INTRODUCTION

The Zone Improvement Plan (ZIP) is a system of numerical codes consisting of five or nine digits to be placed on envelopes as part of the address to expedite the delivery of mail. If the ZIP code is omitted from the address, the correspondence will be delayed.

49–1 ABBREVIATIONS

See also 1–21, State Names, in Chapter 1, Abbreviations and Symbols.

 DO   use the two-letter state abbreviations approved by the United States Postal Service for both inside and envelope addresses. See Table 1–2 in Chapter 1 for abbreviations for the United States and for Canadian provinces and territories.

 DON'T   use the state abbreviations without the city name and ZIP code.

49–2 ADDRESS FORMAT

See also 2–3, Address, and 2–12, Complete Address Appearance, in Chapter 2, Address Formats for Letters and Forms of Address, and 13–2, Mailing Address, in Chapter 13, Envelope Preparation.

 DO   leave one space between the state name and the ZIP code.

529

49–3   CANADIAN POSTAL CODE

☑ DO   place the Canadian code on a line by itself or after the abbreviation for the province *(separated by a two-character space)*.

Dr. Thomas B. Larchmont   *or*   Dr. Thomas B. Larchmont
1858 Haversley Court   1858 Haversley Court
Vancouver, British Columbia   Vancouver, BC V3J 1W1
V3J 1W1

49–4   CITY, STATE, AND ZIP CODE

☑ DO   type the city, state, and ZIP code on one line, after the street address.

New York, NY 10158   *or*   New York, NY 10158-0012

49–5   ENVELOPE PREPARATION

See 13-2, Mailing Address, in Chapter 13, Envelope Preparation.

49–6   REFERENCE SOURCES

☑ DO   use the Internet to quickly obtain a ZIP code. Go to http://www.usps.com/zip4/. Then key in the street address and the city and state names.

☑ DO   obtain a missing ZIP code by calling 800-275-8777. A book entitled *ZIP + 4 Code State Directory* is available for purchase from the United States Postal Service. These are also available on CD-ROM if you have reason to use this information frequently.

49–7   SENTENCE STYLE

☑ DO   insert a comma after the street address and after the name of the city when keying an address in a sentence. There is one space between the state name and the ZIP code.

Dr. Hancock's new address will be 3300 West Main Street, Suite 505, Miami, Florida 33144-2728, but this will not be effective until June 1.

49–8   WORD DIVISION

 DO   in narrative copy, divide between the names of the city and the state or between the state name and the ZIP code. If the name of the city or state contains two or more words, divide between the words.

New York,/New York 10004
or
New York, New York/10004
or
New/York, New York 10004

49–9   ZIP + 4 CODES

 DO   use the nine-digit ZIP code to expedite and reduce mailing costs when using bulk mail delivery service. There is a hyphen between the first set of five numbers and the second set of four numbers.

San Francisco, CA 94120-7168
Portland, OR 97204-2628
New York, NY 10005-4101

Appendix A

Abbreviations Commonly Used

This brief list contains some abbreviations that are commonly used in office chart notes and hospital records. This list is arranged in alphabetical order by abbreviation. A reverse list of selected abbreviations, in which the meanings or terms are arranged alphabetically, is found in Appendix B to help in locating a specific abbreviation.

Abbreviation	Meaning
@	at
A, B, AB, O	these are blood types and can also be dictated with subscript numbers
A_1 or A1	first aortic sound
A_2 or A2	second aortic sound
AB/ab	abortion
ABGs	arterial blood gases
a.c.	before meals
ACh	acetylcholine
ACTH	adrenocorticotropic hormone
a.d. or AD	right ear
a.d.	alternating days
A&D	ascending and descending
ad lib.	freely (usually refers to drug or modality)
ADH	antidiuretic hormone; vasopressin
ADL	activities of daily living
ADT	admission, discharge, transfer
AFB	acid-fast bacillus (tuberculosis organism)
Ag	silver
AIDS	acquired immunodeficiency syndrome
a.m. or AM	in the morning or before noon
AMA	against medical advice; American Medical Association
AP	anteroposterior; apical pulse
A&P	auscultation and percussion
APC	acetylsalicylic acid (aspirin), phenacetin, and caffeine
aq.	water
ARC	AIDS-related complex
ARD	acute respiratory disease
ARDS	adult respiratory disease syndrome
a.s. or AS	left ear

ASAP	as soon as possible (*see* STAT)
ASCVD	atherosclerotic cardiovascular disease
ASD	atrial septal defect
Au	gold
AV	atrioventricular
A&W	alive and well
Ba	barium; basophils
BBB	bundle-branch block
BCC	basal cell carcinoma
BE	barium enema
bib	drink
b.i.d.	twice a day
BLE	both lower extremities
BM	bowel movement
BP or B/P	blood pressure
BPH	benign prostatic hypertrophy
BRP	bathroom privileges
BS	blood sugar; bowel sounds
BTL	bilateral tubal ligation
BUN	blood urea nitrogen
BUS	Bartholin, urethral, and Skene (glands)
BVE	bachelor of vocational education
Bx	biopsy
$\bar{c}$	with
C or °C	Celsius, centigrade
C_1 or C1	first cervical vertebra (continues through C7)
Ca	calcium
Ca or CA	carcinoma
Ca^{++} or Ca^{2+}	calcium ion
CABG	coronary artery bypass graft (surgery)
CAD	coronary artery disease
CAT	computed axial tomography
CBC	complete blood count
CC	chief complaint
cc	cubic centimeter (same as mL)
CCU	coronary care unit; critical care unit
CDC	Centers for Disease Control and Prevention
CF	complement fixation
CHD	coronary heart disease; chronic heart disease; congestive heart disease
CHF	congestive heart failure
Cl	chlorine (in compounds it may represent chloride)
cm	centimeter
CMA	certified medical assistant
CMT	certified medical transcriptionist
CNS	central nervous system
CO	carbon monoxide
Co	cobalt

CO2 or CO$_2$	carbon dioxide
COD	condition on discharge
COPD	chronic obstructive pulmonary disease
CPAP	continuous positive airway pressure
CPR	cardiopulmonary resuscitation
CPX	complete physical examination
CR	cardiorespiratory
C-section	cesarean section
CSF	cerebrospinal fluid
C&S	culture and sensitivity
CT	computed tomography
Cu	copper
CVA	costovertebral angle; cerebrovascular accident
CXR	chest x-ray
D&C	dilation and curettage
DD	differential diagnosis
D$_5$W or D5W	dextrose and water
DOA	dead on arrival
DOB	date of birth
DOE	dyspnea on exertion
DPM	doctor of podiatric medicine
DPT	diphtheria-pertussis-tetanus (vaccine)
DRG	diagnosis-related group
DSM	*Diagnostic and Statistical Manual of Mental Disorders*
DTR	deep tendon reflexes
D/W	dextrose and water
Dx or DX	diagnosis
EAC	external auditory canal
EBL	estimated blood loss
ECG	electrocardiogram
ECMO	extracorporeal membrane oxygenation
ED	emergency department
EDC	estimated date of confinement (due date for baby)
EEG	electroencephalogram
EENT	eyes, ears, nose, throat
e.g.	example given
EKG	electrocardiogram (ECG is preferred)
ELISA	enzyme-linked immunosorbent assay
EMG	electromyogram
EMI	*see* CAT
EMS	emergency medical services
EMT	emergency medical technician; emergency medical treatment
ENT	ear, nose, throat
EOM	extraocular movements
eos	eosinophils
eq.	equivalent
ER	emergency room

Esq.	esquire
ESR	erythrocyte sedimentation rate
et al.	and others (notice punctuation)
F or °F	Fahrenheit
FB	foreign body
FBS	fasting blood sugar
Fe	iron
FH	family history
FHR	fetal heart rate
FHT	fetal heart tone
fl oz	fluid ounce
FSH	follicle-stimulating hormone
ft	foot
5-FU	5-fluorouracil (chemotherapy drug)
FUO	fever of unknown origin
Fx	fracture
G	gravida (pregnant)
g or gm	gram (gm preferred by some to avoid misunderstanding value)
G neg.	gram-negative
G pos.	gram-positive
GB	gallbladder
GC	gonorrhea
GH	growth hormone
GI	gastrointestinal
GP	general practitioner
GSW	gunshot wound
gtt	drop(s)
GTT	glucose tolerance test
GU	genitourinary
GYN or Gyn	gynecology/gynecologist
h.	hour
H	hour or hydrogen
H^+	hydrogen ion
H_2O or H2O	water
Hb	hemoglobin (also hgb)
HCG	human chorionic gonadotropin
HCl	hydrochloric acid
Hct or hct	hematocrit
HDL	high-density lipoprotein
HEENT	head, eyes, ears, nose, and throat
Hg	mercury
hgb	hemoglobin
H&H	hemoglobin and hematocrit (test on rbcs)
HIV	human immunodeficiency virus
HOPE	Health Opportunities for People Everywhere
H&P	history and physical
HPF or hpf	high-power field
HPI	history of present illness

h.s.	bedtime (hour of sleep)
Hx or HX	history
I	iodine
ibid.	in the same place
ICD-9-CM	*International Classification of Diseases, Ninth Revision, Clinical Modification*
ICU	intensive care unit
I&D	incision and drainage
i.e.	that is
IgA	immunoglobulin A (also IgD, IgE, IgG, and IgM)
IM	intramuscular
IMP	impression
in.	inch
I&O	intake and output
IOP	intraocular pressure
IPPB	intermittent positive-pressure breathing
IV	intravenous
IVP	intravenous pyelogram
K	potassium
K+	potassium ion
kg	kilogram
km	kilometer
KUB	kidneys, ureters, bladder
L	liter
L&A	light and accommodation
L1 or L_1	first lumbar vertebra (continues through L5)
lb	pound
LBBB	left bundle-branch block
LDL	low-density lipoprotein
LH	luteinizing hormone
LLQ	left lower quadrant
LMP	last menstrual period
LOC	loss of consciousness
LP	lumbar puncture
LPN	licensed practical nurse
LSH	lutein-stimulating hormone
LTH	lactogenic hormone, prolactin
LUQ	left upper quadrant
LVN	licensed vocational nurse
L&W	living and well
m	meter
MDR	minimum daily requirement
mEq	milliequivalent
mg	milligram
Mg	magnesium
Mg^{++} or Mg^{2+}	magnesium ion
mg%	milligrams percent
MI	myocardial infarction
mL or ml	milliliter

MM	mucous membrane
mm	millimeter
mmHg or mm Hg	millimeters of mercury
MOPP	nitrogen mustard, Oncovin, prednisone, procarbazine (chemotherapy)
mOsm	milliosmole
MR	mitral regurgitation
MRI	magnetic resonance imaging
MS	master's degree in science
MS	multiple sclerosis
MVA	motor vehicle accident
N	nitrogen
N^+	nitrogen ion
NA	not applicable
Na	sodium
Na^+	sodium ion
NG	nasogastric
NKA	no known allergies
NMI	no middle initial
NOS	not otherwise specified
NPC	near point of convergence (eyes); no previous complaint
NPH	no previous history
n.p.o.	nothing by mouth
NS	not significant
NSAID	nonsteroidal anti-inflammatory drug
NSR	normal sinus rhythm
NTP	normal temperature and pressure
NYD	not yet diagnosed
O_2 or O2	oxygen
OB	obstetrics
OB-GYN	obstetrics and gynecology
O&P	ova and parasites
OR	operating room
oz	ounce
P	phosphorus; pulse
P_1 or P1	pulmonic first sound (P1, P2, and so on)
P1	para 1 (and so on)
PA	posteroanterior
P&A	percussion and auscultation
Pap	Papanicolaou (test/smear)
PBI	protein-bound iodine
p.c.	after meals
pCO_2 or pCO2	partial pressure of carbon dioxide
PDR	*Physicians' Desk Reference* (drug reference)
PE	physical examination (also PX)
PERL	pupils equal, reactive to light
PERLA	pupils equal and reactive to light and accommodation

PERRLA	pupils equal, round, reactive to light, and accommodation
PET	positron emission tomography
PFT	pulmonary function test
PH	past history
pH	hydrogen ion concentration (degree of acidity or alkalinity)
PI	present illness
PICU	pediatric intensive care unit
PID	pelvic inflammatory disease
PIP	proximal interphalangeal (joint)
PKU	phenylketonuria (test given to newborns)
PM or p.m.	afternoon
PMH	past medical history
PMI	point of maximal impulse
PMS	premenstrual syndrome
PO	postoperative
p.o.	by mouth
pO_2 or pO2	partial pressure of oxygen
POC	products of conception
p.r.n.	as required or needed; as the occasion arises
PSA	prostate-specific antigen
pt	patient
PTA	prior to admission
PTSD	posttraumatic stress disorder
PVC	premature ventricular contraction
PX	physical examination (also PE)
Px	prognosis
q.	every
q.h.	every hour
q.2 h.	every two hours
q.3 h.	every three hours
q.4 h.	every four hours
q.i.d.	four times a day
QRS	complex in electrocardiographic study
qt	quart
R	respiration
r	roentgen
Ra	radium
RBBB	right bundle-branch block
rbc	red blood cell
RBC	red blood cell count
Rh (factor)	blood type (negative or positive factor antigen on the rbc)
RhoGAM	drug given to Rh-negative women to avoid risk of Rh immunization
RLQ	right lower quadrant
RN	registered nurse
R/O	rule out

ROM	range of motion
ROS	review of systems
RUQ	right upper quadrant
Rx	prescription or treatment
S1 or S_1	first sacral vertebra (also S2, S_2)
s̄	without
SG	specific gravity
SGOT	serum glutamic oxaloacetic transaminase
SI	seriously ill
SIDS	sudden infant death syndrome (crib death)
Sig.	directions
SMAC	automated analytic device for testing blood
SOAP	Subjective, Objective, Assessment, Plan (used for patient notes)
SOB	shortness of breath
SP	status post
sp. gr.	specific gravity
stat or STAT	immediately
SS	signs and symptoms
STD	sexually transmitted disease
T1 or T_1	first thoracic vertebra (continues through T12)
T&A	tonsillectomy and adenoidectomy
TAB	therapeutic abortion
TB	tuberculosis
TIA	transient ischemic attack
t.i.d.	three times a day
TM	tympanic membrane
TNTC	too numerous to count
TPR	temperature, pulse, respiration
TSH	thyroid-stimulating hormone
TURP	transurethral resection of the prostate gland
Tx	treatment
U	uranium
UA	urinalysis
URI	upper respiratory infection
UTI	urinary tract infection
UV	ultraviolet
VA	visual acuity; Veterans Administration
VDRL	Venereal Disease Research Laboratory (test for syphilis)
VF	visual fields
viz	that is; namely
VO	verbal order
vs	versus
VS	vital signs
VSD	ventricular septal defect
V&T	volume and tension (pulse)
wbc	white blood cell

WBC	white blood cell count
w-d	well-developed
WF	white female
WM	white male
w-n	well-nourished
WNL	within normal limits
x	times
X match	cross-match

Appendix B

Selected Abbreviations

Term	Abbreviation
acetylcholine	ACh
after meals	p.c.
after	p
alternating days	a.d.
and others	et al.
as much as desired or needed	ad lib.
as much as needed	q.s.
as needed	p.r.n.
atomic weight	z
barium	Ba
bedtime	h.s.
before meals	a.c.
biopsy	Bx
by mouth	p.o.
calcium	Ca
calcium ion	Ca^{++} or Ca^{2+}
cancer, carcinoma	CA or Ca
carbon dioxide	CO2 or CO_2
centimeter	cm
chief complaint	CC
cobalt	Co
complete physical examination	CPX
copper	Cu
cross-match	X match
cubic centimeter	cc
dextrose (5%) and water	D5W or D_5W
diagnosis	Dx
dilation and curettage	D&C
directions	sig.
drink	bib
drop(s)	gtt
equivalent	eq.
every day	q.d.

every four hours	q.4 h.
every hour	q.h.
every night	q.n.
every other day	q.o.d.
every	q.
every two hours, etc	q.2 h., etc.
example given	e.g.
foot	ft
for example	e.g.
four times a day	q.i.d.
fracture	Fx
freely	ad lib.
followup	F/U
grain	grain (spell out)
gram	gm or g
hematocrit	hct or Hct
hemoglobin and hematocrit	H&H
hemoglobin	hgb or Hb
history	Hx
hour	h. (Latin), h (English), also H (English)
hour of sleep	h.s.
hydrochloric acid	HCl
hydrogen	H
hydrogen ion concentration	pH
hydrogen ion	H^+
if necessary	SOS
immediately	STAT or stat
immunoglobulin	Ig
immunoglobulin A	IgA
immunoglobulin D	IgD
immunoglobulin E	IgE
immunoglobulin G	IgG
immunoglobulin M	IgM
impression	IMP
in the same place	ibid.
inch	in.
iodine	I
iron	Fe
kilogram	kg
kilometer	km
let it be labeled	sig.
liter	L
magnesium	Mg
magnesium ion	Mg^+
mercury	Hg
meter	m
milliequivalent	mEq

milligram	mg
milliliter	mL or ml
millimeter	mm
millimeters of mercury	mmHg or mmm Hg
namely	viz
not otherwise specified	NOS
nothing by mouth	n.p.o. or NPO
ointment	ung.
ounce	oz
oxygen	O2 or O_2
patient	pt
phosphorus	P
physical examination	PX or PE
potassium	K
potassium ion	K^+
pound	lb
prescription	Rx
pressure (partial) of carbon dioxide	pCO2 or pCO_2
prognosis	Px
radium	Ra
red blood cell	rbc
red blood cell count	RBC
Rhesus blood factor	Rh
roentgen	r
rule out	R/O
signs and symptoms	S/S
silver	Ag
sodium chloride	NaCl
sodium	Na
specific gravity	sp. gr.
temperature	T
that is	i.e. or viz
thoracic vertebrae	T1, T2, and so on (also T_1, T_2, and so on)
three times a day	t.i.d.
thyroxin	T_4 also T4
times three	$\times 3$
times	x or $\times$
treatment	Rx or Tx
twice a day	b.i.d.
ultraviolet	UV
unit	unit (spell out)
uranium	U
volt	V
water	aq.

water	$H2O$ or H_2O
watt	W
well-developed	w-d
well-nourished	w-n
white blood cell	wbc
white blood cell count	WBC
wine	vin.
with	c̄
without	s̄
without	w/o

Appendix C

Brief Forms, Short Forms, and Medical Slang

An asterisk indicates that the short form should be written out. The remainder can be used as is, according to usage in one's employment venue.

Brief Form	Meaning
abd*	abdomen
abs*	abdominal muscles
adm*	admission
afib*	atrial fibrillation
alb*	albumin
alk*	alkaline
amb*	ambulatory
amp*	ampule
amp and gent*	ampicillin and gentamicin
amt*	amount
anes*	anesthesia
ant*	anterior
approx*	approximately
appy*	appendectomy (also *hot appy,* meaning an acute appendicitis)
art*	arterial line
bact*	bacteria (pronounced *back-tee*)
bands	band neutrophils
basos	basophils (one of the family of white blood cells)
benzos*	benzodiazepine
bili*	bilirubin
bili light*	billirubin light
bio*	biology
brady*	bradycardia
cap gas*	capillary blood gas
caps	capsules
cath*	catheter
cathed*	catheterized
cauc*	Caucasian
chemo*	chemotherapy
coags*	coagulation studies

consult	consultation
cords*	vocal cords
cric*	cricothyrotomy
crit*	hematocrit
crypto*	Cryptosporidium
c-section	cesarean section
cysto*	cystoscopy
decub*	decubitus
defib*	defibrillated
dex*	dexamethasone
diff*	differential
dig* or dij*	digitalis, digitoxin, digoxin
dispos & admits*	discharges and admissions
d-stix*	Dextrostix
doc*	doctor
echo*	echocardiogram and so on
echs*	ecchymoses (bruises)
emerg*	emergency
eos	eosinophils (one of the family of white blood cells)
epi*	epidural anesthesia
equiv*	equivalent
esp*	especially
e-stim*	electrical stimulation
eval*	evaluation
exam	examination
ex lap*	exploratory laparotomy
fib*	fibula
flu	influenza
fluoro*	fluoroscopy
frac*	fracture
frag*	fragment
freq*	frequency or frequent
glob*	globulin
head post*	examination of brain
H&H*	hemoglobin and hematocrit
hep lock*	heparin lock
H flu*	Haemophilus influenzae
hosp*	hospital
hot appy*	acute appendicitis
hypo*	hypodermic or injection
imp*	impression
infarct	infarction
inoc*	inoculate (pronounced *in-ock*)
inop*	inoperable (pronounced *in-op*)
kilo*	kilogram (kg; e.g., 6 kg, not 6 kilos)
lab	laboratory
lap*	laparotomy
lap chole*	laparoscopic cholecystectomy

lymphs	lymphocytes (one of the family of white blood cells)
lytes*	electrolytes
mag plus	magnesium plus
max*	maximum
meds*	medications
mets*	metastases
metz*	Metzenbaum scissors
milli*	milligram or milliliter
mikes*	micrograms
monos	monocytes (one of the family of white blood cells)
multip*	multipara (a woman who has borne more than one child)
narcs*	narcotics
neg*	negative
nick you*	NICU (neonatology intensive care unit)
nitro*	nitroglycerin
norm	normal
nullip*	nullipara (a woman who has never borne a child)
ODd*	overdosed
Oh neg*	O-negative blood
ox sat*	oxygen saturation
Pap smear/test	Papanicolaou smear or test
path*	pathology
path lab*	pathology laboratory or department
pecs*	pectoral muscles
peds*	pediatrics
plates*	platelets
pneumo*	pneumothorax
polys	polymorphonuclear leukocytes/granulocytes
pos*	positive
post*	postmortem examination or autopsy
postop*	postoperative
preemie	premature infant
preop*	preoperative
prep	to prepare
prepped	prepared
pressors*	vasopressors (blood pressure medications)
primip*	primipara (a woman who is bearing her first child)
pro time	prothrombin time (blood clotting time)
procto*	proctoscopy
pulse ox*	pulse oximetry or oximeter
psych*	psychology or psychiatry or mental health unit
psych eval*	psychiatric evaluation
quads*	quadriceps muscle
rehab*	rehabilitation

reg*	regular
romied*	rule out myocardial infarction (ROMI)
Rx	prescription
sats*	oxygen saturations
scrim*	discrimination
script*	prescription
sec*	second or secondary
sed rate	sedimentation rate
segs	segmented neutrophils
sick you*	surgical intensive care unit (SICU)
sinus tack*	sinus tachycardia
snif unit*	skilled nursing facility (SNF)
spec*	specimen
stabs	stab cells (band cells)
staph	Staphylococcus (a bacterium)
strep	Streptococcus (a bacterium)
succs and fent*	succinylcholine and fentanyl
subcu*	subcutaneous (usually refers to an injection)
surg*	surgery or to perform surgery
tabby*	therapeutic abortion
tabs*	tablets
tachy*	tachycardia
temp*	temperature
tibs, fibs, pops*	tibial, fibular, and popliteal
tics*	diverticula
t max*	maximum temperature
tox screen*	toxicology screen test
trach*	tracheostomy
vanc*	vancomycin
V fib*	ventricular fibrillation
V tach*	ventricular tachycardia

Add to the List:

Appendix D

French Words Used in Medical Records

It is often difficult to locate the correct spelling for French words that may be dictated in a medical document. We have included the general pronunciation to help in your word search.

French Term	Pronunciation
au courant	oh-koo-RAHN
ampule	AM-pul
ballottement	bah-LOT-maw or bah-lot-ment or bah-lot-MAW
barbotage	bar-bow-TAHZH
bas-fond	bah-FON
beaux arts	bow ZAR
belle indifférence	bel ahn-de-fa-RAHNS
belles lettres	bel LET-ehr
bequerel	beck-REHL
berdache	bear-DASH
berloque	bear-LOKE
bête noire	bait NWAR
blancmange	blah-MANZH
bouche	boosh
bouche de tapir	boosh duh tah-PEER
bougie	boo-ZH or BOO-zh or BOO-je
bougienage	boo-zhe-NAHZH
bourdonnement	boor-don-MAW
bouton	boo-TON
brisement	breeze-MON
bruissement	broo-ez-MON
bruit	brew-E or broot
bruits	brew-EZ
cachet	kah-SHAY
cafe-au-lait	kah-FAY-o-LAY
capeline	kap-LEEN
capotement	kah-poht-MAW
carte blanche	KART blansh
caul	KAWL or COWL
cerclage	sair-KLAGE
chancre	SHANG-ker
charbon	shar-BAW

chaude-pisse	shohd-PEES
chordee	kor-DAY
coifed	kwaft
coiffure	kwah-FEWR
contrecoup	kon-tr-KOO
corps	core
coudé	koo-DAY
coup de fouet	kood-fooAY
coup de grace	kood-GRAS
coup de sang	kood-SANG
coup de soleil	kood-so-LAY
coup	koo
coup sur coup	koo-ser-KOO
courbature	koo-bah-TUHR
couvercle	koo-VER-kl
cri du chat	kree-de-SHAH
cuirass	kwe-RAS
cul-de-sac	KUL-de-sahk
curettage	ku-re-tahzh
curette, curet	ku-RET, kuray
de'collement	day-koal-MOH
debride	day-BREED
débridement	da-BREED-maw or de-BRIDE-ment
debris	day-BREE
déclassé	day-clawSAY
déjà entendu	day-zha ahn-tohn-DOO
déjà éprouvé	day-zha aye-proo-VAY
déjà fait	day-zha FAY
déjàa pensé	day-zha pon-SAY
déjà raconté	day-zha rak-on-TAY
déjà vécu	day-zha vay-KOO
déjà voulu	day-zha voo-LOO
déjà vu	day-zha VOO
délire	day-LEER
délire de toucher	day-LEERD-too-SHAY
demibain	dem-ee-BAHN
descemetitis	day-sem-titis
descemetocele	day-sem-to-SEEL
double entendre	dew-blanTANND
douche	doosh
douloureux	doo-loo-RUH
Dupuytren	du-pwe-TRAHN
effleurage	ef-flu-RAHZH
égoïsme à deux	eh-go-ism ah-DOO
en coup de sabre	ahn-koo-duh-SAHBR
en face	ahn-FAHS
enfant	ah-FAHN
état criblé	ay-TAH kree-BLAY
état mamelon	a-TAH maah-mel-un

état vermoulu	a-TAH vayr-moo-LU
facette, facet	fah-SET, fa-SAY
fait accompli	fai-tah-com-PLEE
faux pas	foe PAH
fiche	feesh
fleur de lis	flured-LEE
folie à deux	folee ah-DUH
folie du doute	folee duh-DOOT
folie du pourquoi	folee duh pur-KWAH
folie gemellaire	folee jeh-mel-LAIR
folie raisonnante	folee ray-sohn-AHNT
forage	fo-RAZH
forme fruste	form FROOST
fossette	foh-SET
fourchet	foor-SHAY
fourchette	foor-SHET
frôlement	frohl-MAW
gastrolavage	gas-tro-lah-VAHZH
gatism	GA-tizm
gauche	gohsh
gauntlet	GAWNT-let
gavage	gah-VAHZH
genre	JAWHN-re
grand mal	grahn MAHL
grattage	grah-TAHZH
hachement	ash-MAW
idée fix	ee day FEEKS
idiot savant	id-ee-OH sah-VAHNT
jamais vu	zha-may VOO
joie de vivre	ZHWA duh veev
la belle indifference	lah bel ahn-de-fa-RAHNS
la grippe	lah GRIP
laissez-faire	lay-say FAIR
lavage	lah-VAHZH
loupe	loop
lozenge	LOZ-enj
main d'accoucheur	mahn da-coo-SHUHR
main de tranchées	mahn de trahn-SHAY
main en crochet	maa nah kro-SHAY
main en griffe	maa nah GREEF
main en lorgnette	maa nah lor-NYET
main en pince	maa nah PINCE
main en singe	maa nah SEENGE
main en squelette	maa nah skel-ET
main fourché	mahn foor-SHA
main succulente	mahn suck-cu-LAHNT
mal	MAHL
maladie bronzée	mal-ah-DEE brawn-ZAY
maladie-de-Roger	mal-ah-DEED roe-ZHAY

malaise	mal-AYZ
mal de mer	mahld mare
mamelon	mahm-LON
marche à petis pas	marsh-ah-peh-TEE PAH
masseur	mah-SER
masseuse	mah-SUHZ
ménage	may-NAZH
ménage à trois	meh-NAZH ah TWAH
milieu	mee-LOO
moiety	moi-eh-TEE or mwah-eh-TEE
moiré	mwah-RAY
mouche	MOOHSH
moulage	moo-LAHZH
niche	NEESH
noblesse oblige	naw-blehs oh-BLEEZH
Parrot's	par-OHZ
Pasteur	pas-TER
patois	PAT-wah
peau d'orange	poh-DORAHNJ
pelage	peh-LAHZH
perleche	per-LESH
petit mal	peh-TEE MAHL
petit pas	peh-TEE PAH
Petit's	peh-TEES
pétrissage	pay-tree-SAHZH
Peyronie's	pay-row-NEEZ
pince-ciseaux	panz-see-ZOH
pincement	pans-MAW
plaque	plahk
plombage	plohm-BAZH
pointillage	pwan-tee-YAZH
pouce flottant	poos floh-TAHN
poudrage	poo-DRAHZH
Poupart's	poo-PARZ
prie-dieu	pree-DYUH
raison d' être	ray-zon-DETre
rale	rahl
rale de retour	rahld-raytoor
rale indux	rahl-ahn-DOO
rale redux	rahl-rey-DOO
Riolan's	re-o-LAHNZ
rongeur	raw-ZHUR
rouleau	roo-LOW
Roux-en-Y	ROOS-ah-nee
saccade	za-CAHD
saccadic	sah-KAH-dek
sciage	see-AHZ
serrefine	sayr-FEEN
serrenoeud	sayr-NOH-youd

tache	tahsh
tache blanche	tahsh blahnsh
tache bleuatres	tahsh bleu-AHTR
tache cérébrale	tahsh say-ray-BRAHL
tache laiteuses	tahsh lay-TOOZ
tache méningéeale	tahsh may-nin-zhay-AL
tache motrice	tahsh mo-TRE-eece
tache noire	tahsh nwahr
tache spinale	tahsh spee-NAHL
tambour	tam BOOR
tamponade	tam-pohn-AD
tapotement	tah-poht-MAW
thèque	tech
timbre	TIM-ber or TAM-br
tic	TICK
tic douloureux	tick doo-loo-ROO or tick doo-loo-RUH
tiqueur	te-KER
torsades de pointes	tor-sahd PWAHNT
tour de mître	tourd MEE-tr
triage	tree-AHZH
trocar	TRO-kar
ventouse	vaw-TOOZ
verdigris	ver-dee-GREE

Appendix E

Genus and Species Names, Clinically Significant Current Taxonomy

Even though genus and species names are italicized in print, they are generally typed in a regular font (called roman) in everyday transcription. Do italicize the names when transcribing an article for publication. The genus name is always capitalized. When it is abbreviated, it is a single capital letter followed by a period. The species epithet is not capitalized, nor is the common term. For example, Candida albicans is the full name, genus and species. C. albicans is the genus name abbreviated with species given. The term albicans is the specific epithet; it is not used alone. The common term is candidiasis; it can be used alone.

In the following list, some of the common terms and disease names have been provided.

Acanthamoeba astronyxis
Acanthamoeba castellani
Acanthamoeba culbertsoni
Acanthamoeba keratitis
Acanthamoeba polyphaga
Acanthamoeba rhysodes
Achromobacter lwoffi
Acinetobacter baumannii
Acinetobacter calcoaceticus
Acinetobacter haemolyticus
Acinetobacter junii
Acinetobacter lwoffi
Acinetobacter wolfii
Actinobacillus ureae
Actinobacillus yewk
Actinomadura madurae
Acremonium falciforme
Acremonium kiliense
Acremonium recifei
Acremonium restrictum
Actinobacillus
    actinomycetemcomitans

Actinobacillus equuli
Actinobacillus lignieresii
Actinobacillus suis
Actinomadura pelletieri
Actinomyces bovis
Actinomyces israelii
Actinomyces meyeri
Actinomyces naeslundii
Actinomyces odontolyticus
Actinomyces pyogenes
Actinomyces viscosus
Aerococcus viridans
Aeromonas caviae
Aeromonas hydrophila
Aeromonas hydrophila/caviae
Aeromonas sobria
Aeromonas veronii biovar sobria
Aeromonas veronii biovar veronii
Afipia felis
Agrobacterium radiobacter
Agrobacterium tumefaciens
Ajellomyces capsulatus

Ajellomyces dermatitidis
Alcaligenes bookeri
Alcaligenes faecalis
Alcaligenes xylosoxidans
Altermonas putrefaciens
Alternaria alternata
Amanita bisporigera
Amanita cokeri
Amanita cothurnata
Amanita gemmata
Amanita muscaria
Amanita ocreata
Amanita pantherina
Amanita phalloides
Amanita verna
Amanita virosa
Amblyomma americanum
    (Lone Star tick)
Anaerobiospirillum
    succiniciproducens
Anaerorhabdus furcosus
Ancylostoma braziliense
Ancylostoma caninum
Ancylostoma duodenale
    (hookworm)
Angiostrongylus cantonensis
Angiostrongylus costaricensis
Anisakis marina
Aquaspirillum itersonii
Arachnia propionica
Arcanobacterium haemolyticum
Ascaris lumbricoides (ascariasis)
Aspergillus flavus
Aspergillus fumigatus
Aspergillus glaucus
Aspergillus niger
Aspergillus terreus
Aureobasidium pullulans
Babesia bovis
Babesia microti
Bacillus alvei
Bacillus anthracis
Bacillus brevis
Bacillus cereus (bacillosis)
Bacillus circulans
Bacillus coagulans
Bacillus firmus
Bacillus laterosporus
Bacillus lentus

Bacillus licheniformis
Bacillus macerans
Bacillus megaterium
Bacillus polymyxa
Bacillus pumilus
Bacillus sphaericus
Bacillus stearothermophilus
Bacillus subtilis
Bacillus thermoliticus
Bacillus thuringiensis
Bacteroides bivius
Bacteroides caccae
Bacteroides capillosus
Bacteroides corrodens
Bacteroides distasonis
Bacteroides eggerthii
Bacteroides forsythus
Bacteroides fragilis (bacteroidosis)
Bacteroides merdae
Bacteroides oralis
Bacteroides stercoris
Bacteroides thetaiotaomicron
Bacteroides uniformis
Bacteroides ureolyticus
Bacteroides vulgatus
Balantidium coli
Bartonella bacilliformis
Bartonella elizabethae
Bartonella hensalae
Bartonella quintana
Basidiobolus ranarum
Bdellovibrio
Bifidobacterium bifidum
Bifidobacterium breve
Bifidobacterium dentium
Bifidobacterium infantis
Bipolaris australiensis
Bipolaris hawaiiensis
Bipolaris spicifera
Blastomyces dermatitidis
Blastoschizomyces
    pseudotrichosporon
Bordetella bronchiseptica
Bordetella parapertussis
Bordetella pertussis
Borrelia anserina
Borrelia burgdorferi (Lyme
    disease)
Borrelia mazzottii

Borrelia parkeri
Borrelia recurrentis
Borrelia turicatae
Botryodiplodia theobromae
Branhamella catarrhalis
Brevibacterium linens
Brevundimonas vesicularis
Brucella abortus
Brucella canis
Brucella melitensis (brucellosis)
Brucella suis
Brugia malayi
Budvicia aquatica
Burkholderia cepacia
Burkholderia mallei
Burkholderia pickettii
Burkholderia pseudomallei
Burkholderia thomasii
Calymmatobacterium
  granulomatis
Campylobacter cinaedi
Campylobacter fennelliae
Campylobacter fetus
Campylobacter jejuni
Campylobacter laridis
Campylobacter sputorum
Candida albicans (candidiasis)
Candida glabrata
Candida guilliermondi
Candida kefyr
Candida krusei
Candida lambica
Candida lusitaniae
Candida parapsilosis
Candida paratropicalis
Candida rugosa
Candida stellatoidea
Candida tropicalis
Candida zeylanoides
Cannabis sativa (marihuana)
Capnocytophaga canimorsus
Capnocytophaga ochracea
Cardiobacterium hominis
Cedecea neteri
Cedecea davisae
Cedecea lapagei
Chilomastix mesnili
Chlamydia pneumoniae
Chlamydia psittaci

Chlamydia trachomatis
Chromobacterium violaceum
Chryseobacterium gleum
Chryseobacterium indologenes
Chryseobacterium
  meningosepticum
Chryseomonas luteola
Chrysosporium parvum
Citrobacter amalonaticus
Citrobacter braakii
Citrobacter diversus
Citrobacter farmeri
Citrobacter freundii
Citrobacter youngae
Cladophialophora bantiana
Cladophialophora boppii
Cladophialophora carrionii
  (chromomycosis)
Cladophialophora devriesii
Cladosporium bantianum
Cladosporium cladosporioides
Cladosporium trichoides
  (cladosporiosis)
Cladosporium werneckii
Clonorchis sinensis
  (liver fluke)
Clostridium barati
Clostridium bifermentans
Clostridium botulinum
  (botulism)
Clostridium butyricum
Clostridium cadaveris
Clostridium clostridioforme
Clostridium difficile
Clostridium hastiforme
Clostridium histolyticum
Clostridium innocuum
Clostridium limosum
Clostridium novyi
Clostridium paraputrificum
Clostridium perfringens
Clostridium putrificum
Clostridium ramosum
Clostridium septicum
Clostridium sordellii
Clostridium sphenoides
Clostridium sporogenes
Clostridium subterminale
Clostridium tertium

559

Clostridium tetani (tetanus)
Coccidioides immitis
   (coccidioidomycosis)
Comamonas acidovorans
Comamonas terrigena
Comamonas testosteroni
Conidiobolus coronatus
Conidiobolus incongruus
Coprinus cinereus
Corynbacterium minutissimum
Corynebacterium bovis
Corynebacterium diphtheriae
   (diphtheria)
Corynebacterium jeikeium
Corynebacterium
   pseudotuberculosis
Corynebacterium ulcerans
Corynebacterium xerosis
Coxiella burnetii
Cryptococcus albidus
Cryptococcus laurentii
Cryptococcus luteolus
Cryptococcus neoformans
Cryptococcus terreus
Cryptococcus uniguttulatus
Curtobacterium flaccumfaciens
Curvularia pallescens
Curvularia senegalensis
Curvularia verruculosa
Cysticercus cellulosae,
   cysticercosis
Cysticercus ovis
Dermatophagoides farinae
   (dust mite)
Dermatophagoides
   pteronyssinus
Dermatophilus congolensis
Dientamoeba fragilis
Diphyllobothrium latum
Diplococcus pneumoniae
   (pneumonia)
Dipylidium caninum
Dirofilaria immitis
Donovania granulomatis
Dracunculus medinensis
E. coli O157:H7
Echinococcus granulosis
   (echinococcosis [tapeworm])
Echinococcus multilocularis

Edwardsiella hoshinae
Edwardsiella tarda
Ehrlichia canis
Eikenella corrodens
Endolimax nana
Entamoeba coli (entamebiasis)
Entamoeba gingivalis
Entamoeba hartmanni
Entamoeba histolytica (amebic
   dysentery)
Entamoeba polecki
Enterobacter aerogenes
Enterobacter amnigenus
Enterobacter asburiae
Enterobacter cloacae
Enterobacter gergoviae
Enterobacter hormaechei
Enterobacter intermedius
Enterobacter liquefaciens
Enterobacter sakazakii
Enterobius vermicularis
   (enterobiasis [pinworm])
Enterococcus avium
Enterococcus casseliflavus
Enterococcus durans
Enterococcus faecalis
Enterococcus faecium
Enterococcus gallinarum
Enterococcus hirae
Enterocytozoon bieneusi
Epidermophyton floccosum
Erwinia chrysanthemi
Erysipelothrix rhusiopathiae
Escherichia coli
Escherichia coli O157:H7
Escherichia fergusonii
Escherichia hermannii
Escherichia vulneris
Eubacterium aerofaciens
Eubacterium alactolyticum
Eubacterium lentum
Eubacterium limosum
Eubacterium moniliforme
Eubacterium multiforme
Ewingella americana
Exophiala jeanselmei
Exophiala moniliae
Exophiala spinifera
Exserohilum rostratum

Fasciola hepatica
Fasciolopsis buski
  (fasciolopsiasis [flukes])
Fibrobacter succinogenes
Flavimonas oryzihabitans
Flavobacterium gleum
Flavobacterium indologenes
Flavobacterium
  meningosepticum
Flavobacterium odoratum
Francisella tularensis
Friedländer's bacillus
Fusobacterium mortiferum
Fusobacterium necrophorum
Fusobacterium nucleatum
Fusobacterium periodonticum
Fusobacterium russii
Fusobacterium varium
Gardnerella vaginalis
Gemella morbillorum
Geotrichum candidum
Geotrichum capitatum
Geotrichum penicillatum
Giardia lamblia (giardiasis)
Haemophilus aegyptius
Haemophilus aphrophilus
Haemophilus ducreyi
Haemophilus haemolyticus
Haemophilus influenzae
Haemophilus
  parahaemolyticus
Haemophilus parainfluenzae
Haemophilus paraphrophilus
Haemophilus segnis
Haemophilus vaginalis
Hafnia alvei
Hansenula anomala
Helicobacter hepaticus
Helicobacter mustelae
Helicobacter pylori
Herellea vaginicola
Heterophyes heterophyes
Histoplasma capsulatum
  (histoplasmosis)
Hymenolepis diminuta
Hymenolepis nana
Iodamoeba buetschlii
Isospora belli
Isospora parasite

Ixodes dammini
Ixodes pacificus
Kingella denitrificans
Kingella kingae
Klebsiella ornithinolytica
Klebsiella oxytoca
Klebsiella ozaenae
Klebsiella pneumoniae
Klebsiella rhinoscleromatis
Kluyvera ascorbata
Kluyvera cryocrescens
Koserella trabulsii
Lactobacillus acidophilus
Lactobacillus catenaforme
Lactobacillus cellobiosus
Lactobacillus fermentum
Lactobacillus jensenii
Lactobacillus minutus
Leclercia adecarboxylata
Lecythophora hoffmannii
Lecythophora mutabilis
Legionella anisa
Legionella bozemanii
Legionella brasiliensis
Legionella brunensis
Legionella dumoffii
Legionella feeleii
Legionella gormanii
Legionella jordanis
Legionella longbeachae
Legionella micdadei
Legionella oakridgensis
Legionella pneumophila
  (legionnaire's disease)
Legionella wadsworthii
Leishmania brasiliensis
Leishmania caninum
Leishmania donovani
Leishmania mexicana
Leishmania peruviana
Leishmania tropica
Leptospira biflexa
Leptospira interrogans
Leptothrix buccalis
Leuconostoc mesenteroides
Listeria monocytogenes
Madurella mycetomatis
Malassezia furfur
Malassezia pachydermatis

Mansonella perstans
Mansonella streptocerca
Metagonimus yokogawai
Micrococcus luteus
Microsporum audouinie
  (microsporosis [ringworm])
Microsporum canis
  (microsporosis [ringworm])
Microsporum cookei
Microsporum equinum
Microsporum ferrugineum
Microsporum fulvum
Microsporum gallinae
Microsporum gypseum
Microsporum nanum
Microsporum persicolor
Microsporum praecox
Microsporum racemosum
Microsporum vanbreuseghemii
Moraxella atlantae
Moraxella catarrhalis
Moraxella lacunata
Moraxella nonliquefaciens
Moraxella osloensis
Moraxella phenylpyruvica
Moraxella urethralis
Morganella morganii
Mortierella wolfii
Mycobacterium abscessus
Mycobacterium africanum
Mycobacterium alvei
Mycobacterium asiaticum
Mycobacterium avium
Mycobacterium avium-
  intracellulare
Mycobacterium bohemicum
Mycobacterium bovis
Mycobacterium branderi
Mycobacterium butyricum
Mycobacterium chelonae
Mycobacterium confluentis
Mycobacterium conspicuum
Mycobacterium flavescens
Mycobacterium fortuitum
Mycobacterium gastri
Mycobacterium genavense
Mycobacterium goodii
Mycobacterium gordonae
Mycobacterium haemophilum

Mycobacterium hassiacum
Mycobacterium heckeshornense
Mycobacterium heidelbergense
Mycobacterium hominis
Mycobacterium immunogenum
Mycobacterium interjectum
Mycobacterium intermedium
Mycobacterium intracellulare
Mycobacterium kansasii
Mycobacterium kubicae
Mycobacterium lentiflavum
Mycobacterium leprae, leprosy
Mycobacterium mageritense
Mycobacterium malmoense
Mycobacterium marinum
Mycobacterium microti
Mycobacterium mucogenicum
Mycobacterium novocastrense
Mycobacterium palustre
Mycobacterium parafortuitum
Mycobacterium paratuberculosis
Mycobacterium phlei
Mycobacterium scrofulaceum
Mycobacterium simiae
Mycobacterium smegmatis
Mycobacterium szulgai
Mycobacterium terrae
Mycobacterium triplex
Mycobacterium triviale
Mycobacterium tuberculosis
Mycobacterium tusciae
Mycobacterium ulcerans
Mycobacterium vaccae
Mycobacterium wolinskyi
Mycobacterium xenopi
Mycocentrospora acerina
Mycoplasma buccale
Mycoplasma faucium
Mycoplasma fermentans
Mycoplasma genitalium
Mycoplasma hominis
Mycoplasma orale
Mycoplasma pneumoniae,
  pneumonia
Mycoplasma salivarium
Mycoplasma urealyticum
Naegleria fowleri
Necator americanus, hookworm
Neisseria cinerea

Neisseria elongata
Neisseria flavescens
Neisseria gonorrhoeae
  (gonorrhea)
Neisseria lactamica
Neisseria meningitidis
  (cerebrospinal meningitis)
Neisseria mucosa
Neisseria sicca
Neisseria subflava
Nocardia asteroides (nocardiosis)
Nocardia brasiliensis
Nocardia caviae
Nocardiopsis dassonvillei
Obesumbacterium proteus
Oligella urethralis
Onchocerca volvulus
  (onchocerciasis [roundworm])
Opisthorchis sinensis
Opisthorchis viverrini
Paecilomyces javanicus
Paecilomyces lilacinus
Paecilomyces variotii
Paecilomyces viridis
Pantoea agglomerans
Paracoccidioides brasiliensis
Paragonimus westermani
Pasteurella aerogenes
Pasteurella haemolytica
Pasteurella multocida
Pasteurella pneumotropica
Pasteurella pseudotuberculosis
Pasteurella ureae
Pediculus humanus capitis
Pediculus humanus corporis
Pediculus pubis
Penicillium chrysogenum
Penicillium citrinum
Penicillium commune
Penicillium expansum
Penicillium marneffei
Penicillium spinulosum
Peptococcus anaerobios
Peptococcus niger
Peptostreptococcus anaerobius
Peptostreptococcus
  asaccharolyticus
Peptostreptococcus indolicus
Peptostreptococcus magnus

Peptostreptococcus micros
Peptostreptococcus prevotii
Peptostreptococcus productus
Peptostreptococcus tetradius
Phaeoannellomyces elegans
Phaeoannellomyces werneckii
Phialophora bubakii
Phialophora dermatitidis
Phialophora parasitica
Phialophora repens
Phialophora verrucosa
Phoma eupyrena
Photobacterium damsela
Phthirus pubis (crab louse)
Pichia ohmeri
Pityrosporum orbiculare
Plasmodium falciparum
Plasmodium malariae (malaria)
Plasmodium ovale
Plasmodium vivax
Plesiomonas shigelloides
Pneumocystis carinii
Porphyromonas asaccharolytica
Porphyromonas gingivalis
Prevotella bivia
Prevotella buccae
Prevotella corporis
Prevotella denticola
Prevotella disiens
Prevotella intermedia
Prevotella loescheii
Prevotella melaninogenica
Prevotella oralis
Prevotella oris
Prevotella ruminicola
Prevotella zoogleoformans
Propionibacterium acnes
Propionibacterium avidum
Propionibacterium granulosum
Propionibacterium propionicus
Proteus mirabilis
Proteus morganii
Proteus penneri
Proteus vulgaris
Prototheca wickerhamii
Prototheca zopfii
Providencia alcalifaciens
Providencia rettgeri
Providencia stuartii

Pseudallescheria boydii
Pseudomonas aeruginosa
Pseudomonas alcaligenes
Pseudomonas diminuta
Pseudomonas exotoxin
Pseudomonas fluorescens
Pseudomonas mallei
Pseudomonas maltophilia
Pseudomonas pseudoalcaligenes
Pseudomonas putida
Pseudomonas stutzeri
Pseudomonas testosteroni
Psorospermium haeckelii
Rahnella aquatilis
Retortamonas intestinalis
Rhinocladiella aquaspersa
Rhinosporidium seeberi
Rhizomucor pusillus
Rhizopus arrhizus
Rhizopus microsporus
Rhizopus nigricans
Rhizopus rhizopodiformis
Rhodotorula glutinis
Rhodotorula pilimanae
Rhodotorula rubra
Rhondococcus aurantiacus
Rhondococcus equi
Rickettsia akari
Rickettsia australis
Rickettsia burnetii
Rickettsia conorii
Rickettsia prowazekii
Rickettsia quintana
Rickettsia rickettsii (Rocky
  Mountain spotted fever)
Rickettsia sibirica
Rickettsia tsutsugamushi
Rickettsia typhi
Rochalimaea henselae
Rochalimaea quintana
Saccharomonospora viridis
Saccharomyces cerevisiae
Saksenaea vasiformis
Salmonella arizonae
Salmonella choleraesuis
Salmonella enteritidis
  (salmonellosis)
Salmonella paratyphi A
Salmonella typhi (typhoid fever)

Salmonella typhimurium
Sarcocystis homonis
Sarcocystis suihominis
Scedosporium apiospermum
Schistosoma haematobium
Schistosoma intercalatum
Schistosoma japonicum
Schistosoma mansoni
Schistosoma mekongi
Scopulariopsis brevicaulis
Serratia liquefaciens
Serratia marcescens
Serratia rubidaea
Shewanella putrefaciens
Shigella boydii
Shigella dysenteriae (shigellosis)
Shigella flexneri
Shigella sonnei
Sphingobacterium multivorum
Sphingomonas paucimobilis
Spirillum minus
Sporothrix schenckii
Sporotrichum pruinosum
Sporotrichum schenckii
Staphylococcus aureus
Staphylococcus auricularis
Staphylococcus capitis
Staphylococcus cohnii
Staphylococcus epidermidis
Staphylococcus equi
Staphylococcus haemolyticus
Staphylococcus hominis
Staphylococcus hyicus
Staphylococcus intermedius
Staphylococcus lentus
Staphylococcus oralis
Staphylococcus saprophyticus
Staphylococcus sciuri
Staphylococcus simulans
Staphylococcus warneri
Staphylococcus xylosus
Stenotrophomonas maltophilia
Streptobacillus moniliformis
Streptococcus acidominimus
Streptococcus agalactiae
Streptococcus anginosus
Streptococcus bovis
Streptococcus constellatus
Streptococcus equinus

Streptococcus faecalis
Streptococcus intermedius
Streptococcus milleri
Streptococcus mitis
Streptococcus mutans
Streptococcus pneumoniae
Streptococcus pyogenes
Streptococcus salivarius
Streptococcus sanguis
Streptococcus uberis
Streptococcus viridans
Streptococcus zooepidemicus
Streptomyces paraguayensis
Streptomyces somaliensis
Strongyloides stercoralis
(strongyloidiasis
[threadworm])
Suttonella indologenes
Taenia lata (tapeworm)
Taenia multiceps
Taenia saginata
Taenia solium
Tatumella ptyseos
Thermoactinomyces candidus
Thermoactinomyces sacchari
Thermoactinomyces vulgaris
Thermomonospora alba
Tissierella praeacuta
Torula histolytica
Torulopsis candida
Torulopsis glabrata
Toxocara canis
Toxoplasma gondii
(toxoplasmosis)
Treponema bryantii
Treponema buccale
Treponema carateum
Treponema pallidum (syphilis)
Treponema pertenue
Treponema vincentii
Trichinella spiralis (trichinosis)
Trichomonas hominis
Trichomonas tenax
Trichomonas vaginalis
(trichomoniasis)
Trichophyton ajelloi
Trichophyton concentricum
Trichophyton equinum
Trichophyton fischeri

Trichophyton gourvilii
Trichophyton longifuscum
Trichophyton megninii
Trichophyton mentagrophytes
Trichophyton rubrum
Trichophyton schoenleinii
Trichophyton simii
Trichophyton soudanense
Trichophyton terrestre
Trichophyton tonsurans
(ringworm)
Trichophyton verrucosum
Trichophyton violaceum
Trichosporon beigelii
Trichuris trichiura (trichuriasis
[whipworm])
Tropheryma whipplei
Trypanosoma brucei gambiense
Trypanosoma brucei rhodesiense
Trypanosoma cruzi
Trypanosoma gambiense
Trypanosoma rangeli
Trypanosoma rhodesiense
Tsukamurella paurometabolum
Ureaplasma urealyticum
Veillonella parvula
Vibrio alginolyticus
Vibrio cholerae
Vibrio fetus
Vibrio fluvialis
Vibrio hollisae
Vibrio metschnikovii
Vibrio mimicus
Vibrio parahaemolyticus
Vibrio vulnificus
Wangiella dermatitidis
Wolinella recta
Wuchereria bancrofti
Xylohypha bantiana
Yarrowia lipolytica
Yersinia enterocolitica
Yersinia frederiksenii
Yersinia intermedia
Yersinia kristensenii
Yersinia pestis
Yersinia pseudotuberculosis
Yokenella regensburgei
Zymomonas mobilis

Appendix F

Homonyms and Sound-alike Words

Watch out for homonyms. These are words that are often misused because we confuse them with something that sounds like it could be the word we want. If you let them, they will fool you and your spell-checker and appear in your voice-recognition documents. This list just warns you what to watch for. You should review this list from time to time so that you will not overlook some subtle substitute for the word you really want. Be sure to check the meaning of your word selection in the dictionary. Those words in the list "English Homonyms Speller" marked with an asterisk are fully explained in Chapter 17, Grammar.

ENGLISH HOMONYM SPELLER

abject object
accede exceed
accent ascent assent except
access excess
adapt adept adopt
addenda agenda
addition edition
adherence adherents
adverse averse
advice advise
affect effect
*aid aide
air heir
aisle isle
ale ail
alimentary elementary
allowed aloud
*all ready already
all right alright
*all together altogether
allude elude
*allusion illusion elusion
all ways always
alter altar
*alumna alumnus
anecdote antidote

annual annul
anonymous unanimous
any one anyone
anytime any time
any way anyway
*apposition opposition
*appraise apprise
area aria
ascent assent
assistance assistants
*assure insure ensure
ate eight
attendance attendants
aught ought
avert evert invert overt
*awhile a while
*bad badly
baited bated
bale bail
bare bear Bayer
base bass
bases basis
bazaar bizarre
been bin
beet beat
berth birth

567

*beside besides
biannual biennial
billed build
bizarre bazaar
bloc block
blue blew
boarder border
bolder boulder
bolus bullous
bore boor boar
born borne
bow beau
bow bough
bowl bole
*breach breech
bread bred
breadth breath breathe
break brake
breathe breath breadth
*bridle bridal
build billed
bury berry
but butt
buy bye by
*callous callus
canopy canape
canvas canvass
capitol capital Capitol
carat caret carrot karat
cash cache
casual causal
cease seize
cede seed
cell sell
censer censure sensor
census senses
cent scent sent
cereal serial
choose chews chose
*chord cord
*cite sight site
click clique
coarse course
collision collusion
complacent complaisant
*complement compliment
complementary complimentary
compose comprise
concur conquer

confident confidant
conscience conscious
consul council counsel
    console
*continual continuous
corps corpse
correspondence corespondent
credible creditable
crews cruise
cue queue
current currant
curser cursor
dairy diary
Dane deign
decent descent dissent
decision discission
deer dear
defer differ
deference difference
defuse diffuse
deluded dilute
deposition disposition
descent dissent decent
desperate disparate
device devise
die dye
*dilate dilation dilatation
disburse disperse
disc disk
*discreet discrete
diseased deceased
dissension distention
dissent decent
do dew due
done dun
dough doe
earn urn
edition addition
*effect affect
ejection injection
elementary alimentary
*elicit illicit
eligible illegible
elude allude
elusive illusive
emanate eminence
*emigrate immigrate
*eminent imminent immanent
*enervated innervated

envelop envelope
erasable irascible
evert avert overt invert
*every day everyday
*every one everyone
eves eaves
ewes use
exceed accede
excess access
expand expend
explicit implicit
extant extent
fair fare
facetious factious fictitious
*farther further
faze phase
fecal cecal thecal
feet feat
fiber fibrous
finally finely
fir fur
fiscal physical
flare flair
flaunt flout flute
flee flea
flounder founder
flow floe
flue flew flu
*followup follow up follow-up
foreword forward
*formally formerly
forth fourth
founder flounder
four for
fowl foul
freeze frieze
gage gauge gouge
gait gate
gaited gated
genius genus
gouge gauge gage
graft graph
great grate
guarantee guaranty
guessed guest
hail hale
hair hare
heal heel

hear here
hear sheer
heard herd
heart hart
heir air
him hymn
hoarse horse
hole whole
holey holy wholly
hour our
hue hew
human humane
ideal idle idol
illegible eligible
illicit elicit
*illusion allusion
illusive elusive
*immigrate emigrate
imminent immanent
inapt inept
*incidence incidents
incite insight
indigent indignant indigenous
inequity iniquity
ingenious ingenuous
inherent inherit
insight incite
insure assure
invert evert avert overt
isle aisle
*its it's
knead need
knew new
knot not
know no
knows nose
lacks lax
lapse relapse
*lay lei lie
lead led
lean lien
leased least
leek leak
lesson lessen
lessor lesser
liable libel
lice lyse slice
lichen liken

lie lay
lightening lightning
load lode
loath loathe
loop loupe
*loose lose
lye lie lay
lysed sliced
made maid
mail male
main mane
marital martial
material matériel
maul mall
*maybe may be
maze maize
mean mien
medal meddle
median medium
meet meat
might mite
miner minor
mist missed
modeling mottling
moot mute
moral morale
*mucus mucous mucosa
muse mews
*nauseated nauseous
*naval navel
need knead
new knew
no know
nose knows
not knot
oar ore
object abject
one won Juan
ought aught
our hour
overdo overdue
overt avert evert invert
owed ode
pain pane
pair pare pear
*palate pallet palette
pale pail
pare pear
*passed past

pause paws
peace piece
peak peek
peal peel
pearl purl
pedal petal
peer pier
peer pier
penance pennants
phase faze
pie pi
piece peace
plane plain
pole poll
pour pore purr
pray prey
*precede proceed
precedent president
precedents precedence
prescribe proscribe
preventive preventative
*principle principal
proceed precede
pupal pupil
queue cue
quiet quite
rain reign
raise raze rise
ravage ravish
real reel
red read
reed read
regime regimen
relapse lapse
respectably respectfully
    respectively
resume résumé
rhyme rime
right rite wright write
ring wring
road rode
roll role
*root route
row roe
rows rose
rude rood
rye wry
sale sail
sax sacks

scene seen
seas seize
see sea
seed cede
seeks Sikhs
seem seam
seen scene
sell cell
sensor censor censure censer
*set sit sat
sew so sow
shone shown
sick sic
*sight cite site
sleight slay
slight sleight
so sow sew
sole soul
some time sometime
    sometimes
sore soar
staid stayed
stationary stationery
statue stature statute
steal steel
straight strait
subtle supple
suit suite sweet
sum some
sweet suite
tack tact
tale tail
tare tear tier
tea tee
team teem
tenet tenant
thecal fecal cecal
theirs there's
their there they're
*then than
there their

there their they're
tick tic
time thyme
tortuous tortuous
tow toe
track tract
turn tern
two too
unanimous anonymous
urn earn
vane vain vein
vary very
veil vale
vein vane vain
vial vile
vice vise
wail whale
wait weight
waive wave
ware wear where
way weigh
we wee
week weak
when wen
whether weather
while wile
whine wine
*who whom
whole hole
wholly holy
who's whose
wit whit
would wood
wring ring
write right rite
wrote rote
wry rye
yolk yoke
you yew
your you're yore

MEDICAL HOMONYM SPELLER

a cult occult
a febrile (patient) an afebrile
   (patient)
abasia aphagia aphakia
abdominal abominable
abduction addiction adduction
   subduction
aberrant afferent apparent
   efferent inferent
aberration abrasion erasion
   erosion operation
abject object
ablation oblation
abscess aphthous absence
absorption adsorption sorption
access axis excess
acetic acidic aesthetic ascitic
   asthenic esthesic esthetic
achymosis ecchymosis echinosis
   chemosis
addiction abduction adduction
adherence adherent adherents
adsorption absorption sorption
adverse averse
aerogenous erogenous
affect effect
afferent aberrant efferent
affusion effusion infusion
agonist against
alfa alpha
alkalosis ankylosis
allude elude elute
allusion elution illusion
alpha alfa
alveolar alveolate alveoli
   alveolus alveus alvus areolar
amenorrhea dysmenorrhea
   menorrhagia menorrhea
   metrorrhagia
anecdote antidote
anergia inertia
anesthetic anesthesia
antiseptic asepsis aseptic sepsis
   septic
anuresis enuresis
aphagia abasia aphakia aphasia
aphakia aphagia aplasia

aphthous abscess apophysis
   epiphysis hypophysis
   hypothesis
apposition opposition
areolar alveolus alveolar
arrhythmia erythema
   eurhythmia
arteriostenosis atherosclerosis
   arteriosclerosis
astasia ectasia
atherosclerosis arteriosclerosis
   arteriostenosis
attacks Atarax ataxia
aural aura ora oral orale
auscultation oscillation oscitation
   osculation escalation
avert evert invert overt
axillary auxiliary
axis access
bizarre bazaar
bolus bullous
bowel bile vowel
breath breadth breathe breed
bronchoscopic proctoscopic
bruit brute
calculous calculus caliculus
   callous callus talus
caliber calipers
calices calyces
callous callus
cancellous cancellus
cancer canker chancre cancerous
cancerous cancellus cancellous
carbuncle caruncle furuncle
carotene keratin
carotid parotid
carpus corpus
caudal coddle Cottle
cease seize
cecal fecal thecal
celiotomy ciliotomy
cella sella
cellular sellar
chancre cancer canker
chemosis achymosis ecchymosis
cholic colic
chordae chordee

cilium psyllium
cirrhosis cillosis xerosis psilosis
   sclerosis
climatic climactic climacteric
colic cholic
collum column
complaisant complacent
complement compliment
continence continents
contusion concussion confusion
   convulsion
cor corneal cranial
cord chord
core corps corpse
corollary coronary
corpus carpus copious
cranial corneal
creatine creatinine
creatine creatinine keratan
   keratin
cremation crenation
crepitance crepitus
crus crux
cytology psychology sitology
Cytoxan sitotoxin
decision discission
denervation enervation
   innervation
dental dentia denticle identical
dentinocemental
   dentinoenamel
desperate disparate
diaphysis apophysis diastasis
diarrhea diuria diuresis
diathesis diastasis diaphysis
dilate dilation dilatation
disk disc
dissension distention
ductal ductile
dysphagia dysbasia dyscrasia
   dysphasia dysplasia dyspragia
   dysphonia
dyspraxia dystaxia dyspragia
   dystectia
ecchymosis achymosis echinosis
   chemosis
ectasia astasia
eczema exemia
effect affect defect

efferent aberrant afferent
effusion affusion infusion
ejection ingestion injection
elude elute allude
elution illusion
emanate eminence eminent
   imminent
embolus embolism thrombus
endemic ecdemic epidemic
   pandemic
enema intima intimal
enervated innervated
enervation denervation
   innervation
enfold infold
enteric icteric
enuresis anuresis
epidemic ecdemic endemic
epiphysis apophysis hypophysis
   hypothesis
epiphysis hypophysis
   hypothesis aphthous abscess
   apophysis
erasable irascible
erasion erosion operation
   abrasion aberration
erogenous aerogenous
erythema arrhythmia erythremia
   eurhythmia
escalation oscillation osculation
   auscultation
eschar a scar escharotic scar
ethanal ethinyl ethanol ethenyl
etiology ideology
everted inverted
excess access axis
facial basal fascial faucial racial
   fascicle
falx false
fascicle vesical vesicle
fashion faucial fauces facies
   feces foci
faze phase phrase
fecal cecal fetal focal thecal fatal
fibers fibrose fibrous
filiform phalliform piliform
fissula fistula
flanges phalanges
flexor flexure

foci fossae loci
fontanel fontanelle
fornication formication
fornix pharynx
fossa fossae
fovea folia phobia
fundi fungi
furuncle carbuncle caruncle
gaited gated
gastroscopy gastrostomy
   gastrotomy
gavage lavage
gibbus gibbous
glands glans
glucoside glycoside
hemolysis homolysis
heroin heroine
heterotopia heterotrophia
   heterotropia
homogenous homogeneous
humeral humoral
humerus humorous
hypercalcemia hyperkalemia
hyperinsulinism
   hypoinsulinism
hyperkalemia hypercalcemia
   hyperkinemia hypokalemia
hypertension Hypertensin
   hypotension
hypoinsulinism
   hyperinsulinism
hypokalemia hypercalcemia
   hyperkinemia
hypophysis apophysis epiphysis
   hypothesis
hypotension hypertension
icteric enteric mycteric
ideology etiology
ileac iliac
ileum ilium
illicit elicit
illusion allusion
in toto total
inanimate innominate
inanition inattention inhibition
incidence incidents instance
incision schism scission
inertia anergia

infarction infection infestation
   infraction injection inflection
inflection inflexion in flexion
   injection ingestion
infold enfold
innervated enervated
innervation enervation
innominate inanimate
installation instillation
insulin inulin
intima enema
intralocular intraocular
inverted everted
irascible erasable
irradiate radiate
jewel joule jowl
karyon kerion
keloid keroid
keratin carotene
keratin keratan
keratitis keratosis ketosis
knuckle nuchal
labial labile libel
laceration maceration
   masturbation
lassitude latitude
lavage gavage
libido livedo
lice lyse
linea linear
lipoma fibroma lipomyoma
   lymphoma
lithotomy lithotony
liver livor sliver
loci foci fossae
lymphoma lipoma
lyse lice slice
maceration laceration
   masturbation
mastitis mastoiditis
masturbation maceration
meiosis miosis mitosis mycosis
   myiasis
menorrhagia menorrhea
   metrorrhagia
menorrhea amenorrhea
   dysmenorrhea
metacarpal metatarsal

metastasis metaphysis
  metastases metastasize
  metastatic
metatarsal metacarpal
metrorrhagia menorrhagia
  menorrhea
mnemonic pneumonic
modeling mottling
mucoid Mucor mucosa mucosal
  mucosin
mucous mucus
mucous mucus mucosal
myoclonic myotonic
myogram myelogram
necrosis narcosis nephrosis
  neurosis urosis
nuchal knuckle
nucleide nuclide
object abject
oblation ablation
obstipation constipation
  obfuscation
occult a cult
opposition apposition
oral ora aura aural orale
organism orgasm
oscillation auscultation
  oscitation osculation
osteal ostial
palpable palpebral
palpation palliation palpitation
  papillation
papilledema papal edema
paracytic parasitic
paraesthesia paresthesia
  pallesthesia
parietitis parotiditis parotitis
parotic perotic porotic
parous Paris pars porous
pectineal perineal peritoneal
  peroneal peronia
pedicle medical particle
  peduncle pellicle
pediculous pediculus
perfusion profusion protrusion
perineal pectineal peritoneal
  peroneal
perineum peritoneum
phalanges flanges

phenol phenyl
phobia fovea
phthisis ptosis
pleural plural
pleuritis pruritus
pneumonic mnemonic
prescribe proscribe
profusion perfusion
proptosis ptosis
prostate prostrate rostrate
prostatic prosthetic
protein protean
psoriasis siriasis
psychology cytology sitology
psychosis sycosis
psychotic saccadic
psyllium cilium
pterygium pterygoid
ptosis proptosis phthisis
pupil pupal
purinemia pyuria
pyelonephrosis pyonephrosis
pyuria paruria pyorrhea
  purinemia
racial fascial facial falcial
radical radicle
recession resection
rectus rhexis rictus ructus
refection reflection refraction
reflex efflux reflux
resection recession
RH factor (rheumatoid) Rh
  factor (blood)
rhonchi bronchi
scar a scar eschar scarf
scatoma scotoma
scirrhous cirrhosis cirrus scirrhus
  sclerous serious serous
sedentary sedimentary
seize cease
sella cella
sellar cellular
separation suppression
  suppuration
sepsis antiseptic asepsis aseptic
  septic threpsis
septal septile skeptic
serial sural
serious serosa xerosis

serosa cirrhosis xerosis
serous cirrus scirrhous scirrhus
   sclerous serious
shoddy shotty
sight cite cyte side site slight
sign sine
silicon silicone
sliver livor liver
stasis bases basis
status staxis stasis
stroma soma stoma struma
   trauma
suppression suppuration
   susurration
sural serial
taenia tenia tinea
talus callus calculous calculus
   cancellus
thecal fecal cecal fetal
thenar thinner
tic tick
tortuous torturous

total in toto
trachelotomy tracheophony
track tract
tympanites tympanitis
ureter ureteral
ureterorrhagia urethra uterus
vaccinate vacillate
vagus vagitus valgus
variceal varicella varicose variola
   variolar
varus vastus
venipuncture venepuncture
venous Venus varus
verrucose verrucous very close
   very coarse
vesica vesical vesicle
vicious villose villous villus
viscera visceral
viscose viscous viscus vorticose
wheal wheel
womb wound
xerosis cirrhosis

Appendix G

Laboratory Terminology and Normal Values

This appendix is from Diehl MO: *Medical Transcription Techniques and Procedures*, 5th edition. Saunders, Philadelphia, 2002.

LABORATORY TERMS AND SYMBOLS

The following are some of the more common laboratory terms and symbols.

Term or Symbol	Meaning
10^1	"Ten to the power of one"; shorthand for 10
10^2	Shorthand for 100
10^3	1000
10^4	10,000 (if you cannot write superscript, you can write 10 exp 4.)
10^{10}	A shorthand symbol so that we don't have to write out 10,000,000,000
ABG	Arterial blood gases
C&S	Culture and sensitivity
cm^3	Cubic centimeter
cu cm	Cubic centimeter
cu mm	Cubic millimeter
dL (dl)	Deciliter
dm^3	Cubic decimeter
ESR	Erythrocyte sedimentation rate
IU	International units
MCH	Mean corpuscular hemoglobin (divide the total hemoglobin by rbc)
MCV	Mean corpuscular volume (divide the hematocrit by rbc count)
mm^3	Cubic millimeter
pH	Alkalinity or acidity of a solution; hydrogen ion concentration
PT	Prothrombin time, test to check for one of the blood-clotting factors
RBC	Red blood cell count
rbc	Red blood count
WBC	White blood cell count
wbc	White blood cell

Term or Symbol	Meaning
μg	Microgram (1/1,000,000, gram)
μL (μl)	Microliter
μm	Micrometer
acid-fast bacilli	Organisms that cause tuberculosis and leprosy; bacteria from which acid doesn't wash out stain (e.g., Mycobacterium tuberculosis and M. leprae)
agar	Stiffening agent in media
agglutination	Clumping together, as of blood cells that are incompatible
anisocytosis	Unequal erthrocytes in size and shape
assay	Measure of biologic activity
baseline	Denotes a test result obtained before onset of symptoms
basocyte	Undifferentiated or basophilic leukocyte
basophil(e)	Leukocyte that readily takes up basic (alkaline) dyes
battery	A group of tests performed together
blood gas analysis	Measure of the exchange and transport of gases in the blood and tissues
borderline	Result lies on the margin between normal and abnormal
buffy coat	A layer of white blood cells found between the plasma and the red cells in centrifuged samples of anticoagulated blood
concentration	Amount of a substance per unit volume
critical level	See "panic level"
electrolytes	Sodium, potassium, chloride, and bicarbonate (also called CO2)
en bloc	In one piece
erythrocytosis	Increase in the number of red blood cells
false-negative	Denotes the absence of a condition or disease that is actually present
false-positive	Denotes the presence of a condition or disease that is not actually present
Gram stain	The standard staining procedure for the classification of bacteria
gram-negative	Loses the stain
gram-positive	Takes up the stain
granulocyte	A granular leukocyte
greater	Technical jargon for "more" or "higher"
in vitro	In the laboratory
in vivo	In the body
inoculation	Introduction of infectious material into a medium
level	See "concentration"

Term or Symbol	Meaning
medium	Substance in which a culture is grown
negative	Showing no reaction
normal range	Based on its own previous test results
normal	Within the normal range or limits
panel	A group of tests performed together
panic level	Markedly abnormal test result
parameter	Anything capable of being measured
plasma proteins	Albumin, globulin, fibrinogen, and prothrombin
plating	Placing infectious material onto a solid medium in a petri dish
positive	Having a reaction
profile	A group of tests performed together
rate	Change per unit of time
reference range	See "normal range"
serology	Study of antigen-antibody reactin by a variety of immunologic methods
shift to the left	An increase in the percentage of band cells
smear	Thin, translucent layer of material spread on a microscope slide and stained
stat	Immediately
streaking	See "plating"
therapeutic range	Optimum range for medication resulting in best health benefits
time	Interval required for reaction to take place
titer	Highest dilution in a series that gives a positive result
turnaround time	Time that elapses between the ordering of a test and receiving the report of the results
value	Quantitative measurement of the concentration, activity, and so forth of specific substances

Remember the following when transcribing laboratory data and values. Some physicians dictate the word lab as a short form for laboratory, which is acceptable except in headings and subheadings.

COMPUTERIZED EXAMINATIONS

When laboratory tests are ordered, it is common to hear, for example, "Dr. Mendez ordered a SMAC test on Mrs. Garcia." The equipment that is used, the Sequential Multiple Analyzer Computer, may be abbreviated and typed as SMAC, SMA, or Chem (for chemistry). This study is a panel of chemistry tests; from 4 to as many as 22 tests may be performed on the blood specimen (e.g., SMAC-8, SMA-5, Chem-9).

WRITING LAB VALUES

Use numbers to express laboratory values, but avoid beginning a sentence with a number. As discussed in Chapter 27, always place a zero (0) before a decimal (e.g., 0.6, not .6). Do not use commas to separate a laboratory value from the name of the test (e.g., hemoglobin 14.0). When typing several laboratory tests, separate related tests by commas, and separate unrelated tests by periods. If you are uncertain whether the tests are related, use periods. Use semicolons when a series of internal commas are present.

EXAMPLES

Red blood count 4.2, hemoglobin 12.0, hematocrit 37, urine specific gravity 1.003, pH 5, negative glucose.

Differential showed 60 segs, 3 bands, 30 lymphs, 5 monos, and 2 basos; hemoglobin 16.0; and hematocrit 46.1.

NORMAL VALUES

Because normal values vary slightly from one laboratory to another depending on the type of equipment that is used, the figures given throughout this section are approximate. Many values increase from threefold to tenfold during pregnancy. The brief forms and abbreviations given in parentheses throughout the section are acceptable for use in laboratory data sections of medical documents. The normal values shown here are expressed in conventional units. It is preferred to express a value as normal for age rather than as simply normal.

The following material has to do with the tests and interpretations of the results of the tests on the specimens of blood (plasma, red blood cells, white blood cells, and platelets), urine, and stool.

HEMATOLOGY VOCABULARY

Blood consists of the following components.

- *Formed elements: red blood cells (erythrocytes, which carry oxygen), white blood cells (leukocytes, which fight infection), and platelets or thrombocytes (aid in blood coagulation)*
- *Fluid part: plasma contains 90% to 92% water and 8% to 10% solids (e.g., carbohydrates, vitamins, hormones, enzymes, lipids, salts)*

Various methods are used to collect blood samples, including capillary tubes and venipuncture (phlebotomy, the usual method).

HEMATOLOGY TESTS AND VALUES

The following information will introduce you to laboratory terms used in medical reports that contain patient blood data.

Test or Component	Normal Values	Clinical Significance or Purpose
Haptoglobin	16 to 200 mg/dL	Decreases in hemolytic anemia; increases with certain infections

Test or Component	Normal Values	Clinical Significance or Purpose
Hemoglobin (H, Hg, HGB)	Male: 14.0 to 18.0 gm/dL Female: 12.0 to 16.0 gm/dL 10-year-old: 12 to 14.5 gm/dL	Increases with polycythemia, high altitude, chronic pulmonary disease, decreases with anemia, hemorrhage
Methemoglobin	0% to 1.5% of total hemoglobin	Used to evaluate cyanosis
Hematocrit (crit, H, HCT)	Male: 40% to 54% Female: 37% to 47% Newborn: 50% to 62% 1-year-old: 31% to 39%	Increases with dehydration and polycythemia; decreases with anemia and hemorrhage
White blood cell count (leukocyte count, WBC)	4,200 to 12,000/mm³ Birth: 9.0 to 30.0 × 1000 cells/mm³	Increases with acute infection, polycythemia, and other diseases; extremely high counts in leukemia; decreases in some viral infections and other conditions
Red blood cell count (erythrocyte count, RBC)	Male: 4.6 to 6.2 million/mm³ Female: 4.2 to 5.4 million/mm³	Increases with polycythemia and dehydration; decreases with anemia, hemorrhage, and leukemia

CORPUSCULAR VALUES OF ERYTHROCYTES (INDICES)
Note: normal values are different at different ages.

Test or Component	Normal Values	Clinical Significance or Purpose
Mean corpuscular volume (MCV)	80 to 105 μm	Increases or decreases in certain anemias
Mean corpuscular hemoglobin (MCH)	27 to 31 pg/RBC	Increases or decreases in certain anemias
Mean corpuscular hemoglobin concentration (MCHC)	32% to 36%	Increases or decreases in certain anemias

BLOOD GASES
Blood gas values are used to measure the exchange and transport of the gases in the blood and tissues. Many disorders will cause imbalances, such as diabetic ketoacidosis.

	Arterial	Venous
pH	7.35 to 7.45	7.33 to 7.43
Oxygen (O_2) saturation	94% to 100%	60% to 85%
Carbon dioxide (CO_2)	23 to 27 mmol/L	24 to 28 mmol/L

	Arterial	Venous
Oxygen, partial pressure (PO_2 or pO_2)	80 to 100 mm Hg	30 to 50 mm Hg
Carbon dioxide, partial pressure (PCO_2 or pCO_2)	35 to 45 mm Hg	38 to 55 mm Hg
Bicarbonate (HCO_3)	22 to 26 mmol/L	23 to 27 mmol/L
Base excess	−2 to +2 mEq/L	

COAGULATION TESTS

Test or Component	Normal Values	Clinical Significance or Purpose
Sedimentation rate (ESR or sed rate)	*Wintrobe method* Male: 0 to 5 mm/hr Female: 0 to 15 mm/hr *Westergren method* Male: 0 to 15 mm/hr Female: 0 to 20 mm/hr	Increases with infections, inflammatory diseases, and tissue destruction; decreases with polycythemia and sickle cell anemia
Prothrombin time (PT)	12.0 to 14.0 sec	Indicates ability of blood to clot for patients receiving blood-thinning drugs (e.g., Coumadin or heparin)
Partial thromboplastin time (PTT)	35 to 45 sec	Used to monitor heparin therapy
Fibrin split products (fibrin)	Negative at 1:4 dilution	Increases with disseminated intravascular coagulopathy
Fibrinogen	200 to 400 mg/ 100 mL	Increases with disseminated intravascular coagulopathy
Fibrinolysis	0	Increases with disseminated intravascular coagulopathy
Coombs test	Negative	Used to test infants born to Rh-negative mothers
Bleeding time		
Duke	1 to 5 min	Used to test platelet function
Ivy	<5 min	Used to test platelet function
Simplate	3 to 9.5 min	Used to test platelet function
Clot lysis time	None in 24 hr	Used to test for excessive fibrinolysis
Clot retraction time	30 to 60 min	Used to test platelet function
Coagulation time (Lee-White)	5 to 15 min	Used to test for abnormalities in clotting

Test or Component	Normal Values	Clinical Significance or Purpose
Factor VIII	50% to 150% of normal	Becomes deficient in classic hemophilia
Tourniquet test	Up to 10 petechiae	Used to detect vascular abnormalities

DIFFERENTIAL

This blood smear study determines the relative number of different types of white blood cells present in the blood; the total should equal 100%. A blood smear contains red blood cells, platelets, and white blood cells. The size and shape (morphology) of these cells are also reported.

Test or Component	Normal Values	Clinical Significance or Purpose
Polymorphonuclear neutrophilis (polys, segs, stabs, bands)	45% to 80%	Increases with appendicitis, myelogenous leukemia, and bacterial infections
Lymphocytes (lymphs)	20% to 40%	Increases with viral infections, whooping cough, infectious mononucleosis, and lymphocytic leukemia
Eosinophils (eos or eosin)	1% to 3%	Increases with allergenic reactions, allergies, scarlet fever, parasitic infections, and eosinophilic leukemia
Monocytes (monos)	1% to 10%	Increases with brucellosis, tuberculosis, and monocytic leukemia
Basophils (basos)	0% to 2%	
Myelocytes (myelos)	0%	
Platelets	150,000 to 350,000/mm^3	Increases with hemorrhage
Reticulocytes	25,000 to 75,000/mm^3	Decreases with leukemias

MORPHOLOGY

The shape of the cells can be described with the following terms: aniso (anisocytosis), poik (poikilocytosis), macro (macrocytic), micro (microcytic), and hypochromia.

CHEMISTRY

Test or Component	Normal Values	Clinical Significance or Purpose
Albumin/globulin (A/G) ratio	1.1 to 2.3	
Albumin	3.0 to 5.0 gm/dL	Decreases with kidney disease and severe burns

Test or Component	Normal Values	Clinical Significance or Purpose
Blood urea nitrogen (BUN)	10.0 to 26.0 mg/dL	Used to diagnose kidney disease, liver failure, and other diseases
Calcium (Ca)	8.5 to 10.5 mg/100 mL	Used to assess parathyroid functioning and calcium metabolism and to evaluate malignancies
Cholesterol, total serum	Normal: 120 to 200 mg/dL High: 200 to 240 mg/dL High risk: >240 mg/dL	Increases with diabetes mellitus and hypothyroidism; decreases with hyperthyroidism, acute infections, and pernicious anemia
HDL (high-density lipoproteins)	30 to 85 mg/dL	Has best correlation with development of coronary artery disease; decreased level indicates increased risk
LDL (low-density lipoproteins)	62 to 186 mg/dL	Greater than normal levels may be associated with increased risk of heart disease
Creatinine, serum	0.7 to 1.5 mg/100 mL	Used to screen for abnormalities in renal function
Electrolyte panel		
Bicarbonate, serum (bicarb or HCO_3)	23 to 29 mEq/L	
Chloride (Cl)	96 to 106 mEq/L	Used to diagnose disorders of acid/base imbalance
Potassium (K)	3.5 to 5.0 mEq/L	Used to diagnose disorders of water balance and acid/base imbalance
Sodium (Na)	136 to 145 mEq/L	Used to diagnose acid/base imbalance
Fasting blood sugar	70 to 110 mg/100 mL	Used to screen for abnormalities in carbohydrate metabolism
Gamma-glutamyl transpeptidase (GGTP)	Male: < 40 IU/L Female: <30 IU/L	
Globulin	1.5 to 3.7 gm/dL	

Test or Component	Normal Values	Clinical Significance or Purpose
Glucose-tolerance test (GTT), fasting blood sugar	70 to 100 mg/dL 30 min: 120 to 170 mg/dL; 1 hr: 120 to 170 mg/dL 2 hr: 100 to 140 mg/dL; 3 hr: <125 mg/dL	Used to detect disorders of glucose metabolism
Magnesium, serum	1.5 to 2.5 mEq/L	
Phosphate	2.5 to 4.5 mg/dL	

IMMUNOGLOBULINS (Ig), SERUM

Test or Component	Normal Values	Clinical Significance or Purpose
IgA	60 to 333 mg/dL	Involved in antibody responses
IgD	0.5 to 3.0 mg/dL	Involved in antibody responses
IgE	>300 ng/mL	Involved in antibody responses
IgG	550 to 1900 mg/dL	Involved in antibody responses
IgM	45 to 145 mg/dL	Involved in antibody responses
Iron, serum	75 to 175 µg/dL	
Lipid panel (includes total cholesterol, triglycerides, HDL, and LDL)	See separate tests for normal values	
Liver functions		
Acid phosphatase (ACP)	0 to 0.8 IU/L	
Alkaline phosphatase, serum (ALP or alk. phos.)	30 to 130 IU/L	Used to diagnose liver and bone diseases
Bilirubin (total)	0.3 to 1.1 mg/dL	Increases with conditions causing red blood cell destruction or biliary obstruction
Direct bilirubin	<0.2 mg/dL	
Lactate dehydrogenase (LDH)	25 to 175 IU/L	Used to diagnose myocardial infarction and in differential diagnosis of muscular dystrophy and pernicious anemia

Test or Component	Normal Values	Clinical Significance or Purpose
Alanine-aminotransferase (ALT [SGPT*])	10 to 45 IU/L	Used to detect liver disease; increases with acute pancreatitis, mumps, intestinal obstructions
Aspartate aminotransferase (AST [SGOT†])	10 to 45 IU/L	Used to detect tissue damage; increases with myocardial infarction; decreases in some diseases; becomes elevated in liver disease, pancreatitis, excessive trauma of skeletal muscle
Total protein	6.0 to 8.0 gm/dL	Increases with liver diseases
Triglycerides, serum (TG)	10 to 170 mg/dL	Becomes elevated in atherosclerosis, liver disease, hypothyroidism, and diabetes mellitus
Uric acid	2.2 to 7.7 mg/dL	Used to evaluate renal failure, gout, and leukemia

*SGPT (serum glutamic-pyruvic transaminase) is no longer in use and has been replaced by ALT (alanine aminotransferase).
†SGOT (serum glutamic-oxaloacetic transaminase) is no longer in use and has been replaced by AST (aspartate aminotransferase).

RADIOASSAYS FOR THYROID FUNCTIONS

Test or Component	Normal Values
Tri-iodothyronine (T_3)	25% to 38%
Thyroxine (T_4)	4.4 to 9.9 µg/100 mL
Thyroid-stimulating hormone (TSH)	0 to 3 ng/mL or 2 to 8 µIU/mL

SEROLOGY

Test or Component	Normal Values	Clinical Significance or Purpose
Antinuclear antibody (ANA)	Negative	Used to diagnose certain autoimmune diseases
C-reactive protein (CRP)	Negative	Increases in inflammatory diseases
Rheumatoid arthritis (RA) latex	Negative	Used to detect arthritis
Rapid plasma reagin (RPR)	Negative	Used to diagnose venereal disease
Venereal Disease Research Laboratory (VDRL)	Nonreactive	Used to diagnose venereal disease (syphilis)

URINALYSIS VOCABULARY

In a routine urinalysis, four types of examinations are performed:
1. Physical examination, consisting of volume, color, character, and specific gravity.
2. Chemical examination for determining alkalinity or acidity (pH), glucose, and albumin (protein) content.
3. Chemical tests, including tests for acetone, diacetic acid, urobilinogen, and bilirubin.
4. Microscopic examination for counting the white and red blood cells and identifying casts, cylindroids, epithelial (skin) cells, crystals, amorphous urates and phosphates, bacteria, and parasites.

URINALYSIS TESTS AND VALUES

The following are laboratory terms used in medical reports that contain data on results of urinalysis.

PHYSICAL EXAMINATION AND CHEMICAL TESTS

Test or Component	Normal Values	Clinical Significance or Purpose
Color	Yellow, straw, or colorless	Red may mean blood
Turbidity (clarity)	Clear	Cloudy may mean bacteria or pus
Specific gravity (spec. grav.)	1.002 to 1.030	
pH	4.5 to 8.0	Indicates the acidity or alkalinity of the urine
Nitrite	Negative	Indicates if a bacterial infection is present
Protein or albumin	Negative	Indicates that the kidneys are not functioning properly
Glucose (sugar)	Negative	Indicates that carbohydrates are not being metabolized properly
Hemoglobin	Negative	Indicates that the kidneys are not functioning properly
Acetone or ketones	0 or negative	Indicates that fats are not being metabolized properly
Blood, occult	Negative	Indicates that the kidneys are not functioning properly
Bilirubin (bili)	0.02 mg/dL; negative	Indicates that the liver is not functioning properly
Urobilinogen	0.1 to 1.0 Ehrlich Units/dL	Indicates that the liver is not functioning properly

MICROSCOPY

Test or Component	Normal Values	Clinical Significance or Purpose
Cells		
Red blood cells per high-power field (RBC/hpf)	0 to 2/hpf	Increases with infections
White blood cells per high-power field (WBC/hpf)	5/hpf	Increases with infections
Epithelial cells per high-power field (renal, caudate cells of renal pelvis, urethral, bladder, vaginal)	Few or moderate	Increases with infections
Bacteria per low-power field (yeast and bacteria)	Few or moderate	Increases with infections
Casts (and Artifacts)		
Casts per low-power field (granular, fine, coarse, hyaline, leukocyte, epithelial, waxy, blood)	Negative	
Cylindroids		
Mucous threads	Few or moderate	
Spermatozoa	None	Presence indicates recent intercourse
Trichomonas vaginalis	None	Presence indicates infection with this organism
Cloth fibers and bubbles	None	Presence indicates poor collection
Crystals Found in Acid Urine		

Note: Most crystals are normal; a few are considered abnormal and may be associated with diseases (e.g., cystine, tyrosine, leucine, and some drug crystals)

Crystals per low-power field (uric acid, amorphous urates, hippuric acid, calcium oxalate, tyrosine needles, leucine spheroids, cholesterin plates, cystine)	Few	

Test or Component	Normal Values	Clinical Significance or Purpose

Crystals Found in Alkaline Urine

Crystals per low-power field (triple phosphate, ammonium and magnesium, triple phosphate going in solution, amorphous phosphate, calcium phosphate, calcium carbonate, ammonium urate) — Few

Appendix H

Latin Phrases

Common Latin phrases used in medical dictation are shown here. However, there are well over five thousand Latin words for arteries, bones, muscles, nerves, and veins. Those terms may be found in a good medical dictionary and are not presented here.

abruptio placentae
acanthosis nigricans
acne neonatorum, rosacea,
　vulgaris
Actinomyces bovis, hominis,
　israelii
adenoma sebaceum
adiposis dolorosa
ala nasi
alopecia areata, generalisata,
　totalis
ansa hypoglossi
appendix testis
arcus senilis
Blastomyces dermatitidis
calamus scriptorius
calcinosis cutis
cancrum nasi, oris
caput medusae
caput succedaneum
cauda equina
chondromalacia patellae
chordae tendineae
chordae tympani
cisterna chyli
Coccidioides immitis
condyloma acuminatum, latum
corpus cavernosum, luteum,
　spongiosum, striatum
coxa valga, vara
crista galli
cutis anserina, laxa, marmorata

dermatitis herpetiformis,
　medicamentosa, venenata
Diplococcus pneumoniae
ductus deferens
dystrophia unguium
Epidermophyton floccosum
erythema marginatum,
　multiforme, nodosum
Escherichia coli
facies hippocratica
falx cerebelli, cerebri
fetus papyraceus (s)
fetus papyracei (p)
foramen magnum
foramen ovale cordis
formatio reticularis
fossa navicularis
fovea capitis, femoris
fovea centralis retinae
fragilitas ossium
genu valgum, varum
glans clitoridis
glans penis
glomus caroticum
glomus choroideum
glomus coccygeum
glomus intravagale
glomus vagale
granuloma annulare, inguinale
gubernaculum testis
Haemophilus influenzae
hepar lobatum

herpes gestationis, gladiatorum
herpes simplex, progenitalis,
  zoster
Histoplasma capsulatum
ichthyosis hystrix
impetigo contagiosa
incontinentia pigmenti
keratoconjunctivitis sicca
keratosis follicularis, pilaris
Klebsiella pneumoniae
lichen simplex chronicus,
  planus
limbus corneae
livedo reticularis
Loxosceles reclusa
lupus erythematosus, pernio,
  vulgaris
lusus naturae
lymphedema tarda
lymphogranuloma venereum
molluscum contagiosum
mons pubis, veneris
musculus interosseus dorsalis
Neisseria gonorrhoeae
nevus araneus, flammeus
os calcis, coxae, pubis
pars interarticularis
pectus carinatum, excavatum
periarteritis nodosa
pes anserinus, valgus, varus
pica gravidarum
pityriasis alba, rosea

placenta praevia, previa
placentae previae
portio vaginalis
Proteus mirabilis, vulgaris
pruritus ani, vulvae
Pseudomonas aeruginosa
pulsus bisferiens
rete testis
rima glottidis
roseola infantum
Salmonella typhi
scala tympani
sclerema neonatorum
stratum corneum, granulosum
Streptococcus pneumoniae
taeniae coli
tendo Achillis
tensor fasciae latae
tinea capitis, corporis, cruris,
  unguium
tinea facialis, versicolor
torus palatinus
Treponema pallidum
Trichophyton rubrum
truncus arteriosus
tunica albuginea
ulcus durum, molle
urticaria pigmentosa
vas deferens
vasa vasorum
verruca vulgaris

Appendix I

Plural Forms

This table lists commonly used foreign singular and plural forms.

Singular	Plural
acetabulum	acetabula
addendum	addenda
adnexum*	adnexa
alga	algae
alto	altos
alumna	alumnae
alumnus	alumni
alveolus	alveoli
ameba	amebas
amicus curiae	amici curiae
analysis	analyses
anastomosis	anastomoses
antrum	antra
apex	apices
aponeurosis	aponeuroses
appendix	appendices, appendixes
areola	areolae
artery	arteries
arthritis	arthritides
atrium	atria
axilla	axillae
bacillus	bacilli
bacterium	bacteria
base	bases
basis	bases
bona fide	bona fides
bon vivant	bons vivant
bronchus	bronchi
brucellosis	brucelloses
bulla	bullae
bursa	bursae
calculus	calculi

* Seldom used.

Singular	Plural
calix	calices
calyx	calyces
cannula	cannulas, cannulae
canthus	canthi
carcinoma	carcinomata, carcinomas
catharsis	catharses
cervix	cervices, cervixes
cicatrix	cicatrices
coccus	cocci
comedo	comedones
compendium	compendiums
conjunctiva	conjunctivae
cornea	corneae, corneas
cornu	cornua
corpus	corpora
cortex	cortices
cranium	crania, craniums
crisis	crises
criterion	criteria
crux	cruxes
datum	data
diagnosis	diagnoses
dialysis	dialyses
dictum	dicta
diverticulum	diverticula
ecchymosis	ecchymoses
embolus	emboli
embryo	embryos
encephalitis	encephalitides
exegesis	exegeses
enteritis	enteritides
epididymis	epididymides
exostosis	exostoses
femur	femurs, femora
fetus	fetuses
fibula	fibulas
fimbria	fimbriae
fistula	fistulae, fistulas
focus	foci
foramen	foramina, foramens
formula	formulas, formulae
fornix	fornices
fossa	fossae
fundus	fundi
ganglion	ganglia
genius	geniuses
genus	genera

Singular	Plural
gyrus	gyri
helix	helices
hernia	herniae, hernias
hilum	hila
humerus	humeri
ileum	ilea
ilium	ilia
index	indexes, indices (for numeric expressions)
ischium	ischia
keratosis	keratoses
labium	labia
lacuna	lacunae
lamina	laminae
larva	larvae
larynx	larynges
leiomyoma	leiomyomata
locus	loci
lumen	lumina, lumens
madam	mesdames
matrix	matrices
maxilla	maxillae, maxillas
maximum	maxima
meatus	meatuses
media	mediae (middle)
medium	media
medulla	medullae, medullas
memorandum	memoranda, memorandus
meningitis	meningitides
meniscus	menisci
metastasis	metastases
miasma	miasmas
milieu	milieux, milieus
millennium	millennia
mitosis	mitoses
mucosa	mucosas, mucosae
neurosis	neuroses
nucleus	nuclei
mycelium	mycelia
naris	nares
nevus	nevi
nucleus	nuclei
optimum	optima
os	ora (meaning mouths)
os	ossa (meaning bones)
ovary	ovaries
ovum	ova

Singular	Plural
papilla	papillae
paralysis	paralyses
pelvis	pelves
petechia	petechiae
phalanx	phalanges
phenomenon	phenomena
placebo	placebos
pleura	pleurae
plexus	plexuses
pons	pontes
prognosis	prognoses
prospectus	prospectuses
prosthesis	prostheses
protozoon	protozoa
proviso	provisos
psychosis	psychoses
pubis	pubes
pudendum	pudenda
pupa	pupae
quantum	quanta
quorum	quorums
radius	radii
ratio	ratios
residuum	residua
rhinoplasty	rhinoplasties
rhonchus	rhonchi
ruga	rugae
sarcoma	sarcomata, sarcomas
sclera	sclerae
sclerosis	scleroses
sepsis	sepses
septum	septa
sequel	sequels
sequela	sequelae
serum	sera
sinus	sinuses
spermatozoon	spermatozoa
sputum	sputa
sternum	sternums
stigma	stigmata
stimulus	stimuli
stoma	stomata, stomas
stratum	strata
sulcus	sulci
surgeon general	surgeons general
syllabus	syllabuses, syllabi
symposium	symposia, symposiums

Singular	Plural
synopsis	synopses
testis	testes
therapy	therapies
thesis	theses
thorax	thoraces, thoraxes
trachea	tracheae
ulna	ulnas
ultimatum	ultimatums
ureter	ureters
urethra	urethras
urinalysis	urinalyses
uterus	uteri
uvula	uvulas
vas	vasa
vena cava	venae cavae
verruca	verrucae
vertebra	vertebrae, vertebras
vesicle	vesicles
villus	villi
virus	viruses
viscus	viscera
zygion	zygia

Appendix J

Sound Variations of Syllables

Listed here are some common examples of how English and medical terms sound phonetically, together with clues as to how they would be spelled to help you locate them in the medical dictionary. If you cannot find a word when you look it up, refer to this table and use another combination of letters that has the same sound. For example: Look up the sound *n* in the word *pneumonia*. Notice that the *n* sound as in *no* could be spelled *cn, gn, kn, mn, nn, pn*. Thus, you have some clues as to how to locate the word in the dictionary. (*See also Chapter 43, Spelling.*)

If the Phonetic Sound is Like . . .	Try the Spelling as in . . .	Examples
a in fat	ai	pl<u>ai</u>d
	al	h<u>al</u>f
	au	dr<u>au</u>ght
a in sane	ai	p<u>ai</u>n
	ao	g<u>ao</u>l
	au	g<u>au</u>ge
	ay	p<u>ay</u>, x-r<u>ay</u>, T<u>ay</u>-Sachs
	ue	s<u>ue</u>de
	ie	p<u>ie</u>dra
	ea	br<u>ea</u>k
	ei	v<u>ei</u>n
	eigh	w<u>eigh</u>
	et	sach<u>et</u>
	ey	th<u>ey</u>, p<u>ey</u>ote
a in care	ai	<u>ai</u>r, cl<u>ai</u>rvoyant
	ay	pr<u>ay</u>er
	e	th<u>e</u>re
	ea	w<u>ea</u>r
	ei	th<u>ei</u>r
a in father	au	<u>au</u>ral, <u>au</u>ricle, <u>au</u>scultation
	e	s<u>e</u>rgeant
	ea	h<u>ea</u>rt
a in ago	e	ag<u>e</u>nt
	i	san<u>i</u>ty
	o	c<u>o</u>mply

If the Phonetic Sound is Like . . .	Try the Spelling as in . . .	Examples
a in ago—*cont'd*	u	foc<u>u</u>s
	iou	vic<u>iou</u>s
aci in acid	acy	<u>acy</u>stia
ak	ac	<u>ac</u>cident
	ach	<u>ach</u>romatic
	acr	<u>acr</u>omegaly
ark	arch	<u>arch</u>icyte
b in big	bb	ru<u>bb</u>er
	pb	cu<u>pb</u>oard
bak sound in back	bac	<u>bac</u>teremia
bee	by	pres<u>by</u>opia
ch in chin	c	<u>c</u>ello
	Cz	<u>Cz</u>ech
	tch	sti<u>tch</u>
	ti	ques<u>ti</u>on
	tu	den<u>tu</u>re, fis<u>tu</u>la
d in do	dd	pu<u>dd</u>le
	ed	call<u>ed</u>
die	di	<u>di</u>agnosis, <u>di</u>arrhea
dis	dis	<u>dis</u>charge
	dys	<u>dys</u>pnea
dew	deu	<u>deu</u>teropathy
	dew	<u>dew</u>lap
	du	<u>du</u>ra
e in get	a	<u>a</u>ny
	ae	<u>ae</u>sthetic
	ai	s<u>ai</u>d
	ay	s<u>ay</u>s
	e	<u>e</u>dema
	ea	h<u>ea</u>d
	ei	h<u>ei</u>fer
	eo	l<u>eo</u>pard
	ie	fr<u>ie</u>nd
	oe	r<u>oe</u>ntgen
	u	b<u>u</u>rial
e in equal	ae	h<u>ae</u>moglobin
	ay	qu<u>ay</u>
	ea	l<u>ea</u>n
	ee	fr<u>ee</u>
	ei	dec<u>ei</u>t
	eo	p<u>eo</u>ple
	ey	k<u>ey</u>
	i	hem<u>i</u>cardia
	ie	s<u>ie</u>ge
	oe	am<u>oe</u>ba
	y	tracheotom<u>y</u>

If the Phonetic Sound is Like . . .	Try the Spelling as in . . .	Examples
e in here	ea	<u>ea</u>r
	ee	ch<u>ee</u>r
	ei	w<u>ei</u>rd
	ie	b<u>ie</u>r
ek	ec	l<u>ec</u>totype, <u>ec</u>zema
	ek	<u>ek</u>phorize
er in over	ar	li<u>ar</u>
	ir	elix<u>ir</u>
	or	auth<u>or</u>, lab<u>or</u>
	our	glam<u>our</u>
	re	ac<u>re</u>
	ur	aug<u>ur</u>
	ure	meas<u>ure</u>
	yr	zeph<u>yr</u>
eri, ere, aire	ery	<u>ery</u>throcyte, <u>ery</u>thema
you	eu	<u>eu</u>phoria, <u>eu</u>genic
ex	ex	<u>ex</u>travasation
	x	<u>x</u>-ray
f in fine	ff	cli<u>ff</u>
	gh	lau<u>gh</u>, slou<u>gh</u>
	lf	ha<u>lf</u>
	ph	<u>ph</u>ysiology, pro<u>ph</u>ylactic
fizz	phys	<u>phys</u>ical
floo, flu	flu	<u>flu</u>oride, <u>flu</u>oroscopy
g in go	gg	e<u>gg</u>
	gh	<u>gh</u>ost
	gu	<u>gu</u>ard
	gue	prolo<u>gue</u>
gli in glide	gly	<u>gly</u>cemia
grew	grou	<u>grou</u>p
guy (also see jin)	gy	<u>gy</u>necomastia
h in hat	g	<u>G</u>ila monster
	wh	<u>wh</u>o, <u>wh</u>ooping cough
he	he	<u>he</u>matoma
	hae (British spelling)	<u>hae</u>matology
hi in high	hy	<u>hy</u>drocele
i in it	a	us<u>a</u>ge
	e	<u>E</u>nglish
	ee	b<u>ee</u>n
	ia	carri<u>a</u>ge
	ie	s<u>ie</u>ve
	o	w<u>o</u>men
	u	b<u>u</u>sy
	ui	b<u>ui</u>lt
	y	lar<u>y</u>ngeal, n<u>y</u>stagmus

If the Phonetic Sound is Like . . .	Try the Spelling as in . . .	Examples
i in kite	ai	guaiac
	ay	aye
	ei	height, meiosis
	ey	eye
	ie	tie
	igh	nigh
	is	island of Langerhans
	uy	buy
	y	myograph
	ye	rye
ik or ick	ich	ichthyosis
ink	inc	incubator
j in jam	d	gradual
	dg	judge
	di	soldier
	dj	adjective
	g	register, fungi
	ge	vengeance
	gg	exaggerate
jin	gyn	gynecology
k sound in keep	c	eczema
	cc	account
	ch	chronic, tachycardia
	ck	tack
	cq	acquire
	cu	biscuit
	lk	walk
	qu	liquor
	que	plaque
key	che	chemotherapy
	chy	ecchymosis
ko	cho, co	cholecyst, colon
kon	chon	chondroma
	con	condyloma
kw sound in quick	ch	choir
	qu	quintuplet
l in let	ll	call
	sl	isle
la in lay	lay	layette
	le	lei
lack	lac	lacrimal
loo	leu	leukocyte
	lew	lewisite
m in me	chm	drachm
	gm	phlegm
	lm	balm

If the Phonetic Sound is Like . . .	Try the Spelling as in . . .	Examples
m in me	mb	limb
	mm	hammer toe
	mn	hymn
mass	mac	macerate
mix	myx	myxedema
n in no	cn	cnemial
	gn	gnathic
	kn	knife
	mn	mnemonic
	nn	tinnitus
	pn	pneumonia
ng in ring	ngue	tongue
new	neu	neurology
	pneu	pneumococcus
o in go	au	mauve
	eau	beau
	eo	yeoman
	ew	sew
o in go	oa	foam
	oe	toe
	oh	ohm
	oo	brooch
	ou	shoulder
	ough	dough
	ow	row
o in long	a	all
	ah	Utah
	au	fraud
	aw	thaw
	oa	broad
	ou	ought
off	oph	exophthalmos, ophthalmology
oi in oil	oy	boy
oks	occ	occiput
	ox	oxygen
oo in tool	eu	leukemia
	ew	drew
	o	move
	oe	shoe
	ou	group
	ough	through
	u	rule, tularemia
	ue	blue
	ui	bruise
oo in look	o	wolffian
	ou	would
	u	pull, tuberculosis

If the Phonetic Sound is Like . . .	Try the Spelling as in . . .	Examples
ow in out	ou	m<u>ou</u>th
	ough	b<u>ough</u>
	ow	dr<u>ow</u>n
p in put	pp	ha<u>pp</u>y
pack	pach	myo<u>pach</u>ynsis, <u>pach</u>yderma
pi in pie	py	nephro<u>py</u>osis
r in red	rh	<u>rh</u>abdocyte
	rr	be<u>rr</u>y
	rrh	ci<u>rrh</u>osis, hemo<u>rrh</u>oid
	wr	<u>wr</u>ong, <u>wr</u>ist
re in repeat	rhe	<u>rhe</u>ostosis
	ri	mala<u>ri</u>a
	rrhe	oto<u>rrhe</u>a
rew	rheu	<u>rheu</u>matism
	rhu	<u>rhu</u>barb
rom	rhom	<u>rhom</u>boid
rye	rhi	<u>rhi</u>noplasty
s in sew	c	<u>c</u>yst, fo<u>c</u>i
	ce	ri<u>ce</u>
	ps	<u>ps</u>ychology
	sc	<u>sc</u>iatic, vis<u>c</u>era
	sch	<u>sch</u>ism
	ss	mi<u>ss</u>
	sth	i<u>sth</u>mus
sh in ship	ce	o<u>ce</u>an
	ch	<u>ch</u>ancre
	ci	fa<u>ci</u>al
	s	<u>s</u>ugar
	sch	<u>Sch</u>wann's cell
	sci	fa<u>sci</u>a
	se	nau<u>se</u>ous
t in tea	pt	<u>pt</u>erygium, <u>pt</u>osis
zh sound in azure	ge	gara<u>ge</u>, massa<u>ge</u>, curetta<u>ge</u>
	s	vi<u>s</u>ion
	si	fu<u>si</u>on
	zi	gla<u>zi</u>er
zi	zy	<u>zy</u>goma, <u>zy</u>gote, enzyme
(rhymes with sigh)	x	<u>x</u>iphoid
zz	ss	sci<u>ss</u>ors
	zz	bu<u>zz</u>

As an additional spelling aid, here is a group of letter combinations that can cause problems when you are trying to locate a word.

If You Have Tried . . .	Then Try . . .
pre	per, pra, pri, pro, pru
per	par, pir, por, pur, pre, pro
is	us, ace, ice
ere	ear, eir, ier
wi	whi
we	whe
zi	xy
cks, gz	x
tion	sion, cion, cean, cian
le	tle, el, al
cer	cre
si	psi, ci
ei	ie
x	eks
z	xe
dis	dys
ture	teur
tious	seous, scious
air	are, aer
ny	gn, n
ance	ence
ant	ent
able	ible
fizz	phys

Unusual Medical Terms

acorn-tipped catheter
Adam's apple
aerobic deafness
air-bone gap
ALARM
alligator clamp
Ambu bag
amniotic fluid
anal wink
anchovy
angle of Louis
apple peel syndrome
argyle tube
ash leaf spots (eye)
BABYbird respirator
BabyFace ultrasound
BackBiter instrument
bagged
balloon-on-a-wire
banana blade knife
banjo-string adhesions
baseball stitch
basement membrane
Battle's sign
beat knee syndrome
beaver fever
berry aneurysm
Best clamps
bikini bottom
Billroth II (procedure)
Bird machine (on the Bird)
Bird's Nest filter
birdcage splint
bird-like facies
bishop's nod
black comet's artifact
black doggie clamps
black hairy tongue

black heel
Blessed Information Memory
    Concentration
blown pupil
blowout fracture
blue bloaters
blue diaper syndrome
blue dot sign
blue toe syndrome
blueberry muffin baby
boat hook
boggy uterus
bone wax
bony thorax
boss (surface)
bow-tie sign
boxer's nose
bread-and-butter heart
bronze diabetes
bubble boy disease
bubble hair
bucket-handle tear
buffalo hump
buffy coat
bulldog clamp
bull's-eye lesion
Bunny boot
buried bumper syndrome
butterfly bumper syndrome
butterfly needle
CABG (pronounced "cabbage")
café au lait spots
cake mix kit
CAT scan
chain cystogram
Chance fracture
chandelier sign
charley horse

cherry angioma
chocolate agar
chocolate cyst
choked disc
Christmas disease
cigarette (or cigaret) drain
circle of death
clap (gonorrhea)
clergyman's knee
clog (clot of blood)
clue cell
cobblestoning mucosa
cobra head plate
Coca-Cola–colored urine
coffee-ground stools or emesis
cogwheel breathing
cogwheel gait
cogwheel rigidity or motion
coin test
collar-button abscess
collar-button appearance
comb sign
corn picker's pupil
cottonoid patty
cowboy collar
COWS
cracked pot sound
cracker test
cradle cap
crick (painful spasm in a
    muscle, usually in the neck)
currant jelly stools
DAD
Dandy scissors
dawn phenomenon
devil's grip
devil's pinches
dog-boning complication
doll's eye movements
DOOR syndrome
double bubble sign
double whammy syndrome
drawer sign
dripping candle appearance
duck waddle test
dumbbell tumor
dumping syndrome
echo sign
fat depot

fat pad
fat towels (wound towels)
fern test (an estrogen test)
finger clubbing
finger dissection
fish fancier's finger
fish tank granuloma
fish-mouthed cervix
flashers and floaters (eye exam)
49er brace (a knee brace)
frank breech position
frown incision
gallops, thrills, and rubs
game leg
Gelfoam cookie
gift wrap suture
gimpy (lame)
glitter cells
glove-juice technique
glue ear
glue-footed gait
Goodenough test
goose egg (swelling due to
    blunt trauma)
gull-wing sign
gulper's gullet
gum ball headache
guy suture
haircut (syphilitic chancre)
hair-on-end sign
hammock configuration
hanging drop test
hedgehog molecule
HELLP syndrome
hickey
Hickey-Hare test
His (bundle)
hot cross bun deformity
hot potato voice
incidentaloma
in-the-bag lens implantation
jackstone calculus
jogger's nipples
joint mice
joker (instrument)
kangaroo care
Kerley's B lines (costophrenic
    septal lines)
Kerley's C lines

keyhole surgery
kick counts
kink artifact
kissing spine
kissing-type artifact
lacer cock-up (splint)
leather bottle stomach
lemon squeezer (instrument)
listing gait
little leaguer's elbow
Little lens
locked-in syndrome
locker room syndrome
loofah folliculitis
loose body
maple syrup urine disease
    (MSUD)
march fracture
meat wrapper's asthma
Mercedes sign
Mill-house murmur
moth-eaten appearance
mouse (periorbital ecchymosis)
mouse units
MUGA
mulberry molars
Mule vitreous sphere
musical bruit
Mustard procedure
mute toe sign
napkin-ring obstruction
nutcracker esophagus
nutmeg liver
octopus test
onion peel sensory loss
orphan drug
outrigger (orthopedic)
ox cell hemolysin test
oyster (mass of mucus coughed
    up)
pantaloon hernia
pants-over-vest (technique)
parrot beak tear
past-pointing test
patient flat lined ("expired" is
    preferred)
peanut (a small surgical gauze
    sponge)
pencil-in-cup deformity

PERLA or PERRLA
piggyback probe
pigtail catheter
piles (hemorrhoids)
pill esophagitis
pill-rolling (tremor)
pink puffer (patient showing
    dyspnea but no cyanosis)
pins and needles (paresthesias)
pizza lung
plus disease
polly-beak
pollywogs
POP (plaster of paris)
pop-off needle
porcelain gallbladder
port-wine stain
postage stamp type skin graft
prep or prepped (from the word
    prepared)
prostate, boggy
proud flesh (granulation tissue)
prune-belly syndrome
puddle sign
pulmonary toilet
purse-string mouth
purse-string suture
pyknic habit (short, stocky
    build)
rabbit nose
rabbit stools
raccoon eyes
rice-water stools
rocker-bottom foot
rooting reflex
rubber booties
Rufus and Ruby
rugger jersey sign
runner's rump
running off (diarrhea)
sago spleen
salmon flesh excrescences
sand (encrusted secretions
    about the eyes)
saucerize (refers to suturing a
    cyst inside out so it will heal)
sausage fingers
scotty dog's ear
sea bather's eruption

seagull bruit
setting sun sign
shiner
shoelace suturing
shotty nodes
sick building syndrome
silhouette sign or Golden's S
  sign
silver fork deformity
simian crease (seen in Down
  syndrome)
Sippy diet
skin wheals
skinny needle or Chiba needle
sky suture
sleep (inspissated mucus about
  the eyes)
Slinky catheter
smile or smiling incision
smoker's face
snowball opacities
snowbanks
snuff box
SOAP note
speed dissection
spoon nails
starry-sky pattern
steeple sign (on chest x-ray)
stick-tie
stonebasket
stoved (of a finger; means
  stubbed)
strawberry gallbladder
strawberry hemangioma

strawberry tongue
string sign
sucked candy bone
sugar-tong plaster splint
sugar-tongs (instrument)
surf test
sundown syndrome
swan-neck catheter
swimmer's view
tailor's bunion
tailor's seat
tennis elbow
ThumZ' up (thumbs)
tincture of time
trick (of a joint; means unstable)
trigger finger
tumor plot
two-flight dyspnea
two-pillow orthopnea
vaginal candle
walking pneumonia
washerwoman's skin
watermelon stomach
weaver's bottom
wet mount
whistletip catheter
wing suture
witches' milk
wrinkle artifact
yoga foot drop
yuppie flu
ZEEP (zero end expiratory
  pressure)
zit (comedo)

Bibliography

American Association for Medical Transcription, *The AAMT Book of Style for Medical Transcription*, 2nd ed., Modesto, California, American Association for Medical Transcription, 2002.

American Medical Association, *American Medical Association Manual of Style*, 9th ed., Baltimore, Williams & Wilkins, 1998.

Chicago Manual of Style, 14th ed., Chicago, University of Chicago Press, 1993.

Clark, James L. and Lyn R. Clark, *HOW 10: A Handbook for Office Professionals*, 10th ed., Mason, Ohio, South-Western Publishing, 2004.

Council of Biology Editors, *Scientific Style and Format*, 6th ed., New York, Cambridge University Press, 1994.

Diehl, Marcy O., *Medical Transcription: Techniques and Procedures*, 5th ed., Philadelphia, Saunders, 2002.

Gilman, Mary Louise, *One Word, Two Words, Hyphenated?*, 2nd ed., Vienna, Virginia, National Court Reporters Association, 1998.

Goldstein, Norman (Ed.), *The Associated Press Stylebook and Briefing on Media Law*, Cambridge, Massachusetts, Perseus, 2002.

Huth, Edward J., *Medical Style and Format*, Philadelphia, ISI Press, 1987.

Kessler, Lauren and McDonald, Duncan, *When Words Collide*, 5th ed., Belmont, California, Wadsworth/Thompson Learning, 2000.

Lederer, Richard and Dowis, Richard, *Sleeping Dogs Don't Lay*, New York, St. Martin's Griffin, 1999.

Lederer, Richard and Dowis, Richard, *The Write Way*, New York, Pocket Books, 1995.

Merck Manual of Diagnosis and Therapy of Diseases, 17th ed., Rahway, New Jersey, Merck Publishing Group, 1999.

The Merriam-Webster's Concise Handbook for Writers, 2n., Springfield, Massachusetts, Merriam-Webster, Inc., 199

O'Conner, Patricia, *Words Fail Me*, Orlando, Florida, 1999.

Princeton Review, *Grammar Smart*, New York, New York, 1997.

Pyle, Vera, *Current Medical Terminology*, Health Professions Institute, 2003

Sabin, William A., *The Gregg Ref* Glencoe/McGraw-Hill, 199

Wallach, Jacques, *Handb* Philadelphia, Lippinco

Index

Note: Page numbers in *italics* refer to illustrations; page numbers followed by
t refer to tables. **Boldface** numbers refer to paragraph (rule) numbers.

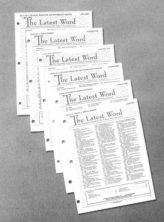

Pocket Guide
to APA Style
2009 UPDATE

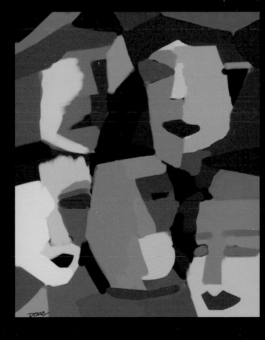

Robert Perrin

Robert Perrin

LAUREATE
EDUCATION INC

Reference-List Entries

Audiovisual Sources 101

Electronic Sources 107

Pocket Guide to APA Style

2009 UPDATE

Robert Perrin

CENGAGE
Learning

Australia • Brazil • Japan • Korea • Mexico • Singapore • Spain • United Kingdom • United States

CENGAGE
Learning™

**Pocket Guide to APA Style
2009 UPDATE
Robert Perrin**

Pocket Guide to APA Style
Robert Perrin
© 2009, 2007 Wadsworth, Cengage Learning. All rights reserved.

Executive Editors:

Maureen Staudt

Michael Stranz

Senior Project Development
Manager:

Linda deStefano

Marketing Specialist:

Courtney Sheldon

Senior Production/
Manufacturing Manager:

Donna M. Brown

PreMedia Manager:

Joel Brennecke

Sr. Rights Acquisition
Account Manager:

Todd Osborne

Cover Image:
Getty Images*

*Unless otherwise noted, all cover
images used by Custom Solutions,
a part of Cengage Learning, have
been supplied courtesy of Getty
Images with the exception of the
Earthviewcover image, which has
been supplied by the National
Aeronautics and Space
Administration (NASA).

For product information and technology assistance, contact us at
Cengage Learning Customer & Sales Support, 1-800-354-9706

For permission to use material from this text or product,
submit all requests online at **cengage.com/permissions**
Further permissions questions can be emailed to
permissionrequest@cengage.com

This book contains select works from existing Cengage Learning resources and
was produced by Cengage Learning Custom Solutions for collegiate use. As such,
those adopting and/or contributing to this work are responsible for editorial
content accuracy, continuity and completeness.

Compilation © 2010. Cengage Learning.

ISBN-13: 978-1-111-72013-1

ISBN-10: 1-111-72013-4

Cengage Learning
5191 Natorp Boulevard
Mason, Ohio 45040
USA

Cengage Learning is a leading provider of customized learning solutions with
office locations around the globe, including Singapore, the United Kingdom,
Australia, Mexico, Brazil, and Japan. Locate your local office at:
international.cengage.com/region.

Cengage Learning products are represented in Canada by Nelson Education, Ltd.

For your lifelong learning solutions, visit **www.cengage.com/custom.**
Visit our corporate website at **www.cengage.com.**

Printed in the United States
of America

Contents

Preface

Pocket Guide to APA Style, in the updated 3rd edition, is designed for students who need to write, document, and present papers in American Psychological Association style. This convenient and easy-to-use guide draws on the principles described in the corrected sixth edition of the *Publication Manual of the American Psychological Association* (2009). What sets *Pocket Guide to APA Style* apart from the lengthy *Publication Manual* is its overriding goal: This text presents the principles in a brief, yet complete and easy-to-use manner. The guide is ideal for undergraduates who are working with APA style for the first time. Yet graduate students and working professionals will also appreciate its user-friendliness. To enhance its use, *Pocket Guide to APA Style* incorporates these helpful features:

- *Writing Scholarly Papers: An Overview* The introductory chapter of *Pocket Guide* describes basic researching and writing methods, serving as a brief review.

- *Manuscript Preparation* In one coherent chapter, *Pocket Guide* describes and illustrates all elements of an APA manuscript.

- *Editorial Style* In one convenient chapter, *Pocket Guide* explains APA guidelines for punctuation and mechanics (periods, quotation marks, capitalization, number style, and so on), general writing style (transitions, verb tense, and so on), and word choice (jargon, biased language, and so on).

- *Separate Documentation Chapters* For easy use, *Pocket Guide* provides separate chapters to explain reference-list entries for periodicals, books, audiovisual sources, and electronic sources.

- *Reference-List Entries and In-Text Citations* Separate reference entries for 119 sources, with updated samples in Chapters 4–8, illustrate the principles of documentation in *Pocket Guide;* all entries are followed by corresponding in-text citations.

- *Sample Papers* Two complete sample papers are included in *Pocket Guide,* one argumentative and one experimental; both include annotations related to manuscript form and issues of writing.

- *A Discussion of Plagiarism*   With its student focus, *Pocket Guide* includes a discussion of plagiarism and ways to avoid it.
- *Appendix*   Included in *Pocket Guide* is an appendix that describes effective ways to prepare poster presentations.

ACKNOWLEDGMENTS

My work on the updated third edition of *Pocket Guide* was pleasant and productive because of the supportive, knowledgeable staff at Wadsworth, Cengage Learning. I also thank Matrix Productions for their careful handling of the production work.

I am also indebted to the following people for their thoughtful reviews of earlier editions of *Pocket Guide to APA:*

Julie Burke, Guilford College

John Chapin, Pennsylvania State University

Larry Z. Daily, Shepherd University

Kathy Earnest, Northwestern Oklahoma State University

Cindy Giaimo-Ballard, University of La Verne

Sandra Petree, Northwestern Oklahoma State University

Finally, I wish to thank Judy, Jenny, Chris, and Kate for their encouragement.

R. P.

1   Writing Scholarly Papers

The research process is a complex combination of thinking, searching, reading, evaluating, writing, and revising. It is, in many ways, a highly personal process because writers approach research activities by drawing on different skills and past experiences. Yet researchers often follow a series of connected phases (which nonetheless occur in a different order for different people).

This chapter reviews, in a brief way, the common steps that most researchers go through; if you are an experienced researcher, you can use this chapter as a "refresher." If your research experiences are limited, consider each discussion carefully as you proceed with your work.

1a   Subject and Topic

Research begins with a subject. In some academic contexts, you may choose the subject yourself, usually with the instructor's approval. But in other contexts, you may be required to choose from a small number of topics or be assigned a topic with a predetermined focus.

GUIDELINES FOR ASSESSING GENERAL SUBJECTS

As you select potential subjects for your research (broad categories such as test anxiety, migrant education, the effects of divorce, and so on), keep these important and practical principles in mind:

- *Interest.* When possible, select a subject that interests you. Do not spend time researching a subject that does not make you curious.
- *Length.* Select a subject that can be adequately treated within the length requirements of the assignment. You may have to expand or reduce the scope of your subject to match these length constraints.
- *Materials.* Select a subject for which you can find materials of the kind identified in the assignment. Be aware that you can use libraries other than your own for your research and that the Internet provides access to a broad range of materials, both traditional and nontraditional.

1

- *Challenge.* Select a subject that challenges you but that does not require technical or other specialized knowledge you may not have time to acquire.
- *Uniqueness.* Select a subject that is not overused. Overly familiar subjects stimulate little interest, and materials are soon depleted.
- *Perspective.* Select a subject you can approach in a fresh, interesting way. Readers will appreciate your efforts to examine subjects from new perspectives.

NARROW TOPIC

In most instances, you will need to narrow your large subject (test anxiety, for example) to a specific topic (test anxiety among middle school students) so that you can research selectively and address the issue in a focused way.

To discover ways to narrow a broad subject to a specific topic, skim general reference materials, paying particular attention to recurrent themes, details, and ideas. Then consider establishing a focus using selected strategies for limiting topics:

- *Time.* Restrict the subject to a specific, manageable time span—for example, school violence in the 1990s.
- *Place.* Restrict the subject to a specific location—for example, teen pregnancy in rural areas of the United States.
- *Special circumstance.* Restrict the subject to a specific context or circumstance—for example, achievement testing for college admissions.
- *Specific population.* Restrict the subject to address its effects on a selected group of people—for example, skin cancer among elderly people.

1b Thesis Statements, Hypotheses, or Stated Objectives

To clarify the central goal of your writing, present your ideas in one of three alternative ways.

THESIS STATEMENT

A thesis statement, sometimes called a problem statement, is a declarative statement (usually one but sometimes two or more sentences) that clarifies your specific topic, presents your opinion of (not merely facts about) the topic, and incorporates qualifications or limitations necessary to understand your views.

> Although the effects of birth order are always evident to some degree, other variables also affect personality, intelligence, and socialization.

HYPOTHESIS

A hypothesis is a conjectural statement that guides an argument or investigation; it can be explored (and potentially proved or disproved) by examining data related to your topic. Conditional in nature, a hypothesis is assessed using available information.

> Students who delay work on major research projects until the last week are more likely to plagiarize than are students who begin their work early.

STATED OBJECTIVE

A stated objective is a brief, well-focused statement that describes a research paper that presents information. Unsubtle and not arguable, it must define the topic clearly and narrow the topic when necessary.

> I will share a brief history of polio in the United States, from early epidemics to the last American case.

1c Research Goals

Although most research is prompted by specific academic or job-related requirements, you should also think broadly about the goals for your work, recognizing that research provides multifaceted learning experiences.

COURSE-RELATED GOALS

Course-related goals are broad in scope and establish the foundation of your research work.

- *Using the library.* Library-based research should take advantage of a full range of sources, as well as the electronic means to locate them (see pages 5–8).

- *Using the Internet for academic purposes.* Research requires that you learn to use the Internet selectively for scholarly purposes, which involves learning to evaluate the credibility and value of online materials (see pages 8–9 and 10–12).

- *Assessing source materials.* In a global way, research depends on evaluating materials critically to ensure that you use sources that credibly support your ideas (see pages 9–14).

- *Taking notes.* Research requires you to record ideas and information from your sources carefully and completely so that you can use them appropriately in your writing (see pages 13–15).

- *Responding effectively to opposing views.* Fair-minded research acknowledges and uses opposing views to maintain a balanced perspective.

- *Synthesizing ideas.* Effective research blends information and ideas from a variety of sources, thereby creating a comprehensive presentation that is better or fairer or clearer than the presentation in individual sources.

- *Incorporating material into writing.* Effective research leads to writing that incorporates ideas and information with clarity, accuracy, and style (see pages 20–24 and section 4f).

- *Citing sources accurately.* Research requires you to give proper credit to the people whose ideas and information you have used; this technically focused process requires attention to detail (see Chapters 4–8).

PROFESSIONAL GOALS

Professional goals develop from the process of establishing a working knowledge in your field of study. As such, they focus on the acquisition of specific skills and knowledge.

- *Learning to use specific sources.* Research in each discipline requires familiarity with the kinds of sources that are respected and commonly used.

- *Using specialized formats.* Each discipline's research incorporates unique formats that you must learn to follow.

- *Using specialized writing styles.* Research in each discipline depends on specific stylistic patterns for presenting ideas and information.

- *Demonstrating discipline-specific knowledge.* Research in each discipline builds upon accepted information that you must be able to incorporate fluently.

PERSONAL GOALS

Personal goals concentrate on degrees of knowledge, improvement, sophistication, and experience. Although they are less easily quantified than goals matched to courses, they are also important.

- *Learning about a subject.* Exploring a subject through research improves your knowledge of your discipline.
- *Improving skills.* Conducting research gives you the opportunity not only to use your early research work but also to develop more sophisticated skills.
- *Expanding experiences.* Research work allows for varied kinds of personal growth.

1d   Research Methods

Methods of research vary depending on the project, but most projects require multidimensional work with a variety of sources. To complete such projects, take advantage of a full range of strategies.

LIBRARY-BASED RESEARCH

Learn to use all of the features of your library, especially familiarizing yourself with the research areas that you will most commonly use:

- *Reference:* General source materials—dictionaries, fact books, encyclopedias, indexes, guides, bibliographies, and so on—that can guide your preliminary research (Many are now available in electronic form.)
- *Catalog (computer):* Computer clusters where you secure the records of library materials
- *Stacks:* Bookcases where print materials (books, bound periodicals, and so on) are stored according to a classification system
- *Current periodicals:* Recent copies of journals, magazines, and newspapers (Many are now available in electronic form.)

- *Government documents:* Printed materials from national, state, and local government departments and agencies—books, monographs, pamphlets, reports, and so on (Many government documents are also available in electronic form through government websites.)
- *Microforms:* Microfilm and microfiche materials
- *Media:* Audiovisual sources—motion pictures, videos, DVDs, CDs, and so on
- *New books:* The area where new books are displayed before being placed in the general collection
- *Special collections:* The area where rare books, archival materials, and other special sources are located
- *Special libraries:* Discipline-specific collections that are housed in sublibraries

PERIODICAL DATABASES AND ONLINE CATALOGS

Periodical databases (online "indexes") allow you to gather technical information about—and very often view full texts of—articles in journals, magazines, and newspapers. Online catalogs (electronic search systems) allow you to gather technical information about books, monographs, government documents, and other materials in the library's collection. Both periodical databases and online catalogs provide access to descriptive material about sources through keyword search techniques.

Keyword searching uses easily recognizable words and phrases (often in combination) to access sources. Computer systems search for keywords in titles, tables of contents, and other descriptive materials and then display "matches." To locate a broad range of materials, use alternative phrases (*collaborative learning, collaboration, team research,* and so on) as you conduct searches. Also explore Library of Congress listings, available online at most libraries, to discover unique category descriptions. For example, the Library of Congress system does not use the fairly conventional expression *medical ethics;* rather, its category notation is *medicine—moral and ethical aspects.*

Information About Periodicals

Periodical databases provide standardized information about articles in journals, magazines, and newspapers. Standardized information includes the following elements:

- *Article title:* Full title and subtitle of the article (listed first because some articles have no attributed author)
- *Author:* Full name of the author (or authors)
- *Periodical title:* Title of the journal, magazine, or newspaper
- *City:* City of publication
- *Date:* Month/year, month/day/year, or season/year of publication
- *Volume and issue number:* Volume (which indicates the number of years that a periodical has been published) and issue number (which refers to the specific issue in which the article appeared) for journals and magazines, but not for newspapers
- *Start page:* Page on which the article begins
- *Number of pages:* Total number of pages of the article (in the original print format)
- *Formats for articles:* Formats available for selected articles: citation/abstract, full text, page image (see page 8)

Information About Books (and Other Library-Based Materials)

All online catalogs provide standardized information about each source in the library's collection:

- *Author:* Full name of the author (or authors)
- *Title:* Full title of the source, including subtitles
- *Facts of publication:* City, publisher, and copyright date
- *Technical description:* Specific features—number of pages, book size, and so on
- *Location:* Location of the source in the library's collection or in a special collection or library
- *Call number:* Classification number assigned to the source (indicating where the source is located in the collection)
- *Number of items:* Number of items (three volumes, one volume with CD-ROM, and so on), if more than one exists
- *Status:* Information on whether the source is checked out, on reserve, on loan, and so on

- *Editions:* Descriptions of editions (second, third, revised, enlarged)
- *Notes:* Descriptions of special features (bibliography, index, appendixes, and so on)
- *Table of contents:* Listing of chapters and section titles and subtitles
- *Subject classification:* Library of Congress classification, both primary and secondary

---

Format Options (Within a Periodical Database)

- *Citation/abstract:* Technical information, plus an abstract (a brief summary of the ideas in an article)
- *Full text:* Technical information and abstract, plus the full text of an article in typed form
- *Page image:* Technical information and abstract, plus scanned images of an article as it appeared in the periodical (often as a pdf file)

INTERNET-BASED RESEARCH

Internet research may lead you to a scholarly project (a university-based, scholarly site that provides a wide range of materials—such as full-text books, research data, and visual materials), an information database (a site that offers statistical information from governmental agencies, research institutions, or nonprofit corporations), or a website (a site designed to share information or ideas, forward a political agenda, promote a product, or advocate a position).

To navigate an Internet site successfully and to gather crucial information for a reference-list entry, learn about the key elements of an Internet home page:

- *Electronic address (URL):* "Uniform resource locator"—the combination of elements that locates the source (for example, http://www.aagpgpa.org/ is the URL for the website of the American Association for Geriatric Psychology)
- *Official title:* Title and subtitle of the site
- *Author, host, editor, or Web master:* Person (or people) responsible for developing and maintaining the site

- *Affiliation or sponsorship:* Person, group, organization, or agency that develops and maintains the material on the site
- *Location:* Place (city, school, organization, agency, and so on) from which the site originates
- *Posting date or update:* Date on which the site was first posted or most recently updated (revised)
- *"About This Site":* Description of how the site was developed, a rationale for it, or information about those involved with the site
- *Site directory:* Electronic table of contents for the site

1e Evaluating Sources

Because not all sources are equally useful, you should analyze them and select the ones best suited to your research. This ongoing process requires continued assessments and reassessments.

PRINT SOURCES

Print sources—journals, magazines, newspapers, books, and so on—have traditionally been the mainstay of most research. Consequently, they are the easiest to evaluate because of their familiarity.

- *Author's credentials.* Determine whether an author's academic degrees, scholarly training, affiliations, or other published work establish his or her authority.
- *Appropriate focus.* Determine whether the source addresses the topic in a way that matches your emphasis. Consider literature reviews to establish scholarly context and empirical studies to incorporate recent primary research.
- *Sufficient coverage.* Determine whether the source sufficiently covers the topic by examining its table of contents, reviewing the index, and skimming a portion of the text.
- *Respected periodicals.* Generally, use journals with strong organizational affiliations; furthermore, note that peer-reviewed journals (those that publish works only after they have been recommended by a panel of expert reviewers) offer more credibility than non-peer-reviewed journals. Choose specialized, rather than

general-interest, magazines. Choose major newspapers for topics of international or national importance, but choose regional or local newspapers for issues of regional or local importance.

- *Reputable publisher.* University, academic, or trade presses publish most of the books you will use, which generally ensures their credibility. Note also that publishers often specialize in books related to particular subjects.

- *Publication date.*   For many topics, sources more than 10 or 15 years old have limited value. However, consider creating a historical context by using older sources.

- *Useful supplementary materials.*   Look for in-text illustrations, tables, charts, graphs, diagrams, bibliographies, case studies, or collections of additional readings.

- *Appropriate writing style.*   Skim a potential source to see how it is developed (with facts, examples, description, or narration); also consider whether the author's style is varied, clear, and persuasive.

AUDIOVISUAL SOURCES

Because of the range of audiovisual sources available, assess each kind individually using specific criteria. Many of the techniques employed for evaluating these sources correspond to those used for print and Internet sources.

- *Lectures and speeches.*   Use criteria similar to those for print sources: speaker, relationship to your topic, coverage, sponsoring group or organization, and date.

- *Works of art, photographs, cartoons, and recordings.* Because these sources are used primarily to create interest in most research papers, consider how well the image or performance illuminates your topic.

- *Maps, graphs, tables, and charts.*   Evaluate these visual sources the same way as traditional print sources.

- *Motion pictures, television shows, and radio programs.* When these sources serve informative purposes, evaluate them as you would assess print sources; when they are used creatively, evaluate them using the same criteria you would apply to other creative audiovisual forms.

INTERNET SOURCES

Although Internet sources provide a fascinating array of materials, much of the material posted on the Internet has not been subjected to scholarly review and is, therefore, not necessarily credible. As a result, you should use only Internet sources that meet important evaluative criteria:

- *Author, editor, host, or Web master's credentials.* A website may or may not have an author, editor, host, or webmaster. If it does, explore the site for information about his or her qualifications to discuss the topic.

- *Appropriate focus.* Skim the website to see whether its focus is suitable for your topic. Sometimes the site's title makes the focus clear; at other times, an entire site has a general focus, but its internal links allow you to locate material on narrower aspects of the larger subject.

- *Sufficient coverage.* Review documents on the website to see whether the coverage is thorough enough for your purposes.

- *Domains.* Examine the website's electronic address (URL) to see how the site is registered with the Internet Corporation for Assigned Names and Numbers (ICANN). The following common "top-level domains" provide useful clues about a site's focus and function:

.com	A commercial site. The primary function of a commercial site is to make money.
.edu	A site affiliated with an educational institution. These sites may be posted by the school or by an individual affiliated with the institution.
.gov	A government site. These sites present trustworthy information (statistics, facts, reports), but the interpretive materials may be less useful.
.mil	A military site. The technical information on these sites is consistently useful, but interpretive material tends to justify a single, pro-military position.
.museum	A site for a museum. Because museums can be either nonprofit or for-profit institutions, consider the purpose that the particular museum serves.
.org	An organizational site. Because organizations seek to advance political, social, financial, educational, and other specific agendas, review these materials with care.

- *Possible biases.* Do not automatically discount or overvalue what you find on any particular kind of website. Rather, consider the biases that influence how the information on a site is presented and interpreted.

- *Affiliation or sponsorship.* Examine the website to see whether it has an affiliation or a sponsorship beyond what is suggested by the site's domain.

- *Posting or revision date.* Identify the date of original posting or the date on which information was updated. Because currency is one of the benefits of Internet sources, look for websites that provide recent information.

- *Documentation.* Review Internet materials to see how thoroughly authors have documented their information. If facts, statistics, and other technical information are not documented appropriately, the information may be questionable as well.

- *Links to or from other sites.* Consider the "referral quality" that Internet links provide.

- *Appropriate writing style.* Skim the website to see how it is written. All sources do not, of course, have to be written in the same style, but it is an issue worth considering when you evaluate a source.

COMBINATIONS OF SOURCES

Although you must first evaluate your sources individually—whether they are print, audiovisual, or Internet—your goal is to gather a set of high-quality sources that together provide a balanced treatment of your topic. Consider these issues:

- *Alternative perspectives.* Taken collectively, does the work of your authors provide a range of perspectives—academic and popular, liberal and conservative, theoretical and practical, current and traditional?

- *Varied publication, release, or distribution dates.* Does your group of sources represent the information, ideas, and interpretations of different periods, when appropriate?

- *Different approaches to the topic.* In combination, your sources should range from the technical (including facts and statistics) to the interpretive (providing commentary and assessments). Also consider literature reviews for secondary analyses and empirical studies for primary research.

- *Diversity of sources.* Incorporate in your work a wide range of sources—periodicals, books, audiovisual sources, and electronic sources—to ensure that you have taken advantage of the strengths of each kind of source. Be aware, however, that in some instances your research must focus on selected kinds of sources.

Evaluating sources is an inexact process. No matter how carefully you review materials, some may later prove unhelpful. Yet early efforts to evaluate sources generally enhance the focus and efficiency of later, more comprehensive work, such as reading and taking notes from the sources.

1f Note-Taking

Note-taking is an individualized process, because different researchers prefer different methods for recording information and ideas from sources. However, all note-taking should be meticulous and consistent, both to avoid plagiarism and to simplify the subsequent writing of the paper. Consider alternative methods for note-taking and remember that note-taking must be complete, consistent, matched to the kind of material being used, and honest.

Before taking notes from a source, create a complete and accurate entry for the reference list. See chapters 4–8 for guidelines and samples.

METHODS OF NOTE-TAKING

Begin your note-taking by analyzing each note-taking system and choosing the one best suited to your specific project, library facilities, work habits, and instructor's expectations.

- *Note cards.* Note cards are easy to handle and to rearrange during planning stages, but they hold only limited amounts of information.
- *Paper.* Paper is easy to handle and has sufficient room for copious notes, but notes on paper are difficult to organize during planning stages.
- *Computers.* Notes on computers do not have to be retyped during the writing process and can be printed multiple times, but on-site note-taking with computers is sometimes awkward.

- *Photocopies and printed texts.* Photocopied and printed materials do not have to be recopied, and they can be marked on. However, photocopying and printing can be expensive.

COMPLETE INFORMATION

Record complete identifying information with each separate note to avoid having to return to a source at a later, and potentially less convenient, time.

- *Author's name.* Record the author's last name (and first initial, if necessary for clarity); for multiauthor sources, record only as many names as are necessary for clarity.
- *Title.* Record only key words from titles but use italics or quotation marks as appropriate.
- *Category notation.* Provide a brief descriptive term to indicate the idea or subtopic that the information supports.
- *Page numbers.* Record the page number(s) from which you gathered information. If material comes from several pages, indicate where the page break occurs. (A double slash [//] is a useful way to indicate a page break.) Also indicate when an electronic source does not include pages.

CONSISTENT FORMAT

Record notes in a consistent format to avoid confusion at later stages of research and writing.

- *Placement of information.* Establish a consistent pattern for placing information so that nothing is omitted accidentally.
- *Abbreviations.* Use abbreviations selectively to save time and space; however, use only standard abbreviations to avoid possible confusion later.
- *Notations.* Note anything unique about the source (for example, no page numbers in a pamphlet or an especially good chart).

KINDS OF NOTES

Four common kinds of notes serve most research purposes. Choose among these kinds of note-taking patterns depending on the sources you use and the kinds of materials they include.

- *Facts.* A fact note records technical information—names, dates, percentages—in minimal form. Record words, phrases, and information in a simple outline or list format and double-check the information for accuracy.

- *Summaries.* A summary note presents the substance of a passage in condensed form. After reading original material carefully, write a summary without looking at the original; this will ensure that the phrasing is yours, not the author's. Double-check the summary note to make sure that your wording is distinct from the original.

- *Paraphrases.* A paraphrase note restates ideas from a passage in your own words, using approximately the same number of words. Write a paraphrase without looking at the original, and then double-check the note to ensure that the phrasing is yours.

- *Quotations.* A quotation note reproduces a writer's words *exactly.* Double-check the quotation note against the original; the copy must be an *exact* transcription of the original wording, capitalization, punctuation, and other elements.

1g Plagiarism

Plagiarism, from the Latin word for kidnapping, is the use of someone else's words, ideas, or line of thought without acknowledgment. In its most extreme form, plagiarism involves submitting someone else's completed work as your own. A less extreme but equally unacceptable form involves copying and pasting entire segments of another writer's work into your own writing. A third form of plagiarism involves carelessly or inadvertently blending elements (words, phrases, ideas) of a writer's work into your own.

- *Whole-paper plagiarism.* This kind of plagiarism is easily discovered. Through experiences with students in class, instructors learn what students are interested in and how they express themselves (sentence patterns, diction, and technical fluency).

- *Copy-and-paste plagiarism.* This kind of plagiarism is also easy to detect because of abrupt shifts in sentence sophistication, diction, or technical fluency.

- *Careless plagiarism.* This form of plagiarism is evident when distinct material is unquoted or when specialized information (dates, percentages, and other facts) is not acknowledged. Even when this is carelessly or inadvertently done, the writer is still at fault for dishonest work, and the paper is still unacceptable.

In all of its forms, plagiarism is academically dishonest and unacceptable, and the penalties for its practice range from failing individual papers or projects to failing courses to being dismissed from college to having degrees revoked. The seriousness of plagiarism cannot be ignored, so you must make a concerted effort to avoid this practice. To avoid plagiarizing, learn to recognize the distinctive content and expression in source materials and take accurate, carefully punctuated, and documented notes.

COMMON KNOWLEDGE

Some kinds of information—facts and interpretations—are known by many people and are consequently described as common knowledge. That Alzheimer's disease is the leading cause of dementia in elderly people is widely known, as is the more interpretative information that Alzheimer's disease is best treated by a combination of drug and psychiatric therapies. But common knowledge extends beyond these very general types of information to include more specific information within a field of study. In medical studies, for example, it is widely known that Prozac is the trade name for fluoxetine hydrochloride; in education, a commonly acknowledged interpretation is that high scores on standardized tests do not uniformly predict academic success. Documenting these facts, beliefs, and interpretations in a paper would be unnecessary because they are commonly known in their areas of study, even though you might have discovered them for the first time.

When you are researching an unfamiliar subject, distinguishing common knowledge that does not require documentation from special knowledge that does require documentation is sometimes difficult. The following guidelines may help.

What constitutes common knowledge

- *Historical facts* (names, dates, and general interpretations) that appear in many general reference books. For example, Sigmund Freud's most influential work, *The Interpretation of Dreams,* was published in 1899.

- *General observations and opinions* that are shared by many people. For example, it is a general observation that children learn by actively doing, rather than passively listening, and it is a commonly held opinion that reading, writing, and arithmetic are the basic skills that elementary school students should acquire.

- *Unacknowledged information* that appears in multiple sources. For example, it is common knowledge that the earth's population is roughly 6.7 billion people and that an *IQ* is a gauge of intelligence determined by a person's knowledge in relation to his or her age.

If a piece of information does not meet these guidelines or if you are uncertain about whether it is common knowledge, always document the material.

SPECIAL QUALITIES OF SOURCE MATERIALS

A more difficult problem than identifying common knowledge involves using an author's words and ideas improperly. Improper use often results from careless summarizing and paraphrasing. To use source materials without plagiarizing, learn to recognize their distinctive qualities.

Special qualities of sources

- *Distinctive prose style:* The author's chosen words, phrases, and sentence patterns
- *Original facts:* Results of the author's personal research
- *Personal interpretations of information:* The author's individual evaluation of his or her information
- *Original ideas:* Ideas that are unique to a particular author

As you work with sources, be aware of these distinguishing qualities and make certain that you do not appropriate the prose (word choices and sentence structures), original research, interpretations, or ideas of others without giving proper credit.

Consider, for example, the following paragraphs from Appleby, Hunt, and Jacob's (1994) *Telling the Truth About History* (New York, NY: Norton):

> Interest in this new research in social history can be partly explained by the personal backgrounds of the cohort of historians who undertook the task of writing history from the bottom up. They entered higher education with the post-*Sputnik* expansion of the 1950s and 1960s, when the number of new Ph.D.s in history nearly quadrupled.

Since many of them were children and grandchildren of immigrants, they had a personal incentive for turning the writing of their dissertations into a movement of memory recovery. Others were black or female and similarly prompted to find ways to make the historically inarticulate speak. While the number of male Ph.D.s in history ebbed and flowed with the vicissitudes of the job market, the number of new female Ph.D.s in history steadily increased from 11 percent (29) in 1950 to 13 percent (137) in 1970 and finally to 37 percent (192) in 1989.

Although ethnicity is harder to locate in the records, the GI Bill was clearly effective in bringing the children of working-class families into the middle-class educational mainstream. This was the thin end of a democratizing wedge prying open higher education in the United States. Never before had so many people in any society earned so many higher degrees. Important as their numbers were, the change in perspective these academics brought to their disciplines has made the qualitative changes even more impressive. Suddenly graduate students with strange, unpronounceable surnames, with Brooklyn accents and different skin colors, appeared in the venerable ivy-covered buildings that epitomized elite schooling.

Now look at the following examples of faulty and acceptable summaries and paraphrases. Questionable phrases in the faulty samples are underlined.

Faulty summary: plagiarism likely

Appleby, Hunt, Jacob   historians' backgrounds

-- A historian's focus is *partially explained* by his or her *personal background*.

-- Because of their experiences, *they have a personal incentive* for looking at history in new ways.

-- Large numbers were important, but the change in viewpoint *made the qualitative changes even more impressive*.

pp. 146–147

Acceptable summary: plagiarism unlikely

Appleby, Hunt, Jacob   historians' backgrounds

-- A historian's focus and interpretations are personal.

-- For personal reasons, not always stated, people examine the facts of history from different perspectives.

-- Large numbers were important, but the change in viewpoint "made the qualitative changes even more impressive."

             pp. 146–147

Faulty paraphrase: plagiarism likely

Appleby, Hunt, Jacob   the GI Bill

-- *Even though ethnic background is not easily found* in the statistics, the GI Bill consistently helped students from *low-income families enter the middle-class* educational system. This was how *democracy started forcing open college education in America*.

             pp. 146–147

Acceptable paraphrase: plagiarism unlikely

Appleby, Hunt, Jacob   the GI Bill

-- Because of the GI Bill, even poor people could attend college. For the first time, education was accessible to everyone, which is truly democracy in action. The GI Bill was "the thin end of a democratizing wedge prying open higher education."

             pp. 146–147

1h Planning

After gathering information, organizing the research paper is an exciting stage because you are ready to bring ideas together in a clear and logical form.

REVIEWING NOTES

Begin by rereading the assignment sheet to reexamine the principles guiding your work. Then review your notes to see the range of materials you have collected and to identify connections among ideas.

THESIS STATEMENT OR STATED OBJECTIVE

After rereading your notes, revise the thesis statement, hypothesis, or objective so that it accurately represents the paper you plan to write. Is the topic clear? Does it express your current (more informed) view? Does it contain appropriate qualifications and limitations? Is it worded effectively?

AN INFORMAL OUTLINE

An informal outline is a structural plan prepared for your own use. Arrange information in logical ways using numbers, arrows, dashes, dots, or other convenient symbols to indicate the order for presentation and the relative importance of ideas.

Using the major headings from the informal outline, sort your notes. If a note fits into more than one group, place it in the most appropriate group and place a cross-reference note (for example, "See Parker quotation, p. 219—in *Childhood*") in each of the other appropriate groups.

A FORMAL OUTLINE

If you choose to develop a formal outline, adhere to the following conventions to establish divisions within the outline:

- *Major topics.*   Use uppercase Roman numerals *(I, II, III)* to indicate major topics.
- *Subdivisions.*   Use uppercase letters *(A, B, C)* to indicate subdivisions of major topics.

- *Clarifications.* Use Arabic numerals *(1, 2, 3)* to indicate clarifications of subdivisions—usually examples, supporting facts, and so on.
- *Details.* Use lowercase letters *(a, b, c)* to indicate details used to describe the examples.

In addition, observe the following conventions:

- Use parallel form throughout. Use words and phrases to develop a topic outline or use full sentences to develop a sentence outline.
- Include only one idea in each entry. Subdivide entries that contain two or more ideas.
- Include at least two entries at each sublevel.
- Indent headings of the same level the same number of spaces from the margin.

1i Writing Strategies

Because incorporating research materials and using in-text documentation extend the time it takes to write a paper, allow ample time to write the draft of your paper. Consider both the general and special circumstances that affect the process of writing and revising any paper, as well as those issues that relate specifically to writing and revising a documented paper.

GENERAL STRATEGIES FOR DRAFTING A PAPER

Because the research paper is in many ways like all other papers, keep these general writing strategies in mind:

- *Gather materials.* Collect planning materials and writing supplies before you begin writing. Working consistently in the same location is also helpful because all materials are there when you wish to write.
- *Work from an outline.* Following an outline, whether informal or formal, develop paragraphs and sections; write troublesome sections late in the process.
- *Keep the paper's purpose in mind.* Arrange and develop only those ideas that your outline indicates are important.
- *Develop the paper "promised" by the thesis, hypothesis, or objective.* Incorporate only the ideas and information that support your thesis, hypothesis, or objective.

- *Attend to technical matters later.* Concentrate on getting your ideas down on paper; you can revise the paper later to correct any technical errors.

- *Rethink troublesome sections.* When sections are difficult to write, reconsider their importance or means of development. Revise the outline if necessary.

- *Reread as you write.* Reread early sections as you write to maintain a consistent tone and style.

- *Write alternative sections.* Write several versions of troublesome sections and then choose the best one.

- *Take periodic breaks.* Get away from your work for short periods so that you can maintain a fresh perspective and attain objectivity.

STRATEGIES FOR DRAFTING A RESEARCH PAPER

Because the research paper has its own peculiarities and demands, keep these special strategies in mind:

- *Allow ample time.* Give yourself plenty of time to write a research paper; its length and complexity will affect the speed at which you work.

- *Think about sections, not paragraphs.* Think of the paper in terms of sections, not paragraphs. Large sections will probably contain several paragraphs.

- *Use transitions.* Although headings can divide your work into logical segments, use well-chosen transitional words to signal major shifts between elements of the paper.

- *Attend to technical language.* Define technical terms carefully to clarify ideas.

- *Incorporate notes smoothly.* Use research materials to support and illustrate, not dominate, your discussion.

- *Document carefully.* Use in-text citations (notes in parentheses) to acknowledge the sources of your ideas and information (see Chapter 4, "Preparing the Reference List and In-Text Citations").

QUESTIONS FOR REVISING CONTENT

Examine the paper's content for clarity, coherence, and completeness. Consider these issues:

- *Title, introduction, headings, conclusion.* Are your title, introduction, headings, and conclusion well matched to the tone and purpose of the paper?

- *Thesis (hypothesis) and development.* Does the thesis accurately represent your current view on the topic, and does the paper develop that idea?

- *Support for thesis.* Do research materials effectively support the paper's thesis? Have you eliminated materials (details, sentences, even paragraphs) that do not directly support your thesis?

- *Organization.* Does your organizational pattern present your ideas logically and effectively?

- *Use of materials.* Have you incorporated a range of materials to develop your ideas in a varied, interesting, and complete way?

- *Balance among sections.* Are the sections of the paper balanced in length and emphasis?

- *Balance among sources.* Have you used a variety of sources to support your ideas?

- *Transitions.* Do transitions connect sections of the paper in a coherent way?

QUESTIONS FOR REVISING STYLE

Achieving coherent, balanced, well-developed content is one aspect of revision. Another consideration is achieving a clear and compelling presentation. Refine the paper's style, keeping these issues in mind:

- *Tone.* Is the tone suited to the topic and presentation?

- *Sentences.* Are the sentences varied in both length and type? Have you written active, rather than passive, sentences?

- *Diction.* Are the word choices vivid, accurate, and suitable?

- *Introduction of research materials.* Have you introduced research materials (facts, summaries, paraphrases, and quotations) with variety and clarity?

QUESTIONS FOR REVISING TECHNICAL MATTERS

Technical revision focuses on grammar, usage, punctuation, mechanics, spelling, and manuscript form. After revising content and style, consider technical revisions to make the presentation correct and precise, giving particular attention to issues related to documentation:

- *Grammar.* Are your sentences complete? Do pronouns agree with nouns, and verbs with subjects? Have you worked to avoid errors that you commonly make?

- *Punctuation and mechanics.* Have you double-checked your punctuation? Have you spell-checked the paper? Have you used quotation marks and italics correctly?

- *Quotations.* Are quotations presented correctly, depending on their length or emphasis?

- *In-text citations.* Are in-text citations placed appropriately and punctuated correctly?

- *Reference list.* Have you listed only the sources actually used in the paper? Is your list alphabetized correctly? Is each entry complete and correct?

- *Manuscript guidelines.* Are margins, line spacing, and paging correct? Does the paper include all necessary elements?

Preparing APA Manuscripts

APA style guidelines for manuscript preparation ensure that manuscripts follow uniform standards and, as a result, present the elements of papers in a generally understood way.

2a Parts of the Manuscript

A manuscript for an APA paper can contain as many as eight separate parts: the title page (with author note), abstract, the text of the paper, reference list, footnotes, tables, figures (with figure captions), and appendices. Not all papers have all of these elements, but when they do, they are arranged in this order.

The first part of this chapter addresses the specific requirements for preparing each element of an APA paper. The last part provides general manuscript guidelines.

TITLE PAGE

The first page of a manuscript is the title page (see pages 119 and 127 for samples), composed of the following elements:

- *Running head with paging.* The first line of the title page contains the running head, a shortened version of the paper's title with the page number. Full instructions for creating the running head appear on page 36, and samples appear on pages 119–136.

- *Title.* Center the title and use headline-style capitalization (see page 48). A good title is descriptive, clarifying both the topic and the perspective of the paper; when possible, the title should create interest through effective wording. APA recommends that titles be no more than 12 words long (a title of this length generally fits on a single line). If the title is longer than one line, divide it logically and center both lines.

- *Author's name.* Two lines below the title, include your name (centered and capitalized normally); APA recommends using your first name and middle initial(s) for additional clarity. Two lines below, list your affiliation; normally, this is your school's name, but you can list the city and state where you live. Some instructors may also ask that you include the title of the course for which you wrote the paper.

- *Author note.* At least four spaces below the affiliation, type the phrase *Author note* (not italicized but centered), followed by a series of clarifying paragraphs: (a) the first paragraph identifies the author's departmental, as well as university, affiliation; (b) the second paragraph identifies changes in affiliation, if any; (c) the third paragraph provides acknowledgments, preceded by any necessary disclaimers or explanations of special circumstances; and (d) the fourth paragraph presents the author's contact information. Use separate, indented, double-spaced paragraphs for each element.

NOTE: Student work—papers for classes, theses, and dissertations—typically do not require an author note.

Parts of an APA Paper

- *Title page.* The opening page incorporates information to label the pages of the paper, highlights the title of the paper, and provides identifying information about the author. An author note may be included at the bottom of the title page.

- *Abstract.* This paragraph presents a brief but detailed overview of the paper, emphasizing key ideas and briefly explaining research procedures.

- *Text.* The text of an argumentative paper or review contains an introduction, body, and conclusion; it is frequently divided using headings that describe the main elements of the discussion. The text of a research study contains an introduction of the problem, an explanation of methodology, a summary of results, and a discussion of the implications of the study.

- *Reference list.* The alphabetically arranged reference list provides technical information about the sources used in the paper.

- *Footnotes.* Content footnotes include clarifying discussions and explanations that might disrupt the flow of the paper. Footnotes may be incorporated within the text of the paper using the footnote function of your word processor.

- *Tables.* Numbered tables include technical data in easily interpreted and comparable forms. References

---

Parts of an APA Paper

---

within the paper correspond to tables that appear on separate pages near the end of the manuscript.

- *Figures.*   Visual images to support ideas in a paper (drawings, graphs, photographs, maps, and so on) appear as numbered figures. References within the paper correspond to the captioned figures that appear on separate pages at the end of the manuscript.

- *Appendices.*   Appendices provide supplementary information that supports the ideas in the paper but would be awkward to include in the paper itself.

ABSTRACT

The abstract (the second page of the manuscript) follows the title page and provides a brief description of the major ideas in the paper (see page 119 for a sample). Because it must summarize the full range of ideas and information in the paper, it is generally written after the manuscript is complete. It must adhere to the following guidelines:

- *Heading*   Three lines below the running head, type the word *Abstract*, centered but not italicized. Two lines below, begin the paragraph.

- *Format.*   The abstract is a single, unindented, double-spaced paragraph.

- *Length.*   Abstracts in APA journals are typically 150–250 words.

- *Concision.*   To save space in the abstract, use standard abbreviations (*AMA,* rather than *American Medical Association*); use digits for all numbers except those that begin sentences; and use active, rather than passive, sentences.

- *Content.*   In the opening sentence, describe the topic or problem addressed in the paper. Use the remaining words in the paragraph to clarify methodology (for a research study), to identify four or five major ideas, and to explain results or conclusions. If a paper is lengthy and multifaceted, describe only the most important elements.

- *Keywords.*   You may include a keyword list with your abstract. Two lines below the abstract, indent, type *Keywords* (italicized, followed by a colon) and provide a brief list of words that best describe the content of your paper.

TEXT

The text of the paper begins on the third page of the manuscript (see pages 120–125 for sample pages). The running head, as always, appears on the top line. Three lines below, center the title, with headline-style capitalization but without special print features (bold, italics, underlining, change in font size, or quotation marks). Two lines below the title, the double-spaced paper begins. The organization of the body of the paper depends on its focus.

An Argumentative Paper, Review, or Meta-Analysis

- *Introduction.*   In this unlabeled section, define, describe, or clarify the topic (problem) and place it within its historical or scholarly context. Present a thesis (a statement of your topic and opinion) to clarify the purpose of your work.

- *Body.*   Examine the facets of the topic (problem) by reviewing current research: evaluate the positions held by others; analyze current data; assess the interpretations of others; synthesize the information and ideas found in other people's work. Use headings and subheadings throughout this section to direct readers through your argument.

- *Conclusion.*   Summarize key points, draw connections among important ideas, and reiterate your thesis.

- *Reference list.*   This labeled section provides a list of sources cited in the paper (see Chapter 4).

- *Additional materials.*   As appropriate, include the following labeled sections: footnotes, tables, figures, and appendices.

A Research Study

- *Introduction.*   In this unlabeled section, describe the problem, state your hypothesis, and describe your research methodology. Consider the importance of the problem and the ways in which the study addresses the problem. Present a historical

---

A Research Study

---

or contextual discussion of what scholars have written, acknowledging alternative perspectives and differing interpretations.

- *Method.* This labeled section should be further divided into labeled subsections that describe participants in the study (and procedures for selecting them), materials used (ranging from standard equipment to custom materials), and procedures (the step-by-step process for conducting the research).

- *Results.* This labeled section summarizes the gathered information. It should be further subdivided into labeled subsections that analyze information that is illustrated by tables, figures, and other statistical material.

- *Discussion.* This labeled section opens with an assertion about the correlation of your data with your original hypothesis. The remaining discussion can address how your findings relate to the work of others, what qualifications are necessary, the value of alternative interpretations, or what conclusions you have reached. End the discussion by commenting on the significance of your research results.

- *Reference list.* This labeled section provides a list of sources cited in the paper (see Chapter 4).

- *Additional materials.* As appropriate, include the following labeled sections: footnotes, tables, figures, and appendices.

REFERENCE LIST

The reference list, which continues the paging of the entire manuscript, provides publishing information for all sources used in the paper (see pages 126 and 134 for samples). Chapter 4 provides a comprehensive discussion of the information required in reference-list entries and the format for presenting the information. Chapters 5–8 provide explanations of 60 kinds of sources, with samples for preparing reference-list entries for periodicals, books and other print materials, audiovisual sources, and electronic sources. Each entry appears with a corresponding in-text citation.

FOOTNOTES

Content footnotes allow writers to provide additional discussion or clarification that, although important, might disrupt the flow of a paper.

Footnotes follow these guidelines for placement and presentation:

- *Heading.*　Three lines below the running head, type the word *Footnotes,* centered but not italicized.

- *Order of notes.*　Footnotes appear on the footnote page in the order in which references appear in the text of the paper. Double-check the numbering.

- *Format.*　Footnotes are typed in paragraph style, double-spaced, with the first line indented and subsequent lines aligned at the left margin. "Tab" once (for a five-space indentation), insert the superscript number, and type the footnote. No space separates the note number from the first letter of the first word of the footnote.

- *Paging.*　Footnotes appear on a new page. Multiple footnotes are placed on the same page, with no additional space between the notes.

NOTE: Footnotes may alternately be incorporated within the text of the paper using the footnote function of your word processor.

Placing Note Numbers in the Paper

- *In-text notes.*　Footnotes are numbered sequentially throughout a paper.

- *Placement of in-text note numbers.*　In the text of the paper, refer to a content note by using a superscript number (a number placed above the line, like this[1]) without additional space. Word-processing programs allow you to achieve this result by using the "Font" feature.

- *Punctuation and note numbers.*　Note numbers follow all punctuation marks, except dashes and parentheses. A note number precedes the dash[2]—without additional space. A note number may appear within parentheses (when it refers only to materials with the parentheses[3]). If the note refers to the entire sentence, however, it follows the parentheses (as in this sample).[4]

TABLES

Because tables present labeled information in columns (vertical elements) and rows (horizontal elements) for easy interpretation or comparison, they are helpful additions to papers that use technical data (see page 135 for a sample). Within the text of the paper, a reference (for example, "see Table 1") directs readers to tables using numerals (which correspond to tables presented near the end of the manuscript). Tables are prepared on separate pages and are presented according to these principles:

- *Table identification.*   Three lines below the running head (flush with the left margin), type the word *Table* and the table's Arabic numeral *(Table 3, Table 4), not* italicized.

- *Title of the table.*   Two spaces below the table heading, also flush left, type the title of the table in italics, with headline-style capitalization. One line below, insert a horizontal, 1-point rule (line); use the graphics or "Insert" feature of your word-processing program to create this element.

- *Column headings.*   Capitalize only the first word of column headings, and center the column heading over the information in each column. One line below the column headings, insert a horizontal rule.

- *Parallel information and style.*   To maintain consistency, headings should appear in parallel grammatical forms (all nouns, all gerunds, and so on), and numbers should appear in similar style (with decimals, rounded to whole numbers, and so on).

- *Spacing.*   The primary elements of tables are single-spaced, and columns should be separated by at least three spaces for visual clarity. However, table notes (general and specific) are double-spaced.

- *Repeated information.*   If information from a table extends beyond one page, repeat the column headings.

- *Table notes (general).*   To provide an explanation of an entire table, include a general note. One line below the body of the table, insert a horizontal rule. Below the rule, type the word *Note* (italicized and flush with the left margin) followed by a period; after one space, type the text of the note, which remains flush left if it extends beyond one line. Place a period at the end of the note, even if it is not a complete sentence. These notes are double-spaced.

- *Table notes (specific).*   To provide an explanation of a specific element within a table, include a specific note. Within the table, insert a superscript lowercase letter—like this[a]—following the element. One line below the body of the table, insert a horizontal rule. Below the horizontal rule and flush with the left margin, insert the corresponding superscript lowercase letter, followed by the explanation. Place a period at the end of the note, even if it is not a complete sentence. If a table also has a general table note, it appears first; the specific table note appears on the line below. If a table has more than one specific note, they continue on the same line, separated by one space. These notes are double-spaced.

- *Paging.*   Each table must begin on a new page.

FIGURES

Figures are visual elements—drawings, graphs, photographs, maps, and so on—that cannot be reproduced by traditional typing (see page 135 for a sample). Each figure is numbered as it is used in the paper; original figures then appear on separate pages at the end of the manuscript, following these guidelines:

- *Figure.*   Three lines below the running head, insert the figure in the highest quality possible, with sharp contrast in photographs, distinct shading in bar graphs, and clear lettering in line graphs. Figures must be scaled to fit appropriately on the page.

- *Label.*   Below the figure, flush left, type the word *Figure*, the number of the figure, and a period. All of these elements are italicized.

- *Caption.*   One space after the figure label, type the caption, using sentence-style capitalization. Place a period at the end of the caption, even if it is not a complete sentence. The caption is *not* italicized.

- *Spacing and indentation.*   Figure captions are double-spaced. If a caption extends beyond one line, it continues flush left.

- *Fonts.*   Printed text that is part of a figure—labels, for example—should use a sans serif font such as Helvetica. The minimum acceptable font size is 8 points, with 14 points being the maximum.

- *Paging.*   Each figure must be presented on a new page.

Special Concerns for Figures

- *Value of the figure.* Consider whether the figure presents information more effectively than would a textual discussion or a table. Because figures are more difficult to prepare than print-based elements, make sure that your time is well spent in creating one.

- *Computer-generated figures.* Today's word-processing programs are capable of creating a wide range of figures, including bar graphs, line graphs, and pie charts. Allow sufficient time to familiarize yourself with the procedures for creating a figure.

- *Visual clutter.* Include only figures that highlight important elements of your discussion. To achieve this goal, eliminate all extraneous detail in graphs, charts, and drawings, and crop (trim) photographs and maps to focus visual attention on key features, not superficial or unrelated elements.

- *Visual clarity.* To ensure that figures achieve maximum impact, make sure that the print quality of graphs and charts is high (best achieved by laser printing). Furthermore, make sure that bar charts, photographs, and maps are sharply focused and have clear tonal contrast.

APPENDICES

One or more appendices can follow figures and continue the page numbering of the entire manuscript. Each appendix should adhere to the following guidelines:

- *Heading.* Three lines below the running head, type the word *Appendix,* centered but not italicized. If more than one appendix is included, label each one with a letter (Appendix A, Appendix B).

- *Appendix title.* Two lines below the heading, type the title of the appendix, centered, with headline-style capitalization.

- *Text.* Begin the text two lines below the appendix title; appended material is double-spaced.

- *Paging.* Each appendix begins on a new page.

2b General Manuscript Guidelines

In preparing a paper in APA style, writers must conform to a variety of principles, each of which is described in the following sections.

PAPER

Use heavy-weight, white bond, $8^{1}/_{2}$" × 11" paper. Avoid onionskin and erasable paper; neither holds up well under review or grading. If you must work on erasable paper, submit a high-quality photocopy on good-quality paper.

FONT SELECTION

Fonts—designed versions of letters, numbers, and characters—appear in different sizes, referred to as *points*. APA encourages the use of serif fonts (those with cross marks on individual letters) for the text of the paper; Times New Roman is the preferred font. Sans serif fonts (those without cross marks) such as Arial or Century Gothic may be used to label figures and illustrations. Font sizes for all elements of the paper except figures should be 12 points, the default size in most word-processing programs.

Use italics *(slanted type),* not underlining, in all parts of your paper. Use your word processor's capabilities to insert accents, diacritical marks, and symbols directly in your paper, rather than adding them by hand.

LINE SPACING

Double-space all parts of the paper except elements within tables and figures, which use single-spacing. For visual clarity, you may triple- or quadruple-space before or after equations or other visual elements. (*NOTE*: Three lines separate the running head from the elements of the paper.)

WORD SPACING

Use two spaces after periods, question marks, and exclamation points (end punctuation). Use one space after commas, colons, and semicolons (internal punctuation); periods with initials (E. V. Debbs); and between elements in citations. No space is required with periods in abbreviations (p.m., e.g., U.S.), with hyphens (first-year student), or with dashes (example: The sounds of vowels—*a, e, i, o, u*—must be transcribed carefully to record speech accurately).

MARGINS AND INDENTATIONS

Leave one-inch margins at the left, right, top, and bottom of each page. If the "default" margins for your word-processing program are not one inch, reset them to one inch. Do not justify the right margin (that is, create a straight text edge on the right); instead, use left justification, which aligns the text on the left but leaves the right margin irregular (ragged). Do not hyphenate words at the ends of lines.

A five- to seven-space indentation ($^1/_2$ inch)—best achieved by using the "Tab" feature—is required at the beginning of paragraphs and for the first line of footnotes. The continuous indentation that is required for long quotations and for second and subsequent lines of reference-list entries is best achieved by using the "Indent" feature.

SERIATION

To indicate series or sequences within a prose paragraph, enclose lowercase letters in parentheses. Although this pattern should not be overused, it has several advantages: (a) it provides visual clarity, and (b) it makes a long sentence with multiple elements easily readable. To achieve a similar effect with a series of set-off sentences or paragraphs, use Arabic numerals followed by periods:

1. Indent the number five to seven spaces from the margin ($^1/_2$ inch).
2. After a period and one space, type the sentence or paragraph.
3. If the item continues beyond one line, subsequent lines can be flush left or indented.

When elements are not presented in chronological order or by order of importance, they may be set off using bullets (typically filled circles or squares):

- This pattern draws attention to each element.
- The order of elements is deemphasized.
- Indentation patterns are the same as for numbered lists.

PAGING (RUNNING HEAD)

On the first line of the title page, flush left, type the words *Running head* (not italicized, but followed by a colon) and an abbreviated version of the paper's title. The title is typed in all capital letters and can contain no more than 50 characters (letters, numbers, symbols, punctuation, and spaces). Flush right, insert the page number. This information must be at least one-half inch from the top of the page; the text begins three lines below the running head (see pages 119 and 127 for samples). On subsequent pages of the paper, use only the running head itself, omitting the label "Running head" (see pages 120 and 128 for samples).

Use the "Header" feature of your word-processing program to type the running head and use codes to insert page numbers automatically throughout the document.

HEADINGS FOR SECTIONS

Use headings to divide and subdivide the paper into logical, and sometimes sequential, sections. APA establishes five potential levels of division for manuscripts, while acknowledging that most writing does not require the use of all five:

- *Level-1 headings* are centered, with headline-style capitalization and boldface.
- *Level-2 headings* are flush left, with headline-style capitalization and boldface.
- *Level-3 headings* are indented, with sentence-style capitalization, boldface, and a period.
- *Level-4 headings* are indented, with sentence-style capitalization, boldface, italics, and a period.
- *Level-5 headings* are indented, with sentence-style capitalization, italics, and a period.

One level of division

> **Level-1 Heading**

Two levels of division

> **Level-1 Heading**
>
> **Level-2 Heading**

Three levels of division

> **Level-1 Heading**
> **Level-2 Heading**
> > **Level-3 heading.**

Four levels of division

> **Level-1 Heading**
> **Level-2 Heading**
> > **Level-3 heading.**
> > ***Level-4 heading.***

Five levels of division

> **Level-1 Heading**
> **Level-2 Heading**
> > **Level-3 heading.**
> > ***Level-4 heading.***
> > *Level-5 Heading.*

When new headings are required, do not begin new pages. Simply type the new heading two lines below the last line of the preceding paragraph.

SUBMITTING THE PAPER

Submit manuscripts according to your instructor's guidelines, acknowledging that alternative formats exist:

- Paper: Secure the pages with a paper clip in the upper-left corner and place them in a manila envelope with your name and affiliation typed or written on the outside. Always keep a photocopy—or another printed copy—of the paper.
- Disk: Submit a copy of the final paper on a separate disk, clearly labeled with your name and affiliation, as

well as a note about the word-processing program you used. Save a copy of the file on another disk for yourself.

- Electronic: Attach the file version of the paper to an e-mail with a clear subject line (Paper 4: Test Anxiety), as well as a note about the word-processing program you used. If you do not receive a confirmation of delivery, resubmit the e-mail and attachment. Print a copy of your e-mail as a record.

3 Following APA Editorial Style

Generally, APA style follows conventions that need little explanation (for example, periods follow sentences that make statements, and question marks follow sentences that pose questions). However, in some situations, agreement about editorial issues is not universal. (Should commas separate *all* elements of listed items? Are prepositions in titles capitalized?) In such special circumstances, follow the APA guidelines in this chapter to ensure that your manuscript meets expectations.

3a Punctuation and Mechanics

PERIODS

Periods most often serve as end punctuation (after sentences), but they are also used with abbreviations and in other specialized contexts.

Uses of periods	*Examples*
End of a complete sentence	Periods end most sentences.
Initials with an author's name	C. S. Lewis
Reference-list abbreviations	Ed., Vol. 6, pp. 34–38, Rev. ed.
After figure captions	*Figure 3.* Student use of computers.
Latin abbreviations	i.e., e.g., vs., p.m.
U.S. when used as an adjective	U.S. government, U.S. economy
Abbreviation for inch	in. (distinct from the preposition *in*)
Decimal points in fractions	2.45 ml, 33.5 lb

COMMAS

Commas are internal forms of punctuation, most often used to separate elements within sentences. However, they also serve a few other purposes.

Uses of commas	*Examples*
Three or more items in a series	men, women, and children
Set off nonessential information	The room, which was well lighted, was on the south corridor.
Clauses of a compound sentence	The first survey was a failure, but the second one was a success.
Years with exact dates	May 25, 2009, the experiment began. *But* May 2009, the experiment began.
Years within in-text citations	(Armstrong, 2008); (Kindervader, 2007)
Numbers of 1,000 or larger	11,205 students, 1,934 books [see "Number Style," page 53, for exceptions]

SEMICOLONS

In APA style, semicolons serve two purposes, one related to compound sentences and one related to elements in a series.

Uses of semicolons	*Examples*
Join clauses of a compound sentence when no coordinating conjunction is used	Males responded positively; females responded negatively.
Separate elements in a series when the elements contain commas	The test groups were from Fresno, California; St. Louis, Missouri; and Raleigh, North Carolina.

COLONS

Colons serve five distinct purposes in APA style. A complete sentence must precede the colon, and if the explanatory material that follows a colon is a complete sentence, the first word is capitalized.

Uses of colons	*Examples*
Introduce a phrase that serves as an explanation or illustration	Two words triggered the strongest reactions: *preferential* and *special.*
Introduce a sentence that serves as an explanation or illustration (the first word of the clarifying sentence is capitalized)	The results are quickly summarized: The experiment was a failure.
Separate elements in a ratio	The ratio was 3:10.
Separate the place of publication and publisher in a reference-list entry	Didion, J. (2005). *The year of magical thinking.* New York, NY: Vintage Books.
Separate the numbered section and page number in a newspaper in a reference-list entry	Rodriguez, A. (2007, September 16). When health care does more harm than good. *The Chicago Tribune,* p. 1:18.

DASHES

Formed by typing two hyphens (with no spaces before and after) or using the em-dash feature of your word-processing program, dashes serve a few selected purposes; however, they should be used sparingly in academic writing. Also note that if a title contains a dash, the word that follows the dash is capitalized.

Uses of dashes	*Examples*
Indicate a break in the thought of the sentence	The national heritage of participants—they identified themselves—proved less important than researchers anticipated.
Insert a series of elements that contain commas	Universities in two small cities—Terre Haute, Indiana, and Bloomington, Illinois—offer similar programs in psychology.

The shorter and more specialized en dash, which can be inserted using your word-processing program, is used to indicate inclusive pages in reference-list entries and in-text citations (102–133, pp. 435–436) and to show equal weight in a compound modifier (parent–teacher conference, doctor–patient relationship).

HYPHENS

Hyphens are most often used to join compound words that precede the noun they modify; this pattern ensures that modification is clear in individual sentences (example: First-person narratives are seldom suitable in academic writing). When the modifiers follow the noun, they are generally written without hyphens (example: The opening paragraphs were written in the first person). When general usage determines that a compound has become a permanent part of the language, it may be spelled either open (high school) or closed (casebook); consult a collegiate dictionary for individual cases.

Uses of hyphens	*Examples*
A compound that functions as an adjective	high-risk behaviors, time-intensive work, all-or-nothing approach
A compound with a number that functions as an adjective	two-part explanation, sixth-grade teacher, 50-word paragraph

Uses of hyphens	*Examples*
A compound using the prefix *self-*	self-help books, self-inflicted injuries, self-imposed limitations
A compound that could be misread	re-form ("form again," not "change"), re-mark ("mark again," not "comment"), re-count ("count again," not "remember")
A compound using a prefix when the base word is capitalized	anti-American sentiment, pseudo-Freudian interpretation, post-Depression regulations
A compound using a prefix when the base word is a number	pre-1960s complacency, post-2005 requirements
A compound using a prefix when the base word is more than one word	non-user-friendly instructions, anti-off-site testing, non-peer-reviewed journals
A fraction used as an adjective	three-fourths majority
A prefix that ends with the first letter of the base word (except *e*)	anti-inflamatory drug, post-traumatic stress (but preexisting condition)

Special cases—No hyphenation	*Examples*
A compound with an adverb ending in *-ly*	newly designed test, recently certified teacher, uncharacteristically exaggerated statement
A compound with a comparative or superlative adjective	less capable practitioner, clearer written instructions, most egregious error
A foreign phrase used as a modifier	ad hoc committee, a priori reasoning, laissez faire attitude

(cont. on next page)

Special cases—No hyphenation	*Examples*
A common fraction used as a noun	two thirds of students, one half of the sample, one quarter of the residents

QUOTATION MARKS

Quotation marks are used within the text of a paper to identify titles of brief works, to indicate a quotation containing fewer than 40 words, and to highlight words used in special ways. Note especially that quotation marks are not used in reference-list entries and that quotations of more than 40 words are indented and use no quotation marks. (See section 4f for additional information on quoted material.)

Uses of quotation marks	*Examples*
Titles of chapters, articles, songs, subsites of websites, and so on (quotation marks are used in the text only; reference-list entries *do not* use quotation marks)	"The High-Risk Child" (chapter), "Grant Writing vs. Grant Getting" (article), "My Vietnam" (song), "Adlerian Web Links" (subsite)
Quoted material (written or spoken) of fewer than 40 words when used word for word	Duncan (2008) asserted, "Normative behavior is difficult to define because community standards apply" (p. 233).
Words used counter to their intended meaning (irony, slang, or coined usage)	Her "abnormal" behavior was, in fact, quite normal.

PARENTHESES

Parentheses are used, always in pairs, to separate information and elements from the rest of the sentence.

Uses of parentheses	*Examples*
Set off clarifying information	We provided parents with four samples (see Figures 1–4).
Set off publication dates in in-text summaries.	Wagner (2008) noted that special-needs students responded well to the protocol.
Set off parenthetical references within the text; they must correspond to entries in the reference list.	First-time offenders are more likely to respond to group therapy sessions than are repeat offenders (Gillum & Sparks, 2008).
Set off page references that follow direct quotations	Rodriguez (2008) noted, "Self-concept is an intangible quality among immigrant children" (p. 34).
Introduce an abbreviation to be used in place of a full name in subsequent sections of a paper	The American Psychological Association (APA) published its first guidelines for manuscript preparation in 1929. Since then, APA has updated its guidelines eight times.
Set off letters that indicate divisions or sequences within paragraphs	The test included sections on (a) vocabulary, (b) reading comprehension, and (c) inferences.

BRACKETS

Brackets are used within parentheses or quotation marks to provide clarifying information. Use brackets sparingly because they can become distracting in academic writing.

Uses of brackets	*Examples*
Clarifying information in a quotation	Thompson (2008) observed, "When [students] work in groups, they perform better" (p. 11). (Used to replace *they* in the original text.)
Parenthetical information already in parentheses	(See Figure 4 [Percentages of students with learning disabilities] for more details.)
Clarifying information in a reference-list entry	*Eternal sunshine of the spotless mind* [Motion picture].

SLASHES

Slashes serve very specialized functions, often related to the presentation of compounds, comparisons, and correlations.

Uses of slashes	*Examples*
Hyphenated compounds in alternatives	first-day/second-day experiences
Fractions (numerator/ denominator)	$3/4$, $X+Y/Z$
Represent *per* in units with numerical value	0.7 ml/L
Indicate phonemes in English	/b/
Separate dual publication dates for reprinted works	Palmer (1995/2008)

CAPITALIZATION

APA follows universally accepted patterns for most capitalization. However, APA uses two distinct capitalization patterns for titles—headline style and sentence style—depending on whether they appear in the text of the paper or in the reference list.

Uses of capitalization	*Examples*
Proper nouns and proper adjectives	Jean Piaget, Robert Coles, Chinese students, Elizabethan drama
Specific departments (and academic units) in universities and specific courses	Department of Psychology, Indiana State University, Criminology 235
Trade and brand names	Prozac, Xerox, WordPerfect 12.0
Specific titles for parts of books	"The Middle-Child Syndrome"
Nouns used with numbers or letters in describing sequenced methods or examples	Day 4, Experiment 6, Table 1, Figure 3
Formal titles of tests	Scholastic Aptitude Test
Table titles: Use headline-style capitalization.	*Grade Ranges of Remedial Students*
First word of a sentence that follows a colon	One challenge could not be met: The cost of the test was too great.
Running head (all capitals)	BEYOND BIRTH ORDER, TEST QUESTIONS

Special cases—No capitalization	*Examples*
Figure captions: Use sentence-style capitalization.	*Figure 1*. Percentages of international students by country of origin.
General references to departments and courses	a number of departments of sociology, a speech pathology course

(cont. on next page)

Special cases—No capitalization	*Examples*
Generic or scientific names of drugs or ingredients	fluoxetine hydrochloride (*but* Prozac)
General names of laws or theories	the empirical law of effect
Common parts of tables	page iv, column 2, row 6
General titles of tests	an achievement test

Capitalization of Titles

APA follows two distinct patterns for the capitalization of titles: one within the text of a paper and one in the reference list and other supporting pages.

* *In-text capitalization.* In the text of a paper, both in your prose and in in-text citations (parenthetical notes), use headline-style capitalization, no matter what kind of source you use.

Headline-style Capitalization

Guiding principles	*Examples*
Capitalize the first and last word; capitalize all other words except articles, *to* (as part of an infinitive phrase), and conjunctions or prepositions of three or fewer letters.	Edwards's *Post-Operative Stress: A Guide for the Family*, "Agent of Change: The Educational Legacy of Thomas Dewey"

Sentence-style Capitalization

Guiding principles	*Examples*
Capitalize the first word of a title or subtitle; otherwise, capitalize only proper nouns and proper adjectives.	*Edwards's Post-operative stress: A guide for the family*, "Agent of change: The educational legacy of Thomas Dewey"

Periodical

Mokhtari and Reichard (2002), in "Assessing Students' Metacognitive Awareness of Reading Strategies," described and analyzed a new self-report instrument used to gauge students' procedures for reading school-related materials.

Book

In *The Mismeasure of Man,* Gould (1981) provided useful insights into the ethical and unethical uses to which intelligence tests can be put.

- *Reference-list (and other) capitalization.* In the reference list, only periodical titles use headline-style capitalization. The titles of articles and all other sources (such as books or broadcasts) use sentence-style capitalization.

Periodical

Mokhtari, K., & Reichard, C. A. (2002). Assessing students' metacognitive awareness of reading strategies. *Journal of Educational Psychology, 94,* 249–259.

Book

Gould, S. J. (1981). *The mismeasure of man.* New York, NY: Norton.

- *Capitalization of special in-text elements.* Headline-style capitalization is used for titles of tables.

NOTE: The running head appears in all capital letters.

ITALICS

APA requires the use of italics (slanted fonts, as in *this example*), rather than underlining, in computer-generated manuscripts.

Uses of italics	*Examples*
Titles of full-length works: periodicals, books, motion pictures, CDs, websites, and so on	*Journal of Cognitive Psychology* (journal), *Wordplay and Language Learning* (book), *A Beautiful Mind* (motion picture), *Back to Black* (CD), *The Victorian Web* (website)

(cont. on next page)

Uses of italics	*Examples*
Genus, species, or varieties	*Pan troglodytes verus* (common chimpanzee)
New terms (when introduced and defined; thereafter, presented without italics)	The term *Nisei,* meaning second-generation Japanese Americans
Words, letters, or phrases used as words, letters, or phrases	Different impressions are created by the words *small, diminutive, minute,* and *tiny.*
Words that could be misread	*more* specific detail (meaning additional detail that is specific)
Letters used as symbols or algebraic variables	$IQ = \dfrac{MA \text{ (mental age)}}{CA \text{ (chronological age)}} \times 100$
Titles of tables	*Factors That Influence School Choice*
Volume numbers for periodicals (in reference-list entries)	*American Psychologist, 123; English Journal, 91*
Anchors for scales	Satisfaction ratings ranged from 1 *(very satisfied)* to 8 *(very dissatisfied).*

NUMBER STYLE

In APA style, numerals are used more frequently than words, whether in written texts or supporting materials; Arabic numerals are preferred in an APA-style text, rather than Roman numerals.

Uses of numerals	*Examples*
Numbers of 10 and larger	14 respondents, 26 chapters, 11th article

Uses of numerals	*Examples*
Numbers smaller than 10 when compared with numbers larger than 10	the 4th chapter of 20; 2 of 30 research subjects; 13 sources: 10 articles, 3 books
Numbers preceding units of measurement	6-in. mark, 300-mg capsule
Numbers used statistically or mathematically	7.5 of respondents, a ratio of 5:2, 9% of the sample, the 3rd percentile
Numbers that represent periods of time	6 years, 5 months, 1 week, 3 hr, 15 min, 7:15 p.m.
Numbers that represent dates	April 1, 2009; November 2005
Numbers that represent ages	4-year-olds, students who are 8 years old
Numbers for population size	1 million citizens
Numbers that refer to participants or subjects	7 participants, 4 rhesus monkeys
Numbers that refer to points or scores on a scale	scores of 6.5 on an 8-point scale
Numbers for exact sums of money	A test costing $4.25, a $5 fee
Numbers used as numbers	a scale ranging from 1 to 5
Numbers that indicate placement in a series	Exam 4, Figure 9
Numbers for parts of books	Chapter 2, page 6
Numbers in a list of four or more numbers	The sample was composed of workgroups with 2, 4, 6, and 8 members.
Numbers in the abstract for a paper	All numbers appear in numeral form.

Uses of words for numbers	*Examples*
Numbers smaller than 10 (see exceptions in the previous table)	two experimental models, three lists, one-topic discussion
Zero and one (when confusion is likely)	zero-percent increase, one-unit design
Numbers that begin sentences	Sixteen authors contributed to the collection. Thirteen people attended.
Numbers that begin titles	"Twelve Common Errors in Research," *Seven-Point Scales: Values and Limitations*
Numbers that begin headings	*Five Common Income Groups* (table heading)
Numbers in common fractions	two thirds of teachers, a reduction of three fourths
Numbers in common names and phrases	the Seven Deadly Sins, the Ten Commandments, the Seven Wonders of the World

Cardinal and Ordinal Numbers

Cardinal numbers (one, two, three, and so on) indicate quantity; ordinal numbers (first, second, third, and so on) indicate order. The principles described in the preceding tables apply whether the numbers are cardinal or ordinal.

Commas in Numbers

In most writing contexts, commas are used in numbers of 1,000 or larger. Place commas between groups of three digits, moving from the right. However, in the following situations, commas are not used.

Numbers without commas	*Examples*
Page numbers	page 1287, pages 1002–1021, (p. 2349)
Degrees of temperature	2044°F
Serial numbers	033776901
Binary digits	01100100
Numbers to the right of decimal points	2.09986
Designations of acoustical frequency	1000 Hz
Degrees of freedom	*F*(31, 1000)

Plurals of Numbers

Whether numbers are presented as numerals or words, form their plurals by adding only *s* or *es*: 1960s, threes, sixes, 25s. Do not use apostrophes to indicate plurality.

Numbered Seriation

To indicate series, sequences, or alternatives in a series of set-off sentences or paragraphs, use Arabic numerals, followed by periods (see page 35).

3b General Style

The way in which a manuscript is written affects the ways in which readers respond. A well-written paper communicates ideas efficiently and effectively, whereas a poorly written paper distracts readers from its central ideas. Consequently, take time to revise your writing to improve its presentation, paying special attention to a few key elements that improve the effectiveness of communication.

TRANSITIONS

Transitions—words or phrases that signal relationships among elements of a paper—facilitate readers' progress through a paper. Use transitional words and phrases to create appropriate links within your work.

Transitional Words and Phrases	
Relationship	*Examples*
Addition	also, and, besides, equally, further, furthermore, in addition, moreover, next, too
Similarity	also, likewise, moreover, similarly
Difference	but, however, in contrast, nevertheless, on the contrary, on the other hand, yet
Examples	for example, for instance, in fact, specifically, to illustrate
Restatements	finally, in brief, in conclusion, in other words, in short, in summary, on the whole, that is, therefore, to sum up
Results	accordingly, as a result, consequently, for this reason, so, therefore, thereupon, thus
Chronology	after, afterward, before, during, earlier, finally, first, immediately, in the meantime, later, meanwhile, next, second, simultaneously, soon, still, then, third, when, while
Location	above, below, beyond, farther, here, nearby, opposite, there, to the left, to the right, under

VERB TENSE

Verbs are primary communicators in sentences, signaling action *(organized, summarized, presented)* or indicating a state of being *(seemed, was)*. Well-chosen, specific verbs make writing direct and forceful. Moreover, tenses of verbs indicate chronology, clarifying the time relationships that you want to express.

In APA style, verbs are used in specific ways to signal ideas clearly.

Uses of verbs	*Examples*
Active voice (to clarify who is doing what)	Respondents completed the questionnaire in 15 minutes. (*Not:* The questionnaire was completed in 15 minutes by the respondents.)
Passive voice (to clarify who or what received the action, not the person or people responsible)	Traditional IQ tests were administered as part of the admissions process. (The use of the tests is emphasized, not the givers of the tests.)
Past tense (to place an action in the past or to describe previous research)	Bradshaw and Hines (2005) summarized their results in one incisive paragraph.
Present perfect tense (to describe an action that began in the past and continues to the present or to describe a concept with continued application)	In the years since, researchers have incorporated Piaget's methods in a variety of studies of children.
Subjunctive mood (to describe a conditional situation or one contrary to fact)	If the sampling were larger, the results might be different.

AGREEMENT

Agreement is the matching of words or word forms according to number (singular and plural) and gender (masculine, feminine, or neuter). Verbs take singular or plural forms depending on whether their subjects are singular or plural.

Subject-Verb Agreement

Special circumstances	*Examples*
Foreign words— *datum* (singular) versus *data* (plural), *phenomenon* (singular) versus *phenomena* (plural), and others: Choose the correct form.	The data suggest that our preconceptions were ill founded. (plural subject/plural verb) The phenomenon is unlikely to occur again. (singular subject/ singular verb)
Collective (or group) nouns: Consider whether members of the group act in unison (singular) or individually (plural).	The couple initiates the counseling sessions. (singular meaning to stress shared action) The couple meet separately with the counselor. (plural meaning to stress individual action)
Singular and plural subjects joined by *or* or *nor:* Match the verb to the nearer subject.	Neither the parents nor the therapist finds their meetings helpful. *Or:* Neither the therapist nor the parents find their meetings helpful.

Pronouns must match their antecedents (the words to which they refer) in both number and gender.

Pronoun-Antecedent Agreement

Common circumstances	*Examples*
Agreement in number: Match the pronoun to its antecedent. (*Also see* "Biased Language," pages 59–62.)	A participant can secure his or her stipend from the controller's office. (singular) Participants can secure their stipends from the controller's office. (plural)

Common circumstances	Examples
Agreement in gender: Match the pronoun to the antecedent. (*Also see* "Biased Language.")	Devon was the first student to complete his booklet. (masculine) The lab rat (subject 3) stopped eating its food during the experiment. (neuter)
Who and *whom:* Use *who* in a subject position; use *whom* in an object position.	Who is responsible for compiling the data? (subject: *He or she* is.) To whom should we address our inquiries? (object: Address them to *him or her.*)

PARALLELISM

Parallelism is the use of equivalent forms when words are used together: nouns, verbs of the same tense or form, and so on.

Parallels	Examples
Elements in a series: Use matching forms.	Even young children are expected to add, to subtract, and to multiply. (parallel verb forms) Reading, writing, speaking, listening, and thinking compose the language arts. (parallel gerund/noun forms)
Correlative conjunctions *(both/and, either/or, neither/nor, not only/but also):* Use matching forms of the words, phrases, and clauses that are linked.	The youngest child in a large family is either the most independent or the least independent of the siblings. (parallel phrases) We found not only that the experiment was too costly but also that it was too time consuming. (parallel clauses)

3c   Word Choice

Word choice makes meaning clear to readers. Specific word choices affect the tone of writing—implying your perception of yourself, your readers, your subject, and your purpose in writing. Consequently, choose words carefully to communicate ideas effectively.

NOUN CLUSTERS

Noun clusters are created when nouns, often in multiples, are used to modify yet another noun. Although the modification patterns may be grammatically correct (nouns *can* function as modifiers), they often create dense clusters of meaning that have to be sorted through carefully.

For example, the phrase *freshman student success ensurance initiative* is overly long, does not read smoothly, and has to be deconstructed. To improve readability, untangle the nouns and place them in easily readable phrases: *an initiative to ensure the success of freshman students.* The reconstructed phrase is easier to interpret than the original and, therefore, communicates the idea more efficiently than does the original.

JARGON

Jargon is the specialized language of a professional group. In some instances, a specific technical term communicates an idea more efficiently than an explanation in everyday language. For instance, the phrase *correlational analyses* explains in two generally understood words a process by which data are both systematically linked and logically compared. However, in many instances, common language that is well selected communicates ideas in a more straightforward and less pretentious way than jargon does. For example, in many instances the phrase *classroom teacher* communicates an idea with greater clarity and less distraction than the more affected phrase *teacher/practitioner,* which is a stilted way of expressing an idea that is implicit in the word *teacher.*

In your writing, choose words with care. Use technical jargon only when it communicates ideas clearly and efficiently—that is, when it is precise and helpful. Never use jargon to impress, because an overreliance on technical terms (especially those that do not communicate ideas precisely and quickly) frustrates readers and clutters prose.

COLLOQUIALISMS

In academic writing, avoid colloquialisms—expressions that are better suited for conversation and other forms of informal communication. Words and phrases such as *write-up* (instead of *report*), *only a few* (rather than *7%*), or *get-together* (in place of *meeting* or *colloquium*) not only lack the specificity of more technical, formal language but also suggest a lack of precision that may make readers question the care with which you have described your research. For these reasons, use precise, professional language in your writing.

SPECIFICITY

Choose specific words to create clear meaning; do not assume that readers will infer meaning from vague language. For example, rather than writing that a survey contained *numerous questions,* be specific and indicate that it contained *75 questions.* Instead of noting that a study was based on the responses of *many Midwestern students,* describe the research group more precisely: *4,000 freshman students in Indiana, Illinois, Missouri, and Iowa.* Even this description could be made more specific by noting the percentage of male/female respondents, the kinds of schools (liberal arts colleges, small state universities, large state universities, and so on), and the locations of the schools (urban, rural, and so on).

The credibility of research depends on using language that communicates clearly. Consequently, choose words that are as specific as possible.

BIASED LANGUAGE

Whether employed consciously or unconsciously, the use of biased language conveys a writer's insensitivity, ignorance, or, in some instances, prejudice—any of which disrupts communication because readers expect to find balance and fairness in what they read. Writing that incorporates biased language reflects badly on the writer, alienates thoughtful readers, and consequently interferes with effective communication.

As a writer, you should make a conscious effort to use accurate, equitable language. Recognizing that your potential readers represent a broad spectrum of society, choose words with care and avoid stereotypes.

Racial and Ethnic Bias

Language that is racially and ethnically biased often relies on dated words related to racial or ethnic groups. In other instances, racially and ethnically biased word choices ignore the distinct groups that exist within larger classifications, thereby perpetuating broad stereotypes. Consequently, it is preferable to refer to racial or ethnic groups as specifically as possible.

Preferred Racial or Ethnic Terms		
Questionable	*Preferred terms for American citizens*	*Preferred terms for non-American citizens*
Arab	Arab American; *or* Saudi American, Iraqi American, and so on	Saudi, Iraqi, Afghan, and so on
Hispanic	Latino/Latina, Chicano/Chicana; *or* Cuban American, and so on	Mexican, Cuban, Costa Rican, and so on
Indian	Native American; *or* Cherokee, Ogallala Sioux, Seminole, and so on	Mesoamerican, Inuit, and so on
Black	African American; *or* Kenyan American, and so on	African; *or* Ugandan, Kenyan, and so on

Questionable	Preferred terms for American citizens	Preferred terms for non-American citizens
White	European American; *or* Italian American, French American, Irish American, and so on	Caucasian, European; *or* German, French, Hungarian, Russian, and so on
Oriental	Asian American; *or* Japanese American, Korean American, Chinese American, and so on	Asian; *or* Korean, Japanese, Vietnamese, and so on

Gender Bias

Language based on stereotypical gender roles—also called *sexist language*—implies through choices of nouns, pronouns, and adjectives that people fall into preassigned roles. Because gender-biased language fails to reflect the diversity of contemporary society, it is inaccurate. Replace nouns that imply gender exclusivity—for example, *chairman* or *spokesman*—with words whose gender meanings are neutral *(chairperson* or *spokesperson)*.

Avoid using gender-specific pronouns when their antecedents are not gender specific. The most common concern is the generic use of a masculine pronoun *(he, him, his, himself)*, as in this sentence: "A psychiatrist is bound by professional oath to keep his patients' records confidential." Although this usage was once acceptable, today's writers and readers expect pronoun use to be inclusive, not exclusionary. Solutions include using alternate pronouns ("A psychiatrist is bound by professional oath to keep his or her patients' records confidential."), plural forms ("Psychiatrists are bound by professional oath to keep their patients' records confidential."), and omission of the pronoun when no confusion is likely ("A psychiatrist is bound by professional oath to keep patients' records confidential.").

Avoid using gender-related adjectives when other modifiers create similar meaning without bias or when gender is not an issue. "The male nurse was both competent and friendly, reassuring the patient and family members" is better presented this way: "The nurse was both competent and friendly, reassuring the patient and family members."

Other Forms of Bias

Be sensitive to the ways in which your language characterizes people by age, class, religion, region, physical and mental ability, or sexual orientation. Do your word choices create stereotypical impressions that disrupt your discussions? Do they convey unintended but negative feelings? Will they offend potential readers and therefore distract them from your ideas? Examine your writing carefully for instances of these kinds of bias and explore alternative ways to convey your meaning.

Biased Language in a Historical Context

Historical texts often contain language that violates today's standards of usage. However, if you quote from such a text, you should retain the original language. The date in the in-text reference will allow readers to place the language in the correct historical context. If the language is particularly troublesome, you may insert an asterisk (*) following the first use of the word or phrase and provide commentary in a footnote.

Preparing the Reference List and In-Text Citations

The reference list provides comprehensive information on each of the sources used in a paper. By listing the author (or authors) of each source—along with publication dates, full titles, and information about publishers (producers, distributors, or websites)—writers ensure that readers can locate sources for further study.

Sources that appear in the reference list must be cited in the paper using parallel information. For example, if a reference-list entry includes two authors, then the in-text citation must also include both authors' names (see "In-Text Citations" later in this chapter). For this reason, writers should prepare reference-list entries for sources before writing the paper.

This chapter includes detailed discussions of the information required for a reference list, as well as its formatting requirements; Chapters 5–8 provide explanations and examples of the most commonly used sources for APA papers. In addition, this book provides information on some sources that are not traditionally used in APA journal articles (the writing done by professionals) but that are potentially useful for students' writing; the principles of APA documentation style have been applied in preparing these sample entries.

4a The Reference List—An Overview

A reference list is an alphabetically arranged list of sources used in a paper. It starts on a new page immediately after the last text page of the paper, continues the page numbering, and is also double-spaced. It is introduced by the word *References* (centered but not italicized); if the reference list continues on a second page, no additional heading is required. Entries in the reference list follow the formats described in this chapter. (See pages 126 and 134 for the reference lists of the sample papers.)

4b Information for APA Entries

Entries for the reference list vary because of the different information they include. All, however, must follow an established order for presenting information:

1. *Authors (and editors).* Take names from the first page of an article or from the title page of a book. Authors' or editors' names are listed in the order in which they appear (not alphabetical order), and initials are used instead of first or middle names. *All* authors' names are inverted (last name first), not just the name of the first author. The names of group, institutional, or organizational authors are spelled out completely.

2. *Publication dates.* For professional journals and books, include the publication year in parentheses. For sources that use specific dates—such as popular magazines, newspapers, television broadcasts, or websites— include the year and the month or the year, month, and day in parentheses. If a source has no author, the entry begins with the title, followed by the date.

3. *Titles.* List titles completely, taking information from the first page of an article or from the title page of a book. Include both titles and subtitles, no matter how long they are.

4. *Additional information.* Include any of the following information in the order presented here if it is listed on the first page of the article, essay, chapter or other subsection, or the title page of the book:

   - Translator
   - Edition number
   - Volume number
   - Issue number (if the journal is paginated separately by issue)
   - Inclusive pages

5. *Facts of publication.* For periodicals, take the volume number, issue number (if needed), and date from the first few pages in journals and magazines, often in combination with the table of contents, or

from the masthead (a listing of information at the top of the first page of newspapers). For books, use the first city listed on the title page and provide a two-letter abbreviation for the state or the full name of the foreign country. Take the publisher's name from the title page, presenting it in abbreviated form (see the following box for explanations of how to shorten publishers' names and Chapters 5–8 for samples within entries). Use the most recent date from the copyright page (which immediately follows the title page).

6. *Retrieval information.* For electronic sources, provide a retrieval statement to direct readers to the electronic copy.

Shortened Forms of Publishers' Names

Use the full names of associations and corporations that serve as publishers.	American Psychological Association, National Council of Teachers of English (These publishers' names appear in their full forms.)
Use the full names of university presses.	Harvard University Press, University of Illinois Press (These publishers' names appear in their full forms.)
Use full names for government publishers.	U.S. Government Printing Office (This name appears in its full form.)
Drop given names or initials.	Harry N. Abrams is shortened to Abrams.
Use the first of multiple names.	Farrar, Straus, and Giroux is shortened to Farrar.

(cont. on next page)

Shortened Forms of Publishers' Names

Drop corporation designations: *Publishers, Company, Incorporated,* and so on.	Doubleday and Co., Inc. is shortened to Doubleday.
Retain the words *Books* and *Press.*	Bantam Books, American Psychiatric Press (These publishers' names appear in their full forms.)

4c Format for APA Entries

To ensure easy reading, entries for the reference list must follow this format:

- *Indentation patterns.* Begin the first line of each entry at the left margin; indent subsequent lines five to seven spaces ($^1/_2$ inch), using the "Indent" feature.

- *Authors' names.* Because entries must be arranged in alphabetical order, invert all authors' names (Haley, R.) and use an ampersand (&), not the word *and*, to join the names of multiple authors (Haley, R., & Taylor, J.).

- *Authorless sources.* When no author is identified, list the source by title. Alphabetize a reference-list entry by using the primary words of the title (excluding *a, an,* or *the*).

- *Article titles.* Include full titles but use sentence-style capitalization. Article titles use no special punctuation in a reference-list entry (although they are placed in quotation marks in in-text citations and in the paper).

- *Periodical titles.* Present the titles of periodicals in headline style (all major words capitalized). Follow the title with a comma and the volume number. Italicize the title *and* the volume number, including the separating comma and the comma that follows the volume number.

- *Issue numbers.* If a journal paginates issues separately, place the issue number in parentheses after the volume number; no space separates the volume number from the issue number, and the parentheses and issue number are *not* italicized. In APA style, both volume and issue numbers are presented as Arabic numbers, not Roman numerals.

- *Titles of books.* Present the titles of books with sentence-style capitalization. The title is also italicized.

- *Publishers' names.* Shorten the names of commercial publishers to a brief but clear form, using only the main elements of their names (*Houghton,* not *Houghton Mifflin*) and dropping descriptive titles *(Publishers, Company, Incorporated).* However, list university presses and organizations and corporations that serve as publishers completely, using the words *Books* and *Press* whenever they are part of a publisher's name. If a work has co-publishers, include both publishers' names, separated by an en dash or a hyphen (Harvard–Belknap Press).

- *Punctuation within entries.* Separate major sections of entries (author, date, title, and publication information) with periods, including elements enclosed in parentheses or brackets; the period used with the abbreviation of authors' first or middle names substitutes for this period. However, separate the place of publication from the publisher's name with a colon. When an entry ends with a DOI or URL, no period is required to close the entry.

- *Spacing within entries.* One space separates elements in APA entries. However, when a journal paginates issues separately, the issue number (in parentheses) follows the volume number without a space.

- *Abbreviations.* Use abbreviations for standard parts of periodicals, books, and other print materials. (See the following box for a list of acceptable abbreviations.)

- *Page numbers.* When citing articles in periodicals or chapters or other portions of complete works, list numbers completely (*176–179,* not *176–9* or *176–79*), separated by an en dash or a hyphen. Journals and magazines list page numbers without page abbreviations; however, page references for newspapers, books, and other print materials use the abbreviations *p.* (for *page*) and *pp.* (for *pages*). No commas are used to separate digits of numbers one thousand or larger when citing pages *(pp. 1295–1298).* When articles appear on nonconsecutive pages, list them all, separated by commas *(34–35, 38, 54–55, 57, 59).*

- *Line spacing.* The entire reference list is double-spaced.

Acceptable Abbreviations

Digital Object Identifier (doi)	DOI *or* doi
edition	ed.
Editor (Editors)	Ed. (Eds.)
no date	n.d.
No place of publication	N.p.
no publisher	n.p.
Number	No.
page (pages)	p. (pp.)
Part	Pt.
Revised edition	Rev. ed.
Second edition	2nd ed.
Supplement	Suppl.
Technical Report	Tech. Rep.
Translator	Trans.
Uniform Resource Locator	URL
Volume (Volumes)	Vol. (Vols.)

4d Alphabetizing the Reference List

The reference list must be in alphabetical order, which seems simple enough. Reality often proves more complicated, however, so use the guidelines in the following box.

Circumstances	*Rule and sample*
Letter-by-letter style	Alphabetize one letter at a time: *Baker, R. L.* precedes *Baker, W. S.*; *Our American Heritage* comes before *Our American Legacy*.
"Nothing precedes something"	The space that follows a name supersedes the letters that follow: *Wood, T. S.* precedes *Woodman, K. F.*

Circumstances	*Rule and sample*
Prefixes	Prefixes are alphabetized as they appear, not as if they appeared in full form: *MacDonald, J. B.* precedes *McDonald, B. V.*
Names with prepositions	Names that incorporate prepositions are alphabetized as if they were spelled closed: *De Forest, A. M.* precedes *Denton, R. L.* (Consult a dictionary regarding patterns for names in different languages.)
Multiple works by the same author	Arrange selections in chronological order: *Sparks, C. G. (2006)* precedes *Sparks, C. G. (2008)*
Single-author and multiple-author works	Single-author works precede multiple-author works: *Kelly, M. J.* precedes *Kelly, M. J., & Dorfinan, P. G.*
Groups, institutions, or organizations as authors	Alphabetize group, institutional, or organizational authors by major words in their completely spelled-out names (omitting *a, an,* or *the*): *American Psychological Association* precedes *Anderson, V. W.*
Authorless works	Authorless works are alphabetized by the first significant words in their titles (omitting *a, an,* or *the*): *The price of poverty* precedes *Stewart, R. P.*

(cont. on next page)

Circumstances	*Rule and sample*
Numerals in titles	Numerals in titles are alphabetized as if they were spelled out: "The 10 common errors of research" precedes *Twelve angry men.*

4e   In-Text Citations

APA documentation has two areas of emphasis: (a) the authors of source materials and (b) the year in which sources were published or presented. This pattern is commonly described as the author–date style.

When incorporating information from a source, provide an in-text citation that includes, at minimum, the author's last name and the year of publication or presentation. The complexity of some sources may require the inclusion of additional information.

PATTERNS FOR IN-TEXT CITATIONS

An in-text citation (also called a parenthetical note) corresponds to an entry in the reference list at the end of the paper. The information in an entry for the reference list determines what information appears in a citation in the text. For example, if a reference-list entry for a book begins with the author's name, then the author's name appears in the in-text citation. If a reference-list citation for a book begins with the title, however, then the title (or a shortened version of it) appears in the in-text citation. If these correlations are clear and consistent, readers can turn from the paper's in-text citation to the reference list and readily locate the full entry for the source.

BASIC FORMS OF IN-TEXT CITATIONS

To avoid disrupting the text, in-text citations identify only the last name of the author or a brief version of the title under which the source appears in the reference list, followed by the year of publication (even when reference-list entries require the month or month and day). For the sake of clarity and smoothness, you may incorporate some of the necessary information in your sentences. After the author and date have been introduced, the date may be omitted in subsequent references within the same paragraph.

> A variety of psychological and social factors influence the likelihood of smoking among adolescents: patterns of rebelliousness and impulsiveness, indications of low self-esteem or poor achievement, and modeled behavior among peers or family members (Young, 2005). Young also noted that attempts to ameliorate these behaviors were not always successful.

OR

> A variety of psychological and social factors influence the likelihood of smoking among adolescents. Young (2005) cited patterns of rebelliousness and impulsiveness, indications of low self-esteem or poor achievement, and modeled behavior among peers or family members. Young also noted that attempts to ameliorate these behaviors were not always successful.

Reference-list entry

Young, T. K. (2005). *Population health: Concepts and methods* (2nd ed.). New York, NY: Oxford University Press.

In special cases, the rule of using only the author's last name and the date is superseded:

Special circumstances	*Rule and sample*
Two authors with the same last name	Include initials with the last name: (Barratt, J. D., 2008), distinct from (Barratt, L. K., 2008).
Multiple works by the same author (same year)	Use letters to distinguish the sources: (Morrison, 2009a), distinct from (Morrison, 2009b). The letters indicate the alphabetical order of the titles.

(cont. on next page)

Special circumstances	*Rule and sample*
Multiple works by the same author (same note)	To cite several works by the same author (all included in the reference list), include the author's name and all dates in chronological order, separated by commas: (Vidich, 2004, 2006, 2008).
Three, four, or five authors	The first notation includes all names (Jarnow, Judelle, & Guerriro, 2007). *Subsequent* citations use the first author's name and *et al.*, not italicized: (Jarnow et al., 2007).
Six or more authors	Beginning with the first notation, use only the first author's name and *et al.*, not italicized: (Austen et al., 2008)
Two or more works by different authors (same note)	To cite several works by different authors in the same note, list each author (in alphabetical order) and date, separated by semicolons: (Bennet, 2008; Greene, 2006; Swift, 2007).
Organization as author	In the first note, present the organization's name in full, with an abbreviation in brackets: (National Council of Teachers of English [NCTE], 2008). Use the shortened form in subsequent notations: (NCTE, 2008).

Special circumstances	*Rule and sample*
No author	Include a shortened version of the title, appropriately capitalized and punctuated, and the year: ("Optimum Performance From Test Subjects," 2008); (*Common Ground*, 2007). If "Anonymous" is the *explicit* attribution of a work, it is used in the author position: (Anonymous, 2006).
Multiple publication dates	Include both dates, separated by a slash: (Jagger & Richards, 1994/2001).
Reference works	List by author if applicable (Angermüller, 2009) or by a shortened form of the title ("Manhattan Project," 2009).
Parts of sources	When citing only a portion of a source—for example, a page to cite a quotation or a chapter in a general reference—include the author or title as appropriate, the date, and clarifying information: (Thomas, 2008, p. 451); (Spindrell, 2007, Chapters 2–3).
Personal communication (*NOTE*: Although cited in the text, personal communications do not have entries in the reference list. Initials are also used with the person's last name.)	Cite e-mail, correspondence, memos, interviews, and so on by listing the person's name, the clarifying phrase *personal communication* (not italicized), and the specific date (L. R. Bates, personal communication, June 7, 2009).

4f   Quotations

When an author's manner of expression is unique or when his or her ideas or language are difficult to paraphrase or summarize, quote the passage in your text. To avoid plagiarism, quoted material must be reproduced word for word, including exact spelling and punctuation, and must be properly separated from your text and accurately cited.

The pattern for incorporating a quotation varies depending on the length of the quotation. In-text citations for quotations also include specific page references.

BRIEF QUOTATIONS (FEWER THAN 40 WORDS)

A quotation of fewer than 40 words appears within a normal paragraph, with the author's words enclosed in quotation marks. The in-text citation, placed in parentheses, follows the closing quotation mark, whether it is in the middle or at the end of a sentence; if the quotation ends the sentence, the sentence's period follows the closing parenthesis. The citation includes the author's name and the publication date (unless they have been previously mentioned in the text), as well as a specific page reference, introduced with the abbreviation *p.* or *pp.* (not italicized). For example:

> The tacit assumption that intelligence is at the heart of success has been called into question: "The memory and analytical skills so central to intelligence are certainly important for school and life success, but perhaps they are not sufficient. Arguably, wisdom-related skills are at least as important or even more important" (Sternberg, 2003, p. 147).

OR

> The tacit assumption that intelligence is at the heart of success has been called into question. Sternberg (2003) observed: "The memory and analytical skills so central to intelligence are certainly important for school and life success, but perhaps they are not sufficient. Arguably, wisdom-related skills are at least as important or even more important" (p. 147).

Reference-list entry

Sternberg, R. J. (2003). *Wisdom, intelligence, and creativity synthesized.* Cambridge, England: Cambridge University Press.

LONG QUOTATIONS (40 OR MORE WORDS)

A quotation of 40 or more words is set off from a normal paragraph in an indented block paragraph. After an introductory statement, start the quotation on a new line, indented five to seven spaces or $^1/_2$ inch (use the "Indent" feature to maintain the indentation throughout the quotation). Quotation marks do not appear at the opening and closing of a block quotation. Like the surrounding text, the quotation is double-spaced. Note that the period precedes the in-text citation with a block quotation. For example:

> Clements and Fiorentino (2004) articulated the value of children's play in their holistic development:
>
>> Play exists at the very heart of childhood. It is the fundamental means through which children learn about themselves, their family members, their local communities, and the world around them. The freedom to explore, experiment, make believe, and make one's choices is a key ingredient in the healthy development of every child. (p. xv)
>
> Current research in countries around the world reinforces this principle, even when the social and moral standards vary greatly from culture to culture.

Reference-list entry

Clements, R. L., & Fiorentino, L. H. (2004). [Introduction]. In R. L. Clements & L. H. Fiorentino (Eds.), *The child's right to play: A global approach* (pp. xv–xvi). Westport, CT: Praeger.

PUNCTUATION WITH QUOTATIONS

Single Quotation Marks

To indicate an author's use of quotation marks within a brief quotation (which is set off by double quotation marks), change the source's punctuation to single quotation marks, as in this example:

> Young (2005) stressed the cautionary and even alarmist nature of current approaches to health management. He asserted, "Each year as many as 40,000 to 50,000 articles are published where the term *risk* appears in the titles and abstracts—this has led some observers to refer to a 'risk epidemic' in the medical literature" (p. 177).

Reference-list entry

Young, T. K. (2005). *Population health: Concepts and methods* (2nd ed.). New York, NY: Oxford University Press.

Because long block quotations do not begin and end with quotation marks, the source's quotation marks remain double, as in this example:

> Borland (2003) posited:
>
> > Giftedness and gifted children are recent inventions in education that can be traced to the advent of psychometrics. It is no coincidence that the person universally regarded as the "father" of gifted education in this country, Lewis M. Terman, was also the developer of the Stanford-Binet Intelligence Scale. Individual differences in test scores, as well as more apparent differences in academic achievement as compulsory education laws became more common and better enforced, can be seen as the direct progenitor of such constructs as those that later became giftedness and mental retardation. (p. 107)
>
> Few scholars would question Terman's central role in assessing intelligence, but some would question the centrality of his role in the development of gifted programs.

Reference-list entry

Borland, J. H. (2003). The death of giftedness: Gifted education without gifted children. In J. H. Borland (Ed.), *Rethinking gifted education* (pp. 105–124). In *Education and Psychology of the Gifted Series.* New York, NY: Teachers College Press.

Brackets

Use brackets to indicate that you have either added words for clarity or introduced a substitution within a quotation. Most often, the words you add are specific nouns to substitute for pronouns that are vague outside the context of the original work. However, you may substitute a different tense of the same verb (for example, *used* for *use*).

> In analyzing the problem-solving skills of creative people, Henderson (2004) observed:
>> [Inventors] recalled the freedom they were given to explore their surrounding environments and the tolerance their parents and educators showed if they made a mess, broke something, or shorted out electrical circuits as a result of their inventive endeavors. (p. 119)
>
> Such forbearance from adults, Henderson's study suggested, is integral to developing creative problem-solving skills.

Out of the context of her chapter, Henderson's original phrase—*The participants*—lacks specificity.

Reference-list entry

Henderson, S. J. (2004). Inventors: The ordinary genius next door. In R. J. Sternberg, E. L. Grigorenko, & J. L. Singer (Eds.), *Creativity: From potential to realization* (pp. 103–125). Washington, DC: American Psychological Association.

NOTE: Do not change dated language or material to make it more acceptable by today's standards; rather, let the material stand on its own and provide your own separate commentary. (See page 62.)

Ellipsis points

Use ellipsis points—three spaced periods—to indicate where words have been omitted within a quotation. Ellipsis points are unnecessary at the beginning or end of a quotation, unless a quotation begins or ends in the middle of a sentence. To indicate an omission between sentences, retain the preceding sentence's punctuation (producing four spaced periods).

Miller (2003) observed that socially constructed self-esteem is inextricably tied to other people's praise: "Flattery is narcotic and addicting. It preys on two desperate and inescapable desires: to be thought well of by others and to think well of ourselves. . . . [T]hey are complexly intertwined" (p. 96).

[Omitted: "The second desire depends on the first more than the first on the second; in any event . . ."; the substitution of a capital letter is indicated with brackets.]

Reference-list entry

Miller, W. I. (2003). *Faking it.* Cambridge, England: Cambridge University Press.

Concerns about Quotations

While quotations can enhance a paper because they present the ideas of other writers in their own words, the overuse of quotations become distracting. Therefore, assess the value of quotations by asking the following questions:

- *Style.* Is the style so distinctive that you cannot say the same thing as well or as clearly in your own words?
- *Vocabulary.* Is the vocabulary technical and therefore difficult to translate into your own words?
- *Reputation.* Is the author so well known or so important that the quotation can lend authority to your paper?
- *Points of Contention.* Does the author's material raise doubts or questions or make points with which you disagree?

If you answer yes to any of these questions, then use of the quotation is appropriate. If not, summarize the material instead.

5 Citing Periodicals

Most often affiliated with professional organizations, journals are scholarly publications whose articles are subjected to careful review. Often called refereed journals, they are the mainstay of much research because they present ideas and information developed by scholars and specialists—and reviewed by scholars—for an audience of scholars. Magazines, by contrast, are commercial publications that present ideas and information for general readers who are nonspecialists; they provide nontechnical discussions and general reactions to issues. Newspapers, published daily or weekly, provide nearly instantaneous reactions to issues in primary stories and more reflective discussions in editorials and feature articles. These periodicals provide discussions of contemporary ideas and issues, as well as reports on research of importance to writers of researched papers.

To cite periodicals in a reference list, follow the guidelines given in this chapter.

5a An Article in a Journal With Continuous Paging

A journal with continuous paging numbers the pages of an entire year's worth of journals consecutively, even though each issue has a separate number. For example, *Educational Psychologist*'s volume 42 (representing 2007) has numbered issues that are continuously paginated: issue number 1 (winter 2007) includes pages 1–78, number 2 (spring 2007) spans pages 79–122, number 3 (summer 2007) continues with pages 123–190, and so on.

When an article comes from a journal with continuous paging, list its authors first, followed by the year of publication and the title of the article with sentence-style capitalization (without quotation marks). Next, include the title of the journal (with headline-style capitalization), a comma, the volume number, and another comma (all italicized). Finish the entry by listing the inclusive page numbers, without a page abbreviation.

Courtois, C. A. (2004). Complex trauma, complex reactions: Assessment and treatment. *Psychotherapy: Theory, Research, Practice, Training, 41,* 412–425.

> ***In-text citation***   (Courtois, 2004)

Nuttman-Shwartz, O. (2007). Is there life without work? *The International Journal of Aging and Human Development, 64,* 129–147.

> ***In-text citation***   (Nuttman-Shwartz, 2007)

5b An Article in a Journal With Separate Paging

A journal with separate paging begins each numbered issue with page 1, even though a year's worth of journals is assigned a single volume number. For example, *Women and Health*'s volume 44 (representing 2006) has numbered issues, each of which has separate paging: issue number 1 includes pages 1–136, issue number 2 spans pages 1–134, issue number 3 covers pages 1–122, and so on.

When a journal has separate paging for each issue, follow the volume number with the issue number, in parentheses; no space separates the volume from the issue, and the issue number and its parentheses are not italicized. All other information in the entry is the same as in an entry for a journal with continuous paging.

Hughes, J. C., Brestan, E. V., Christens, B. D., Klinger, L. J., & Valle, L. A. (2004). Problem-solving interactions between mothers and children. *Child and Family Behavior Therapy, 26*(1), 1–16.

> ***First in-text citation***   (Hughes, Brestan, Christens, Klinger, & Valle, 2004)

> ***Second and subsequent citations***   (Hughes et al., 2004)

McDonald, T. P., Poertner, J., & Jennings, M. A. (2007). Permanency for children in foster care: A competing risks analysis. *The Journal of Social Science Research, 33*(4), 45–56.

> ***First in-text citation***   (McDonald, Poertner, & Jennings, 2007)

> ***Second and subsequent citations***   (McDonald et al., 2007)

5c   An Abstract

Although writers most often refer to entire articles, in very special circumstances (for example, when an abstract's summary of key principles is succinct or quotable), you may want to cite only the abstract. In those rare instances, first prepare a full citation of the article; however, insert the word *Abstract,* not italicized, within brackets after the article's title. The period that normally follows the title follows the closing bracket.

Daniels, J. A., Bradley, M. C., Cramer, D. P., Winkler, A. T., Kinebrew, K., & Crockett, D. (2007). The successful resolution of armed hostage/barricade events in schools: A qualitative analysis [Abstract]. *Psychology and the Schools, 44,* 601–613.

> ***In-text citation***   (Daniels et al., 2007)

Schooler, D., Ward, L. M., Merriwether, A., & Caruthers, A. (2004). Who's that girl: Television's role in the body image development of young white and black women [Abstract]. *Psychology of Women Quarterly, 28,* 38–47.

First in-text citation (Schooler, Ward, Merriwether, & Caruthers, 2004)

Second and subsequent citations (Schooler et al., 2004)

5d An Article in a Monthly Magazine

An article from a monthly magazine is listed by author. The date is given by year and month, separated by a comma, in parentheses. The article title appears next with sentence-style capitalization. The title of the magazine, with headline-style capitalization, is presented with all major words capitalized, followed by a comma, the volume number, and another comma (all italicized). The entry ends with inclusive page numbers listed without page abbreviations. Note that only the year is included in the in-text citation, not the year and month.

Duenwald, M. (2005, January). The psychology of facial expressions. *Discover, 26*(1), 16–17.

In-text citation (Duenwald, 2005)

Martinez-Conde, S., & Macknik, S. L. (2007, August). Windows on the mind. *Scientific American, 297*(2), 56–63.

In-text citation (Martinez-Conde & Macknik, 2007)

5e An Article in a Weekly Magazine

The entry for a weekly magazine is identical to the entry for a monthly magazine except that the date of publication (along with the year and month) is included in parentheses. In the corresponding in-text citation, however, only the year is required.

Gasparino, C. (2005, July 25). Good news: You're fired. *Newsweek, 146*(4), 48.

In-text citation (Gasparino, 2005)

Sacks, O. (2007, September 24). The abyss: Music and
    memory. *The New Yorker, 83*(28), 100–112.

> *In-text citation* (Sacks, 2007)

5f   An Article in a Newspaper

An entry for a newspaper article resembles that for a
magazine, except that section numbers or letters are included, and paging is indicated with a page abbreviation
(*p.* or *pp.*, not italicized).

When sections are indicated by letters, they are
presented along with the page numbers, with no intervening punctuation or space. However, when newspaper
sections are numbered, a colon is used to separate the
section from the page number.

Mayer, C. E. (2005, January 7). Group takes aim at junk-food
    marketing. *The Washington Post*, p. E2.

> *In-text citation*   (Mayer, 2005)

Rodriguez, A. (2007, September 16). When health care
    does more harm than good. *The Chicago Tribune*,
    p. 1:18.

> *In-text citation* (Rodriguez, 2007)

5g   An Article in a Newsletter

The entry for an article in a newsletter follows the pattern
for a magazine: the author, date, title of selection, title of
newsletter, volume number, and inclusive pages (without
page abbreviations). If a newsletter appears seasonally,
include such identifying information along with the year
(2008, spring).

Allen, R. (2007, April). Making science matter: Fresh
    approaches to teaching diverse students. *Education
    Update, 49*(4), 1, 6–8.

> *In-text citation* (Allen, 2007)

When pages are not sequential, list them all, separated
by commas.

Garcia, J. (2004, October). Where are Canada, Latin America, and Africa in the social studies curriculum? *The Social Studies Professional, 183*(4), 3.

> *In-text citation*   (Garcia, 2004)

5h An Editorial

The entry for an editorial—an opinion-based essay—resembles that for a magazine or newspaper article, with one exception: The word *Editorial* (not italicized) is placed within brackets immediately after the title of the essay, if there is one. The period that normally follows the title follows the closing bracket.

Herbert, B. (2007, September 15). The nightmare is here [Editorial]. *The New York Times*, p. A29.

> *In-text citation*   (Herbert, 2007)

Shorris, E. (2005, January 25). The hero within [Editorial]. *The Nation, 280*(3), 8, 26.

> *In-text citation*   (Shorris, 2005)

5i A Letter to the Editor

Following the author's name and the publication date, include the phrase *Letter to the editor* (not italicized) in brackets, followed by a period. The rest of the entry follows the pattern appropriate for the periodical.

Anich, M. D. (2005, January). [Letter to the editor]. *Smithsonian, 35*(1), 16.

> *In-text citation*   (Anich, 2005)

Birch, M. A. (2007, September 3). [Letter to the editor]. *Fortune, 156*, 13.

> *In-text citation*   (Birch, 2007)

5j A Review

After the author, date, and review title (if there is one), include a descriptive phrase that begins "Review of the book (motion picture, music recording, car, computer game)" and ends with the specific product name; enclose this information in brackets, followed by a period. Then continue the entry as is appropriate for the source.

Carson, T. (2005, January/February). The Murdoch touch [Review of the book *The fourth network: How Fox broke the rules and reinvented television,* by D. M. Kimmel]. *The Atlantic, 295*(1), 163, 166–168.

In-text citation   (Carson, 2005)

Fox, B. (2006). [Review of the book *Ghosts of slavery: A literary archeology of black women's lives,* by J. Sharpe]. *African American Review,* 40, 838–839.

In-text citation   (Fox, 2006)

5k An Abstract From *Dissertation Abstracts International*

This specialized entry requires the author's name, the year in parentheses, and the title of the dissertation (without quotation marks or italics). If you obtained the abstract from UMI (formerly University Microfilms), follow the title with *Dissertation Abstracts International* (italicized), the volume number, the issue number, and the page number.

If you obtained the dissertation from a university, place this information in parentheses: the phrase *Doctoral dissertation* (not italicized), the degree-granting university, and the year of completion—all separated with commas. Follow the closing parenthesis with a period. Complete the entry by identifying *Dissertation Abstracts International* (italicized), followed by the volume, issue, and the page number.

Markarian, G. (2005). Analyst forecasts, earnings management, and insider trading. *Dissertation Abstracts International, 66*(1), 237.

In-text citation   (Markarian, 2005)

Vinski, E. J. (2007) Academic dishonesty and cognitive dissonance (Doctoral dissertation, City University of New York, 2007). *Dissertation Abstracts International, 67*(3), 117.

In-text citation   (Vinski, 2007)

51　A Secondary Source

The authors of primary sources report their own research and ideas; the authors of secondary sources report the research and ideas of others. For example, Malecki and Elliott (2002) did a longitudinal analysis of data related to children's social behaviors as indicators of academic performance; it is a primary source. Rimm-Kaufman and Chiu (2007) incorporated material from the original article in an article for *Psychology in the Schools;* it is a secondary source. Although it is best to use the original or primary source (Malecki and Elliott), at times you must use the secondary source (Rimm-Kaufman and Chiu).

If you cite material that appears in a secondary source, the reference-list entry must be for *the source you used,* not the original (even though you might be able to secure full documentation from the secondary source's reference list); for ethical reasons, you must cite the source that was part of your research. Therefore, refer to the original source in the text of the paper. In the in-text citation, however, clarify the use of the original material with the phrase *as cited in* (not italicized). In the reference list, provide an entry for the secondary source you used.

Rimm-Kaufman, S. E., & Chiu, Y. I. (2007). Promoting social and academic competence in the classroom: An intervention study examining the contribution of the *response classroom* approach. *Psychology in the Schools, 44,* 397–413.

In-text reference and citation　Malecki and Elliott (2002) analyzed social behavior as an indicator of academic performance (as cited in Rimm-Kaufman & Chiu, 2007), which adds further dimension to the discussion.

Citing Books and Other Separately Published Materials

Books provide comprehensive, extended discussions of topics. Those published by scholarly or university presses are often targeted to specialists in particular fields and provide a broad range of technical information and complex analyses. Those published by trade (commercial) publishers are often directed to nonspecialists.

Because books take several years to produce, they frequently provide reflective interpretations that have the benefit of critical distance. Consequently, they provide balance in research. To cite books in a reference list, follow the guidelines in this chapter.

6a A Book by One Author

The entry for a book by a single author begins with his or her name, followed by the year in parentheses, the title, the city and state (or country), and the publisher. A book title is presented in italics, with sentence-style capitalization.

Chessick, R. D. (2007). *The future of psychoanalysis.*
New York, NY: State University of New York Press.

> *In-text citation* (Chessick, 2007)

Thornicroft, G. (2006). *Shunned: Discrimination against people with mental illness.* New York, NY: Oxford University Press.

> *In-text citation* (Thornicroft, 2006)

6b A Book by Two or More Authors

When a book has multiple authors, their names appear in the order presented on the title page, not alphabetical order. The names of two to seven authors are listed, with all of their names inverted. An ampersand (&) joins the last two names. If a book has eight or more authors, the first six are listed, followed by ellipsis points (three spaced periods) and the name of the last author.

Wright, J. P., Tibbetts, S. G., & Daigle, L. E. (2008). *Criminals in the making: Criminality across the life course.*
Thousand Oaks, CA: Sage.

> *In-text citation* (Wright, Tibbetts, & Daigle, 2008)

Lazarus, R. S., & Lazarus, B. N. (2006). *Coping with aging.*
New York, NY: Oxford University Press.

> *In-text citation* (Lazarus & Lazarus, 2006)

6c A Book With No Author Named

When no author or editor is named, list the book by title. When an editor is listed, begin with the editor's name. The following source is listed by title.

United Press International stylebook and guide to newswriting (4th ed.). (2004). Herndon, VA: Capital Books.

> ***In-text citation*** (*United Press International*, 2004)

United Press International has each word capitalized because it is an organization. The edition number follows the title, in parentheses; notice that the edition number is not italicized and that the period follows the closing parenthesis. With an authorless book, the year follows the title or edition number. (See 6e for the common pattern of presenting editions.)

The following source is listed by editor.

VandenBos, G. R. (Ed.). (2007). *APA dictionary of psychology.* Washington, DC: American Psychological Association.

> ***In-text citation*** (VandenBos, 2007)

6d A Book With an Organization as Author

When an organization is listed as the author, spell out the name completely in the author position. When the organization is also the publisher, use the word *Author,* not italicized, in the publisher position.

American Medical Association. (2007). *American Medical Association manual of style: A guide to authors and editors* (10th ed.). New York, NY: Oxford University Press.

> ***First in-text citation*** (American Medical Association [AMA], 2007)

> ***Second and subsequent citations*** (AMA, 2007)

The first in-text citation with an organization as an author includes the full name, followed by the abbreviated name within brackets; additional references include only the abbreviated name.

American Psychological Association. (2009). *Publication manual of the American Psychological Association* (6th ed.). Washington, DC: Author.

> **First in-text citation**   (American Psychological Association [APA], 2009)

> **Second and subsequent citations**   (APA, 2009)

6e   An Edition Other Than the First

The edition number, which appears on the title page, follows the title of the book, in parentheses. Note that it is not italicized and that the period that normally follows the title follows the closing parenthesis instead.

Turner, L. H., & West, R. (2006). *Perspectives on family communication* (3rd ed.). Boston, MA: McGraw-Hill.

> **In-text citation**   (Turner & West, 2006)

Young, M. E., & Long, L. L. (2007). *Counseling and therapy for couples* (2nd ed.). Belmont, CA: Brooks/Cole.

> **In-text citation**   (Young & Long, 2007)

6f   An Edited Collection

Present an entire edited collection like a traditional book, with the editor's name in the author position.

Gilde, C. (Ed.). (2007). *Higher education: Open for business.* Lanham, MD: Lexington Books.

> **In-text citation**   (Gilde, 2007)

McAdams, D. P., Josselson, R., & Lieblich, A. (Eds.). (2006). *Identity and story: Creating self in narrative.* Washington, DC: American Psychological Association.

> **In-text citation**   (McAdams, Josselson, & Lieblich, 2006)

6g　An Original Selection in an Edited Collection

To cite an original selection in an edited collection, begin with the name of the author of the selection, followed by the date in parentheses and the selection's title (with sentence-style capitalization and no quotation marks). Introduced by the word *In* (not italicized), the collection editor is listed next (his or her name is in normal order, followed by the abbreviation *Ed.* in parentheses but not italicized), followed by a comma. The title of the collection, italicized, is followed by the inclusive page numbers for the selection, with the abbreviation for pages, listed in parentheses. The entry ends with the facts of publication.

Drewes, A. A. (2005). Play in selected cultures: Diversity and universality. In E. Gil & A. A. Drewes (Eds.), *Cultural issues in play therapy* (pp. 26–71). New York, NY: Guilford Press.

In-text citation　(Drewes, 2005)

Royzman, E. B., McCauley, C., & Rozin, P. (2005). From Plato to Putnam: Four ways to think about hate. In R. J. Sternberg (Ed.), *The psychology of hate* (pp. 3–35). Washington, DC: American Psychological Association.

In-text citation　(Royzman, McCauley, & Rozin, 2005)

6h　A Previously Published Selection in an Edited Collection

When a selection has been reprinted from a work published earlier, provide identifying information in parentheses at the end of the entry. Include the information for the original source, but notice that page numbers appear with the abbreviation for pages—even when the original source is a journal or magazine—and the year follows the page numbers. Also note that the closing parenthesis is not followed by a period.

Bazemore, G., & Day, S. E. (2005). Restoring the balance: Juvenile and community justice. In D. L. Parry (Ed.), *Essential readings in juvenile justice* (pp. 405–414). Upper Saddle River, NJ: Pearson. (Reprinted from *Juvenile Justice, 3*(1), pp. 3–14, 1996)

In-text citation　(Bazemore & Day, 2005)

Pojman, L. (2002). The moral status of affirmative action. In E. Heath (Ed.), *Morality and the market: Ethics and virtue in the conduct of business* (pp. 493–505). Boston, MA: McGraw-Hill. (Reprinted from *Public Affairs Quarterly, 6,* pp. 181–206, 1992)

> ***In-text citation***   (Pojman, 2002)

6i   A Revised or Enlarged Edition

Enclose the description of a revised or enlarged edition in parentheses following the title. As with other editions, the parenthetical information precedes the period that follows the title, and this information is not italicized.

Benardot, D. (2006). *Advanced sports nutrition* (Rev. ed.). Champaign, IL: Human Kinetics.

> ***In-text citation***   (Benardot, 2006)

McCoy, A. W. (2003). *The politics of heroin: CIA complicity in the global drug trade—Afghanistan, Southeast Asia, Central America, Columbia* (Rev. ed.). Chicago, IL: Hall.

> ***In-text citation***   (McCoy, 2003)

6j   A Reprinted Book

The entry for a reprinted book begins with the full entry of the version you have used; the entry ends with a parenthetical description of the original publication date, with no period after the closing parenthesis. Note that the in-text citation includes both dates, presented in chronological order, separated by a slash.

Fukuyama, F. (2006). *The end of history and the last man.* New York, NY: Free Press. (Original work published 1992)

> ***In-text citation***   (Fukuyama, 1992/2006)

Kimmel, A. J. (2007). *Ethical issues in behavioral research: Basic and applied perspectives.* Malden, MA: Blackwell. (Original work published 1966)

> ***In-text citation***   (Kimmel, 1966/2007)

6k　A Multivolume Work

When citing a complete multivolume work, the number of volumes appears in parentheses following the title but before the period; if an edition number is required, it precedes the volume number.

Ignatavicius, D. D., & Workman, M. L. (2006). *Medical–surgical nursing: Critical thinking for collaborative care* (5th ed., Vols. 1–2). St. Louis, MO: Elsevier Sanders.

> *In-text citation*　(Ignatavicius & Workman, 2006)

When citing a separately titled volume of a multivolume work, list the multivolume title first, followed by a colon and one space. Then list the separate volume number, followed by a period, and the single volume title. The multivolume title, volume information, and specific title are all italicized. Note that the names of series editors precede those of volume editors; the order of presentation, then, corresponds to the order of the titles.

Osherson, D. N. (Series Ed.), Sternberg, S., & Scarborough, D. (Vol. Eds.). (1995). *An invitation to cognitive science: Vol. 4. Conceptual foundations* (2nd ed.). Cambridge, MA: MIT Press.

> *In-text citation*　(Osherson, Sternberg, & Scarborough, 1995)

61　An Article in an Encyclopedia or Other Reference Work

To cite an article in an encyclopedia or other reference work, begin with the author's name, when it is available, followed by the date in parentheses. Next list the subject heading under which the material appears (exactly as it appears in the source), without special punctuation. Follow it with the title of the reference work. In parentheses, but before the period that follows the title, include the volume number, if applicable, and the inclusive pages. End the entry with the city and state (or country) and the publisher.

If a reference work has a large editorial board, include the first editor's name and *et al.* (not italicized) to substitute for the other editors' names.

Fluoxetine hydrochloride [Prozac]. (2004). In *2004 Lippincott's nursing drug guide* (pp. 530–532). Philadelphia, PA: Lippincott-Williams.

    In-text citation   ("Fluoxetine Hydrochloride," 2004)

Note that in the in-text citation the article title is enclosed in quotation marks.

Sullaway, F. J. (2007). Birth order and sibling competition. In R. I. M. Dunbar & L. Barrett (Eds.), *Oxford handbook of evolutionary psychology* (pp. 297–311). New York, NY: Oxford University Press.

    In-text citation   (Sullaway, 2007)

6m A Work in a Series

If a book is part of a series, that fact is stated on the title page. The entry follows the pattern for a similar book, except that the series title (italicized, with headline-style capitalization) appears in a phrase preceding the city and publisher.

Levesque, R.T. R. (2007). *Adolescents, media, and the law: What developmental science reveals and free speech requires.* In *American Psychology–Law Society Series.* New York, NY: Oxford University Press.

    In-text citation   (Levesque, 2007)

Nelson, S. J. (2007). *Leaders in the labyrinth: College presidents and the battleground of creeds and convictions.* In *Praeger Series on Higher Education.* Westport, CT: Praeger-Greenwood.

    In-text citation   (Nelson, 2007)

6n A Translation

Under most circumstances, the translator of a text is cited in parentheses immediately after the title of the selection (whether it is an essay, chapter, or complete text) but before the closing period for that element.

de Beauvoir, S. (2003). The married woman (H. M. Parshly, Trans.). In S. Hirschberg & T. Hirschberg (Eds.), *Past to present: Ideas that changed our world* (pp. 188–194). Upper Saddle River, NJ: Prentice Hall.

   In-text citation   (de Beauvoir, 2003)

The previous example indicates that Parshly translated only the selection presented in this entry. Had he translated the entire collection, his name would have appeared after the anthology's title.

Eco, U. (Ed.). (2004). *History of beauty* (A. McEwen, Trans.). New York, NY: Rizzoli.

   In-text citation   (Eco, 2004)

This entry indicates that McEwen translated the entire book.

---

60 A Government Document—Committee, Commission, Department

An entry for a government document follows the pattern used for another similar source. Because many government documents are book-length, that pattern most often applies. Note, however, that APA style requires a publication number for a government document, if available (usually found on the title page or back cover), presented in parentheses after the title; the document number is not italicized. When serving as publisher, the *U.S. Government Printing Office* is spelled out, not abbreviated.

Greenberg, E., Dunleavy, E., & Kutner, M. (2007). *Literacy behind bars: Results from the 2003 national assessment of adult literacy prison survey* (NCES 2007–473). Washington, DC: National Center for Educational Statistics.

   In-text citation   (Greenberg, Dunleavy, & Kutner, 2007)

National Archives and Records Administration. (2004). *Federal records pertaining to Brown v. Board of*

Education of Topeka, Kansas (1954) (Reference
Information Paper 112). Washington, DC: Author.

In-text citation   (National Archives, 2004)

6p   A Preface, Introduction, Foreword, Epilogue, or Afterword

When introductory or closing material is titled, it is presented like a selection in a collection; however, a descriptive word (preface, epilogue, and so on) is enclosed within brackets before the period.

Untitled material is cited separately by providing a descriptive title (within brackets), followed by complete entry information.

Kozol, J. (2007). [Afterword]. In J. Kozol, *Letters to a young teacher* (pp. 243–248). New York, NY: Crown.

In-text citation   (Kozol, 2007)

Nieto, S. (2007). The national mythology and urban teaching [Introduction]. In G. Campano, *Immigrant students and literacy: Reading, writing, and remembering* (pp. 1–6). New York, NY: Teachers College Press.

In-text citation   (Nieto, 2007)

The preceding sample shows an introduction written by someone (Nieto) other than the author of the book (Campano). Notice that page numbers for this selection are indicated in Arabic numerals, rather than the typical Roman numerals of most introductory material.

6q   A Monograph

To create an entry for a monograph (a separately published, essay-length selection that is sometimes a reprint of a journal article and sometimes an independently prepared selection that is part of a series), include traditional publishing information. However, after the title and in parentheses, include the monograph series title and monograph number, if available; the monograph number is introduced by *No.,* the abbreviation for *number.*

Checkoway, H., Pearce, N., & Kriebel, D. (Eds.). (2004).
    Research methods in occupational epidemiology
    (2nd ed.). (Monographs in epidemiology and
    biostatistics No. 34). New York, NY: Oxford
    University Press.

> ***In-text citation***   (Checkoway, Pearce, & Kriebel, 2004)

Seedhouse, P. (2004). *The interactional architecture of the*
    language classroom: A conversation analysis perspec-
    tive (Language Learning Monograph). Malden, MA:
    Blackwell.

> ***In-text citation***   (Seedhouse, 2004)

6r   A Pamphlet or Brochure

When a pamphlet or brochure contains clearly presented
information, it is cited like a book, with a descriptive title
enclosed in brackets. When information is missing, use
these abbreviations: *N.P.* for "No place of publication,"
n.p. for "no publisher," and *n.d.* for "no date." None of
these abbreviations is italicized in an entry.

Loving your family, feeding their future: Nutrition education
    through the food stamp program [Pamphlet]. (2007).
    Washington, DC: Food and Nutrition Service, U.S.
    Department of Agriculture.

> ***In-text citation***   (*Loving Your Family,* 2007)

Strock, M. (2002). *Depression* [Pamphlet]. Bethesda, MD:
    National Institutes of Health. (Original work published
    1994)

> ***In-text citation***   (Strock, 1994/2002)

6s   An Unpublished Dissertation

The entry for an unpublished dissertation begins with
the author's name, the date, and the title, presented in
the pattern used for a book. In parentheses, include the
phrase *Unpublished doctoral dissertation* (not italicized),
followed by a period. Then provide the name of the
degree-granting university, followed by a comma and
the city and state (or country). Published dissertations
are books and should be cited accordingly.

Hall, E. M. (2007). *Posttraumatic stress symptoms in parents of children with injuries.* (Unpublished doctoral dissertation). Boston University, Boston, MA.

> ***In-text citation***   (Hall, 2007)

Killgore, L. (2004). *Beyond the merit of test scores: Gatekeeping in elite college admissions.* (Unpublished doctoral dissertation). Brown University, Providence, RI.

> ***In-text citation***   (Killgore, 2004)

6t Published Proceedings From a Conference

The published proceedings from a conference present revised, printed versions of papers that were delivered at the meeting. If the proceedings are published individually, cite them as books. If they are published regularly, present them as periodicals.

Capitalize the name of the meeting or conference. If the title includes the state, province, or country, do not repeat it in the publishing information.

Le Prohn, N. S. (Ed.). (2002). Assessing youth behavior using the child behavior checklist in family and children's services. In *Proceedings from the Child Behavior Checklist Roundtable.* Washington, DC: CWLA.

> ***In-text citation***   (Le Prohn, 2002)

Zacharacoponlou, E. (2006). Beyond the mind–body dualism: Psychoanalysis and the human body. In *Proceedings of the 6th Delphi International Psychoanalysis Symposium.* Delphi, Greece. San Diego, CA: Elsevier.

> ***In-text citation***   (Zacharacoponlou, 2006)

6u Multiple Works by the Same Author

When citing several sources by the same author, repeat the name completely each time. Alphabetical order takes precedence, with single authors listed before multiple authors. List works by single authors or by the same multiple authors chronologically. If works are published in the same year, arrange them alphabetically by title.

Ehrenreich, B. (1999a, June 20). Looking to put father-
hood in its proper place. *The New York Times*,
p. L14.

Ehrenreich, B. (1999b, June). Who needs men? Addressing
the prospect of a matrilinear millennium. [Interview].
Harper's, 290, 33–46.

Ehrenreich, B. (2002). *Nickel and dimed: On (not) getting by
in America.* New York, NY: Holt.

Ehrenreich, B. (2003, January). The strong, violent type.
Progressive, 67, 12–13.

Ehrenreich, B., Hess, E., & Jacobs, G. (1986). *Re-making love:
The feminization of sex.* Garden City, NY: Anchor-
Doubleday.

Alternative in-text citations

- The *Times* article: (Ehrenreich, 1999a)
- The *Harper's* article: (Ehrenreich, 1999b)
- All four single-author works in the same citation: (Ehrenreich, 1999a, 1999b, 2002, 2003)
- The multiple-author book: (Ehrenreich, Hess, & Jacobs, 1986)

Ehrenreich's four separately written works appear first, arranged in chronological order and then alphabetically by title. The Ehrenreich, Hess, and Jacobs book follows.

6v A Secondary Source

The authors of primary sources report their own research and ideas; the authors of secondary sources report the research and ideas of others. For example, Tomasello (1992) conducted a study of young children's language acquisition and reported it in a journal article; it is a primary source. Nelson (2007) incorporated material from the original article in her book *Young Minds in Social Worlds: Experience, Meaning, and Memory;* it is a secondary source. Although it is best to use the original or primary source (Tomasello), sometimes you must use the secondary source (Nelson).

If you cite material that appears in a secondary source, the reference-list entry must be for *the source you used,* not the original (even though you might be able to secure full documentation from the secondary source's reference list); you must ethically cite the source that was part of your research. Therefore, refer to the original source in the text of the paper. In the in-text citation, however, clarify the use of the original material with the phrase *as cited in* (not italicized). In the reference list, provide an entry for the secondary source you used.

Nelson, K. (2007). *Young minds in social worlds: Experience, meaning, and memory*. Cambridge, MA: Harvard University Press.

> **In-text reference and citation** Tomasello (1992) asserted that children learn words within usage-based, grammatical contexts (as cited in Nelson, 2007).

7   Citing Audiovisual Sources

Audiovisual sources—motion pictures, recordings, speeches, works of art, and other visual images—are used infrequently in APA papers. Nevertheless, they can provide interesting support for discussions and create variety within a paper.

To cite an audiovisual source in a reference list, follow the guidelines in this chapter.

7a   A Motion Picture

An entry for a motion picture begins with the producer's or director's name (with the word *Producer* or *Director* in parentheses but not italicized), followed by the year of the motion picture's release, its title (italicized, with sentence-style capitalization), and a descriptive title (in brackets). The entry ends with the country of origin and the company.

Include other people's contributions after the motion picture title (in brackets), using brief phrases (*Narr. by, With, Written by*—not italicized) to clarify their roles.

Ridberg, R. (Producer). (2006). *Big bucks, big pharma:*
     Marketing disease and pushing drugs [Motion picture].
     [Written by R. Ridberg]. United States: Media
     Education Foundation.

> ***In-text citation***   (Ridberg, 2006)

This documentary has no director.

Pakula, A. J., Barish, K., Gerrity, W. C., & Starger, M.
     (Producers), & Pakula, A. J. (Director). (1982). Sophie's
     choice [Motion picture]. [With M. Streep,
     K. Kline, & P. MacNichol]. United States: Universal.

> ***In-text citation***   (Pakula, Barish, Gerrity, & Starger, 1982)

7b   A Filmstrip or Slide Program

A filmstrip or slide program is cited just as a motion picture
is, with one exception: Include a descriptive title such as
Filmstrip in brackets (but not italicized) after the title.

Blocks to therapeutic communication [Filmstrip]. (1990).
     United States: Concepts Media.

> ***In-text citation***   (*Blocks*, 1990)

Technical Working Group for Eyewitness Evidence. (2003).
     Eyewitness evidence: A trainer's manual for law
     enforcement (NCJ 188678) [Slides]. United States:
     U.S. Department of Justice.

> ***In-text citation***   (Technical Working Group, 2003)

As a government document, this entry incorporates a
publication number after the slide series title.

7c   A Television Broadcast

A regular television program is listed by producer or
director, broadcast date (which may be either a year or a
specific broadcast date), program title (italicized, with
sentence-style capitalization), a descriptive phrase (in
brackets), the city and state (or country), and the network
(spelled out completely). Include other people's contributions after the program title (in brackets), using brief
phrases (*Narr. by, With, Written by*—not italicized) to clar
ify their roles.

Lawrence, B. (Producer). (2007). *Scrubs* [Television series].
[With Zach Braff, Donald Faison, Sarah Chalke, &
Judy Reyes]. New York, NY: National Broadcasting
Company.

> ***In-text citation***   (Lawrence, 2007)

To refer to an individual episode, cite the writer and
director, the specific broadcast date, the episode title
without special punctuation, and a descriptive phrase
in brackets. Then, use the word *In* (not italicized) to introduce the program title. The rest of the entry follows
normal patterns.

Hess, S. (Writer), & Glatter, L. L. (Director). (2007,
November 20). You don't want to know [Television
series episode]. [With Hugh Laurie, Robert Sean
Leonard, & Lisa Edelstein]. In *House*. Los Angeles,
CA: Fox Broadcasting Company.

> ***In-text citation***   (Hess & Glatter, 2007)

7d A Radio Broadcast

An entry for a radio broadcast follows the guidelines for a
television broadcast. If a broadcast does not have an
assigned title, add a descriptive phrase in brackets.

Murrow, E. R. (1940, September 13). [Radio broadcast].
New York, NY: WCBS.

> ***In-text citation***   (Murrow, 1940)

7e A Recording

An entry for an entire recording begins with the
writer–composer's name, the date of the recording, and the
album title (in italics, with sentence-style capitalization),
with the recording format in brackets. The entry ends with
the city and state (or country), and distribution company.

The Beatles. (1969). *Abbey Road* [CD]. Hollywood,
CA–London, England: Capital–EMI.

> ***In-text citation***   (The Beatles, 1969)

To emphasize a single selection on a recording, begin
with the writer–composer and the date, followed by the

title of the brief work (with sentence-style capitalization but without special punctuation). Using the word *On* (not italicized), include the title of the complete recording and other production information. Include the track number in the in-text citation.

Winehouse, A. (2006). Rehab. On *Back to black* [CD]. New York, NY: Universal Records.

>   ***In-text citation*** (Winehouse, 2006, track 1)

7f An Interview

An interview is a personal communication. As such, it is not included in a reference list. However, it is cited in the text of the paper by enclosing the phrase *personal communication* (not italicized) and the date in parentheses.

>   Kalb (personal communication, April 4, 2008)
>   stressed the importance of double-blind studies.

7g A Transcript

A transcript entry describes the source of an original broadcast, with clarifying information in brackets, and information about availability.

Greenberger, D. (2007, December 28). Memories like bits of paper, shaken in a jar. *All things considered* [Radio broadcast]. [Transcript]. Washington, DC: National Public Radio. Available: NPR Transcripts.

>   ***In-text citation*** (Greenberger, 2007)

Whitfield, F. (2006, December 16). Welcome to the future. *CNN presents* [Television broadcast]. [Transcript]. Atlanta, GA: Cable News Network. Available: LexisNexis.

>   ***In-text citation*** (Whitfield, 2006)

7h A Lecture or Speech

An entry for a lecture or speech includes the speaker's name, the date of the speech, the title of the speech

(italicized) or a description title (in brackets), a series title or a description of the speech-making context, and
the location (most often, the city and state or country).

Hofstadter, D. (2006, February 6). *Analogy as the core of
cognition*. Lecture presented for the Stanford
Presidential Lectures in Humanities and Arts,
Stanford University, Stanford, CA.

> ***In-text citation*** (Hofstadter, 2006)

Nixon, R. (1974, August 8). [Resignation speech]. Speech presented at the White House, Washington, DC.

> ***In-text citation*** (Nixon, 1974)

7i   A Work of Art

An entry for a work of art includes the artist's name, the
completion date, the title (either assigned by the artist or
attributed), a description of the medium (enclosed in
brackets), the museum or collection name, and the city
(and state or country, if necessary). When artists assign
titles, they are italicized; do not italicize titles that other
people have assigned to the work.

Gauguin, P. (1891). *The brooding woman* [Oil on canvas].
Worcester Art Museum, Worcester, MA.

> ***In-text citation*** (Gauguin, 1891)

Healy, G. P. A. (1887). Abraham Lincoln [Oil on canvas].
National Portrait Gallery, Washington, DC.

> ***In-text citation*** (Healy, 1887)

Healy, the artist, did not formally title this painting.
"Abraham Lincoln" is the attributed title and, therefore, is
not italicized.

7j   A Map, Graph, Table, or Chart

Often prepared as part of a book, a map, graph, table, or
chart is most often treated like a selection in an edited
collection (or a chapter in a book). If known, include the
name of the author, artist, or designer responsible for the
source, followed by the publication date, in parentheses.

Include the title as it is presented in the source, with sentence-style capitalization but without special punctuation Follow the title with a descriptive label in brackets, followed by a period. Then include entry information required for the source. In those instances when a map, graph, table, or chart is prepared independently, it is treated like a book.

Feistritzer, C. E., & Haar, C. K. (2008). Number of alternative routes to teacher certification in each state (2006) [Map]. In C. E. Feistritzer & C. K. Haar, *Alternative routes to teaching* (p. 4). Upper Saddle River, NJ: Pearson.

   In-text citation   (Feistritzer & Haar, 2008)

Phillips, K. L. (2002). A growing income disparity [Chart]. In K. L. Phillips, *Wealth and democracy: A political history of the American rich* (p. 129). New York, NY: Broadway.

   In-text citation   (Phillips, 2002)

8 Citing Electronic Sources

Many researchers turn to Internet sources—web journals, scholarly projects, websites, blogs and others—because of their easy access. Researchers should note, however, that while electronic sources are sometimes easy to secure, they are often challenging to cite in a paper.

Because sources on the Internet are developed without the rigid standards that exist for print sources, it is sometimes difficult to locate the information that is required for reference-list entries and corresponding in-text citations. Whereas the copyright dates for books can always be found on the copyright page (following the title page), website hosts or developers may include the posting (or revision) date at the top or bottom of the home page; they may locate it on the "About This Site" subpage; or they may not include a date at all. As a result, researchers must be willing to explore online sources thoroughly in order to secure necessary information.

Principles for Citing Electronic Sources

1. *Follow patterns for print sources when possible.* Use reference-list entries for similar print sources as you guide: Include as much of the information that is required for corresponding print versions as you can locate and present the information in the same order and format.

2. *Provide retrieval information.* After providing basi information about an online source—author, date title, and so on—add sufficient retrieval information to allow readers to locate your sources on the Internet Use retrieval dates *only* when sources likely to change (for example, Wikis).

3. *Use a digital object identifier (DOI) when available* Current publications usually display the DOI—a fixed alphanumeric link to an online document—at the top of the first page. When it is available, use it at the end of the citation to identify the source.

4. *Use a uniform resource locator (URL) as an alternative* When a DOI is not available, use the URL of the home page of the online source. A complete URL is necessary *only* when a source is difficult to locate within website.

5. *Present a source's DOI or URL with care.* To ensure that you record a DOI or URL exactly, copy and past it into your reference-list entry.

6. *Present retrieval statements with care.* A retrieval statement ending with a DOI or a URL has no ending punctuation, because a closing period might be misinterpreted as part of the identification number or electronic address.

Kind of source	*Pattern for retrieval statement*
A source with a digital object identifier (DOI)	doi:10.1022/0012-9142.76.3.482

Kind of source	*Pattern for retrieval statement*
A source with a home page URL	Retrieved from http://www .childdevelopmentinfo .com
An abstract (A phrase ending in a database name is followed by a period; a phrase ending in a URL has no closing period.)	Abstract retrieved from Wiley Education database. Abstract retrieved from http://www.ncjrs.gov
A source from an organizational or professional website	Retrieved from the American Psychological Association website: http://www.apa.org/

As you gather entry information to cite electronic sources, your goal should be to gather the most complete set of information possible for each electronic source, following the guidelines in this chapter.

Specialized Online Sources

Online sources exist in many forms. Although they are all designed in approximately the same way—with a home page that directs users to subpages where information can be found—some specialized sites have distinct purposes and applications.

- *Online scholarly projects.* Often affiliated with universities, foundations, and government agencies, these sites are depositories of resources as varied as articles, books, digitized images of original documents, sound recordings, and film clips. Because their affiliations help establish their credibility, that information is sometimes included in reference-list entries.

- *Information databases.* Typically developed by governmental agencies or by information-technology

(cont. on next page)

Specialized Online Sources

firms, these sites provide access to cataloged information that is accessed by using keyword search terms. Periodical databases like ProQuest, EBSCOhost, LexisNexis, JSTOR, and WorldCat make periodical articles available in a variety of formats (see section 1d); other databases provide access to cataloged music, art, historical documents, and so on. Because the database name is usually included in a URL, it does not have to be listed separately in a reference-list entry.

- *Professional websites.* Affiliated with professional organizations in virtually every discipline, these sites make available materials that support or enhance the work of the organization—research documents, online resources, web links, news items, press releases, and so on. Website titles typically include the organization's name, but if they do not, this information may be added for clarity.

8a An Article in an Online Journal

To cite an article in an online journal, first provide the information that is required for the print version of the article (see 5a and 5b). Then close the entry with a retrieval statement. If the article has a digital object identifier (DOI), use that number. If it does not, present a retrieval statement that is appropriate for the kind of online source (see pages 108–109).

Renn, K. A. (2009). Education policy, politics, and mixed-heritage students in the United States. *Journal of Social Issues, 65,* 165–183. doi:10.1111.1540-4560.2008.01593.x

In-text citation   (Renn, 2009)

Pachter, W. S., Fox, R. E., Zimbardo, P., & Antonuccio, D. O. (2007). Corporate funding and conflicts of interest:

A primer for psychologists. *American Psychologist, 62*(9), 1005–1015. Retrieved from http://www.apa.org/journals/

First in-text citation   (Pachter, Fox, Zimbardo, & Antonuccio, 2007)

Second and subsequent citations   (Pachter et al., 2007)

8b   An Article in an Online Magazine

Articles in online magazines are presented in the same ways as online journals, except that dates may also include days and months (see 5d–5e). Follow similar patterns to present reference-list entries.

Dangerfield, W. (2007, February 1). Family ties: African Americans use scientific advances to trace their roots. *Smithsonian*. Retrieved from http://www.smithsonianmag.com

No volume, issue, or page information is available for this source.

In-text citation   (Dangerfield, 2007)

Kluger, J. (2007, October 17). The power of birth order. *Time, 170*(18), 42–48. Retrieved from http://www.time.com

In-text citation   (Kluger, 2007)

8c   An Article in an Online Newspaper

To cite an article in an online newspaper, first provide the information that is required for the print version of the article (see 5f), but exclude section designations and page numbers. Then present a retrieval statement that is appropriate for the kind of online source (see pages 108–109).

Gettleman, J. (2007, December 27). UN says malnutrition in Darfur on the rise. *Boston Globe*. Retrieved from http://www.boston.com

In-text citation   (Gettleman, 2007)

When teachers don't make the grade. (2005, July 31). *Los Angeles Times*. Retrieved from http://www.latimes.com

> ***In-text citation***   ("When Teachers Don't Make the Grade," 2005) or ("When Teachers," 2005)

8d An Article in an Online Newsletter

An entry for an online newsletter follows the same pattern as that for an online newspaper. However, because newsletter articles are sometimes difficult to locate, include the complete URL for your source.

Keith, D. (2007, October). Test your leadership skills: Do you have what it takes? *Team Strategies for Business Leaders*. Retrieved from http://www.mlevelsystems.com /October2007/Newsletter.pdf/

> ***In-text citation***   (Keith, 2007)

Light, T. (2001, May). Canadian tobacco tax measures. *Alcohol & Tobacco Newsletter, 2*(5). Retrieved from http://www.atf.gov/pub/alcatob_pub/may

> ***In-text citation***   (Light, 2001)

8e An Online Book

To cite an online book, first prepare a standard entry (see 6a–6q); however, because the electronic version is the one you are citing, the city and publisher are omitted. Then provide the retrieval statement.

Pierce, R. V. (1895). *The people's common sense medical advisor in plain English, or medicine simplified* (54th ed.). Retrieved from http://www.gutenberg.org /catalog/

> ***In-text citation***   (Pierce, 1895)

Sims, R. R., & Sims, S. J. (Eds.). (1995). *The importance of learning styles: Understanding the implications of learning, course design, and education.* Retrieved from http://www.questia.com

> ***In-text citation***   (Sims & Sims, 1995)

8f An Online Dissertation

To cite an online dissertation, include author, date, and title, followed by the phrase *Doctoral Dissertation* (not italicized) in parentheses. Close the entry with a retrieval statement that includes the name of the database and the accession or order number in parentheses.

Aultman-Bettridge, T. (2007). A gender-specific analysis of community-based juvenile justice reform: The effectiveness of family therapy programs for delinquent girls. Retrieved from ProQuest Dissertations and Theses. (UMI No. AAT 3267887)

> ***In-text citation*** (Aultman-Bettridge, 2007)

Rader, B. R. (2005). The effect of consultation on nursing educators' student ratings of instruction. Retrieved from Digital Library and Archives–Electronic Theses and Dissertations. (Accession No. 10262005-14352)

> ***In-text citation*** (Rader, 2005)

8g An Online Abstract

To cite an abstract of an article in an online journal or an abstract from an online service, first provide the information that is required for the print version of an abstract (see 5c). Then provide a retrieval statement that is appropriate for your source; you may include an accession number in parentheses at the end of the entry.

Boldt, R. C., & Singer, J. B. (2006). Juristocracy in the trenches: Problem-solving judges and therapeutic jurisprudence in drug treatment courts and unified family courts (SSRN No. 923550) [Abstract]. *Maryland Law Review, 65*(1), 82–99. Abstract retrieved from Social Science Research Network abstracts database. (No. 923550)

> ***In-text citation*** (Boldt & Singer, 2006)

Borius, M., Holzapfel, S., Tudiver, F., & Bader, E. (2007, December). Counseling and psychotherapy skills training for family physicians [Abstract]. *Families, Systems, and Health, 25*(4), 382–391. Retrieved from http://www.apa.org/psycharticles/

In-text citation   (Borius, Holzapfel, Tudiver, & Bader, 2007)

Second and subsequent citations   (Borius et al., 2007)

8h An Article in an Online Encyclopedia or Other Reference Work

To cite an article from an online encyclopedia or reference work, first provide the information required for a print source (see 6l). Then include a retrieval statement.

Intelligence. (n.d.). In *Merriam-Webster's online dictionary*. Retrieved from http://www.merriam-webster.com /dictionary/

In-text citation   ("Intelligence," n.d.)

Sternberg, R. J. (2008). Intelligence, human. In *Encyclopaedia Britannica online*. Retrieved from http://search.eb.com/

In-text citation   (Sternberg, 2008)

8i An Online Scholarly Project, Information Database, or Professional Website

If you refer to an entire online scholarly project, information database, or professional website, you do not need to include an entry in your reference list. However, you must identify the title of the source clearly in the text of your paper (capitalized but without special punctuation) and provide a very basic in-text entry (the electronic address), as in these samples:

The Victorian Web presents a wide range of information on the period, ranging from discussions of art to important people, from the history of ideas to the elements of popular culture, from science to philosophy, from technology to social history (http://www .victorianweb.org/).

The UNICEF website provides links to a variety of useful sources that discuss the welfare of children around the world (http://www.unicef.org/).

To cite a source—an article, illustration, map, or other element—from an online scholarly project, information database, or professional website, include the author (or artist, compiler, or editor) of the individual source, if available; the date; and the title of the source, without special punctuation. The retrieval statement includes the name of the project, database, or website (not italicized), a colon, and the site's URL. However, if a website's name is clear from the URL, it is not required in the retrieval statement.

de Vries, S. (2007, November 18). Close encounters with Alfred Adler. Retrieved from Classical Adlerian Psychology website: http://ourworld.compuserve.com

> ***In-text citation***   (de Vries, 2007)

American Library Association. (1986, July 1). Mission, priority areas, goals. Retrieved from http://www.ala.org/ala/

> ***First in-text citation***   (American Library Association [ALA], 1986)

> ***Second and subsequent citations***   (ALA, 1986)

8j An Online Transcript of a Lecture or Speech

To cite an online transcript of a lecture or speech, first provide the information required for a lecture or a speech (see 7h). Then include the word *Transcript*, not italicized and in brackets, and the retrieval statement.

King, M. L., Jr. (1964, December 10). [Nobel Peace Prize acceptance speech]. Speech presented at Nobel Prize Ceremony, Oslo, Sweden. [Transcript]. Retrieved from http://nobelprize.org/

> ***In-text citation***   (King, 1964)

Roosevelt, E. (1948, September 28). [Address]. Speech presented at the United Nations Conference, Paris, France. [Transcript]. Retrieved from http://www.americanrhetoric.com/

> ***In-text citation***   (Roosevelt, 1948)

8k   An Online Map, Graph, Table, or Chart

To cite an online map, graph, table, or chart, first provide the information required for the kind of visual element (see 7j). Then provide the retrieval statement.

United States Geological Survey. (2003, February 6). Colima
    Volcano [Satellite image]. In *Earth as Art Series.*
    Retrieved from the United States Geological Survey
    website: http://eros.usgs.gov/

   In-text citation   (United States Geological Survey, 2003)

This image is part of a series, which is identified after the title.

United States Census Bureau. (2006). School enrollment by
    poverty status, sex, and age [Table]. Retrieved from
    the United States Census Bureau website: http://
    pubdb3.census.gov

   In-text citation   (United States Census Bureau, 2006)

This graph is found on a government website.

8l   A CD-ROM Source

To cite a CD-ROM source, include the author or editor, the release date, and the title, italicized. End the entry with the following information in parentheses: the publisher or distributor; the word *CD-ROM,* not italicized; the release date; and an item number, if applicable.

Centers for Disease Control and Prevention. (2003).
    International classification of diseases (6th ed.).
    (Government Printing Office, CD-ROM, 2003 release).

   In-text citation   (Centers for Disease Control and
   Prevention, 2003)

Chen, J. X. (2003). *Guide to graphics software tools.* (Springer,
    CD-ROM, 2003 release).

   In-text citation   (Chen, 2003)

8m   An E-mail Interview

An interview conducted through e-mail correspondence is considered personal communication. As such, it is not included in the reference list. However, it is cited in the text of the paper by enclosing the phrase *personal communication* (not italicized) and the date of the e-mail in parentheses.

Davis (personal communication, March 13, 2008) noted
that classroom technology is only as good as the
people who use it.

8n An Online Video Podcast

To cite an online video podcast, provide as much as possible of the information required for regularly distributed motion pictures or television broadcasts (see 7a, 7c). Then add a retrieval statement that matches the kind of online source (scholarly project, website, and so on).

The daily English show [Video podcast]. (2006,
July 28). [With Sarah]. Retrieved from http://the
dailyenglishshow.blogspot.com/

    In-text citation   (*The Daily English Show*, 2006)

Ruiz, M. (Producer). (2008, February 21–25). *Autism: The
hidden epidemic* [Video podcast]. New York, NY:
National Broadcasting Company. Retrieved from the
Autism Speaks website: http://www.autismspeaks.org

    In-text citation   (Ruiz, 2008)

8o An Online Audio Podcast

To cite an audio podcast, provide as much as possible of the information required for regular radio broadcasts, recordings, or speeches (7d–7e, 7h). Then add a retrieval statement that matches the kind of online source (scholarly project, website, and so on).

The beep heard round the world: The birth of the space age
[Audio podcast]. (n.d.). [With Jane Platt]. Retrieved from
the National Aeronautics and Space Administration
website: http://www.nasa.gov/

    In-text citation   ("The Beep Heard Round the
World," n.d.)

Rovner, J. (2008, April 5). Eric Cartman: America's favorite
little $@#&*%. In *In character* [Audio podcast].
Retrieved from http://www.npr.org

    In-text citation   (Rovner, 2008)

8p　An Online Posting—Discussion Group or Blog

To cite an online posting to a forum or discussion group, or blog, provide the author, identified by name or screen name; the date of the posting; the title of the posting, with a description of the message; and a retrieval statement that is appropriate to the kind of source.

Lanier, C. (2007, June 20). College would be optional if high school meant something. [Discussion group comment]. Retrieved from the *Washington Post* discussion group: http://www.washingtonpost.com

　　In-text citation　(Lanier, 2007)

Nguyen, K. T. (2007, August 4). Re: Pre-teen body image issues. [Blog message]. Retrieved from http://www.cnn.com/ HEALTH/blogs/

　　In-text citation　(Nguyen, 2007)

1/2 inch

Running head: BEYOND BIRTH ORDER   1

Labeled
running head:
all capitals
(25)

Identifying
information:
centered
(26)

Beyond Birth Order:

Recognizing Other Variables

Elissa Allen and Jeremy Reynolds

Indiana State University

If an author
note is
required, it
appears at the
bottom of the
title page
(26).

1/2 inch

BEYOND BIRTH ORDER   2

Centered label
with normal
capitalization
(27)

Unindented ¶:
250 words or
fewer (27)

Abstract

Although scholars continue to make a case for birth-
order effects in children's development, exclusive
reliance on this useful but one-dimensional criterion
ignores other variables that affect children's personal,
intellectual, and social development. The sex of other
siblings, the time between births, the size of the family,
the age of the mother, the psychological condition
of the children, the absence of a parent, and the
birth order of the parents also influence a child's
development.

BEYOND BIRTH ORDER   3

The text begins on page 3. (28)

Beyond Birth Order:

Recognizing Other Variables

Sigmund Freud, Queen Elizabeth II, Albert
Einstein, William Shakespeare, George Washington,
Jacqueline Kennedy, John Milton, Julius Caesar,
Leontyne Price, and Winston Churchill. What do these
famous people have in common? They were all first-
born children. The fact that so many important people
in all spheres of influence have been first-born children has lent credence to the notion that birth order
helps determine the kind of people we become.

Scientific studies over the years have, in fact,
suggested that birth order affects an individual's
development. For example, studies (Pine, 1995) have
suggested that first-born children acquire language
skills sooner than later-born children. Further, Ernst
and Angst (1983) explained the underlying premise
of birth-order effects this way: "Everybody agrees
that birth-order differences must arise from differential socialization by the parents. There is, however,
no general theory on how this differential socialization actually works" (p. x). Yet other studies
(Herrera, Zajonc, Wieczorkowska, & Cichomski,
2003) suggest that parents' beliefs about birth-order
diffences influence their expectations for their children. Stein (2008) also observed that birth-order
effects are more pronounced in families that are
competitive and democratic. It is not surprising,
then, that a general theory has not emerged because
many other variables besides birth order influence
an individual's personal, intellectual, and social
development.

Marginal notes:

- Centered title with headline-style capitalization (28)
- Allusions as an introductory strategy
- Historical context established
- Past tense to describe scholarship (55)
- General reference: author and date (70–71)
- Specific reference: author, date, and page (73)
- Thesis statement (2–3)

BEYOND BIRTH ORDER   4

Headings
to divide the
discussion
(36–37)

Sex of the Siblings

While acknowledging that birth order plays a part
in an individual's development, scholars have begun to
recognize that it is only one variable. For example,
Sutton-Smith and Rosenberg (1970) observed that even
in two-child families there are four possible variations

Elements in a
series (35)

for sibling relationships based on gender: (a) first-born
female, second-born female; (b) first-born female,
second-born male; (c) first-born male, second-born male;

Common
knowledge
suggests that
the number
increases to
24. (16–17)

(c) first-born male, second-born female. In families with
three children, the variations increase to 24. To suggest
that being the first-born child is the same in all of these
contexts ignores too many variables.

Time Between Births

Summary of
Forer's ideas

Forer (1976) suggested that when the births of
children are separated by five or more years, the
effects of birth order are changed. For example, in a

Comparative
numbers in
the same form
(51)

family with four children (with children aged 12, 6, 4,
and 2 years old), the second child would be more
likely to exhibit the characteristics of an oldest child
because of his or her nearness in age to the younger
children and the six-year separation in age from the
oldest child. The pattern would differ from that of a

Elissa and
Jeremy's own
example: no
documentation
required

sibling in a four-child family if the children were
spaced fewer than three years apart (for example, if the
children were 10, 8, 5, and 3 years old); this second
child would exhibit the characteristics typical of a
second-middle child.

Size of Family

Studies have also suggested that the size of the
family modifies the effects of birth order. Whereas in a
moderate-sized family (two to four children) the

first-born child usually achieves the highest level of education, Forer (1969) observed that "a first-born child from a large family has often been found to obtain less education than a last-born child from such a family" (p. 24). Whether this occurs because large families tend to have lower socioeconomic status or whether it is the result of varied family dynamics, the overall size of the family seems to alter the preconceived notions of birth order and its influence on a child's development.

Last names only

Age of the Mother

Studies have suggested that a mother's age has a strong bearing on the child's learned behavior, regardless of birth order. Sutton-Smith and Rosenberg (1970) offered this perspective:

> On a more obvious level, younger mothers have more stamina and vigor than older mothers. One speculation in the literature is that they are also more anxious and uncertain about their child-training procedures, and that this has an effect of inducing anxiety in their offspring. (p. 138)

Long quotation: 5-space indentation (75)

Set-in quotation: period before the citation (75)

It seems safe to assume, then, that the third child of a woman of 28 will have a different experience growing up than the third child of a woman of 39. They may share the same relational patterns with their siblings, but they will not share the same patterns with their mothers.

Psychological Factors

Early studies on birth order failed to account for psychological differences among children, even among those who shared the same birth status. Forer (1969) asserted, however, that "special conditions involving a child in a family may change the birth-order effect both for him and his siblings" (p. 19). Such conditions as a child's mental retardation, severe hearing loss, blindness, disabling handicaps—or even extreme beauty, exceptional intelligence, or great physical skill—can alter the dynamics of the family and consequently affect the traditionally described effects of birth order. In short, a middle child whose physiological conditions are outside the normal spectrum—because of different potential and opportunity—will not have the same life experiences as a middle child who is considered average.

Summary of ideas

Absence of a Parent

Parents may be absent from family units for a variety of reasons: a parent may die, creating a permanent void in a family unit; a parent may be gone to war or be hospitalized for an extended period, creating a temporary but still notable disruption in the family; or a parent may travel for business or be gone for brief periods to attend school, creating a brief but obvious interruption in the family's normal workings. These conditions affect a child's experiences and can, under certain circumstances, mitigate the effects of birth order. Toman (1993) explained that the effects will be greater

A long quote (75)

   a. The more recently they have occurred,

   b. The earlier in a person's life they have occurred,

   c. The older the person lost is (in relation to the oldest family member),

   d. The longer the person has lived together with the lost person,

   e. The smaller the family,

   f. The greater the imbalance of the sexes in the family resulting from the loss,

BEYOND BIRTH ORDER   7

     g. The longer it takes the family to find a
       replacement for the lost person,

     h. The greater the number of losses, and the
       graver the losses, that have occurred before.
       (pp. 41–42)

Such disruptions—whether major or minor—alter the
family unit and often have a greater influence on the
children than the traditional effects of birth order.

Birth Order of Parents

    A number of scholars have asserted that the birth
order of parents influences to a high degree their inter-
relationships with their children and, consequently,
creates an impact that extends beyond the simple birth
order of the children. Toman (1993) described the
family relationships, based on birth order, that promise
the least conflict and, hence, best situation for children's development:

> If the mother is the youngest sister of a brother
> and has an older son and a younger daughter, she
> can identify with her daughter and the daughter
> with the mother. The daughter, too, is the younger
> sister of a brother. Moreover, the mother has no
> trouble dealing with her son, for she had an older
> brother in her original family and her son, too, is
> an older brother of a sister. (p. 199)

Toman's assumption that parents relate better to their
children when they have shared similar sibling-related
experiences leads to this assumption: When parents
can create a positive and productive home environment (because of familiar familial relationships), the
children will benefit. When conflict occurs

because sibling relations are unfamiliar, everyone suf-
fers. Parent–child relationships—determined, at least
in part, by the parents' own birth orders—would
consequently vary from family to family, even when
children of those families share the same birth order.

Conclusion

According to U.S. Census information, collected
from 92,119 randomly selected mothers, 28% of children are first born, 28% second born, 20% middle
born, and 18% youngest born (cited in Simpson,
Bloom, Newlon, & Arminio, 1994). As long as census
takers, scholars, family members, parents, and children think in terms of birth order, we will have an
oversimplified perspective of why children develop as
they do. Yet studies (Parish, 1990) have suggested that
adolescents recognize that family structure and personal interaction have a stronger bearing on their per-
ceptions of themselves, other family members, and
their families than do birth order or even gender. And,
importantly, websites such as Matthias Romppel's
Birth Order Research (2008) approach the issue cau-
tiously, suggesting that birth-order effects on children
are changeable (http://www.romppel.de/birth-order/).
Perhaps we should take our cues from these young
people and current scholars and recognize that birth
order is but one interesting variable in personality
development.

Percentages in **numeral-symbol** form (51)

Multiple authors: joined by an ampersand (66)

A reference to a complete website occurs in the paper but does not appear in the reference list. (114–115)

BEYOND BIRTH ORDER　　9

References

Ernst, C., & Angst, J. (1983). *Birth order: Its influence on personality.* Berlin, Germany: Springer.

Forer, L. K. (1969). *Birth order and life roles.* Springfield, IL: Thomas.

Forer, L. K. (1976). *The birth order factor: How your personality is influenced by your place in the family.* New York, NY: McKay.

Herrera, N. C., Zajonc, R. B., Wieczorkowska, G., & Cichomski, B. (2003). Beliefs about birth rank and their reflection in reality. *Journal of Personality and Social Psychology 85*(1), 142–150. doi:10.1037/0022-3514.85.1.142

Parish, T. S. (1990). Evaluations of family by youth: Do they vary as a function of family structure, gender, and birth order? *Adolescence, 25,* 353–356.

Pine, J. M. (1995). Variations in vocabulary development as a function of birth order. *Child Development, 66,* 272–281.

Simpson, P. W., Bloom, J. W., Newlon, B. J., & Arminio, L. (1994). Birth-order proportions of the general population in the United States. *Individual Psychology: Journal of Adlerian Theory, 50,* 173–182.

Stein, H. T. (2008). Adlerian overview of birth order characteristics. Retrieved from the Alfred Adler Institute of San Francisco website: http://ourworld. compuserve.com/homepages/hstein/birthord.htm

Sutton-Smith, B., & Rosenberg, B. G. (1970). *The sibling.* New York, NY: Holt.

Toman, W. (1993). *Family constellation: Its effects on personality and social behavior.* New York, NY: Springer.

Sequential page numbers (29, 63)

Descriptive title: centered (63)

Italicized, not underlined (49)

Author names repeated in subsequent citations (98–99)

A DOI is used instead of a full retrieval statement. (108)

First lines at the normal margin; subsequent lines indented (66)

Labeled run
ning head: all
capitals (25)

Identifying
information:
centered
(25–26)

If an author
note is
required, it
appears at the
bottom of
the title page
(26).

Students' Reactions to Kinds of Test Questions:

A Piece in the Test-Anxiety Puzzle

Gabriel Stevenson

Indiana State University

Centered label
with normal
capitalization
(27)

Unindented ¶:
250 words or
fewer (27)

Abstract

The purpose of this brief study was to determine
whether specific kinds of test questions produced anx-
icty in students. The results of a survey of 89 high
school freshmen indicate that true/false, multiple-
choice, and matching are low-anxiety question formats, whereas essay, fill-in-the-blank, and listing are
high-anxiety question formats. However, the study revealed that students' anxiety levels related to question
types do not vary dramatically, either by question type
or by students' performance levels, as indicated by
previous grades.

STUDENTS' REACTIONS

3 The text begins on page 3. (28)

Students' Reactions to Kinds of Test Questions:
A Piece in the Test-Anxiety Puzzle

Centered title with headline-style capitalization (28)

Today's students are faced with an increasing number of tests. Not only do they take tests for their individual classes, but they also take state-mandated competency tests to progress through school and standardized achievement tests to gain admission to colleges and universities. With the emphasis currently being placed on tests, it is no wonder that many students are now experiencing test anxiety.

Unlabeled introduction: contextualizes the paper, clarifies the topic (28–29)

One area, however, has not received sufficient attention: students' reactions to specific kinds of test questions. Consequently, using data collected from a sampling of high school students, this brief study attempts to discover with what types of test questions students are most comfortable and what kinds of questioning techniques produce the greatest amount of insecurity or anxiety.

The nature of students' test anxiety has been—and continues to be—studied by scholars in education, psychology, and related fields. By understanding the forms, causes, and results of test anxiety, they hope to provide the means for students and educators to address the problem in helpful ways.

Spielberger and Vagg (1995) have discussed testing in a large cultural context, cataloging the ever-increasing number of tests used in educational and work-related settings. Wigfield and Eccles (1989) have described the nature of test anxiety, providing useful categories and explanations to enhance the understanding of this multifaceted problem. Hancock (2001) has further contextualized the testing situation by describing the high-stakes environments in which tests are given.

Literature review as part of introduction (29)

Other scholars have explored the cognitive processes that are related to test anxiety. Schutz, Davis, and Schwanenflugel (2002) have distinguished between high and low levels of test anxiety and have discussed the ways students perceive the test-taking process and the ways they cope. Others have addressed students' self-awareness about the emotional nature of the testing process and their own procedures for handling emotion during testing (Weiner 1994; Zeidner 1995a, 1995b).

Yet other scholars have discussed test anxiety among special student populations. Swanson and Howell (1996) have expressed particular concern that test anxiety among disabled students can lead to poor test performance, which in turn can lead to poor overall academic performance and low self-esteem. Further, Nelson, Jayanthi, Epstein, and Bursuck (2000) have presented information on alternatives to and adaptations of traditional testing that can allow special-needs students to demonstrate what they know without the additional burden of test anxiety.

These studies have laid a contextual groundwork for further study, especially in areas such as test design and test preparation.

Method

Participants

The survey group was composed of 89 high school freshmen (44 females and 45 males) from three classes. The students were enrolled in a required (and untracked) freshman English class that included students of varied abilities at a consolidated high school in west-central Indiana. The students had completed one grading period; their grades from the previous term ranged from *A* to *F*.

[Margin notes:]

Multiple references, separated by semicolons (72)

Level-1 headings for major subtopics (36–37)

"Method" subsection: level-2 headings (36–37)

Materials

Students were given a brief questionnaire (see Appendix) that included these elements: (a) an element to determine gender, (b) an element to record their grades in English during the previous nine weeks, and (c) a six-element questionnaire using a Likert-type scale so that students could indicate their anxiety-related responses to six types of test questions.

In-text reference to an appendix (33)

Procedures

The students' teacher distributed the questionnaire at the beginning of each of the three class periods and read the instructions aloud, emphasizing that students should respond to the types of questions based on their entire testing experiences, not just those on English tests. Students were then given 10 minutes to complete the questionnaire; most completed the questionnaires in fewer than 5 minutes.

Description of materials and procedures (29)

Results

The most general analysis of the data involved computing students' ratings of question types using the Likert-type scale (1–2 = *secure,* 3–4 = *no reaction,* 5–6 = *insecure*). Percentages of students' responses appear in Table 1.

"Results" section: summarizes the data (29)

In-text reference to a table (31–32)

Low-Anxiety Question Types

The findings indicate that true/false test questions create the least anxiety, with 31.4% of students giving it a 1 rating; in addition, 81.9% rated true/false as a 1, 2, or 3, indicating little anxiety. Matching and multiple-choice questions also achieved low anxiety ratings, with 25.8% of students giving them a 1 rating; 79.7% rated matching as a 1, 2, or 3, indicating little anxiety. Interestingly, 84.3% rated multiple-choice questions as a 1, 2, or 3, making it the question type that produces the least anxiety in the greatest percentage of students.

High-Anxiety Question Types

The findings indicate that essay questions create the most anxiety, with 49.4% of students giving them a 6 rating; further, 71.9% rated essay questions as a 4, 5, or 6, indicating a high degree of anxiety. Fill-in-the-blank questions also achieved a high-anxiety rating, with 24.6% of students giving them a 6 rating; 65.1% rated fill-in-the-blank questions as a 4, 5, or 6, indicating a high degree of anxiety. Finally, 21.4% of students rated listing questions as a 6; 65.3% rated them as a 4, 5, or 6, making this a high-stress question type.

Mean Responses

The mean responses to the question types (1–2 = *secure;* 3–4 = *no reaction;* 5–6 = *insecure*) correlate with the individual low-anxiety and high-anxiety ratings given by students, as shown in Figure 1. True/false (2.35), multiple-choice (2.43), and matching (2.53) remain in the low-anxiety category, but multiple-choice and matching reverse their rating order. Essay (4.56), fill-in the blank (4.27), and listing (4.16) remain in the high-anxiety category; they retain the same rating order.

As Figure 1 illustrates, mean responses by students' grade categories show slightly varied preferences among high-performing and low-performing students: *A* students (1: matching; 2: multiple-choice; 3: true/false; 4: fill-in-the-blank; 5–6: listing and essay), *B* students (1: multiple-choice; 2: matching; 3: true/false; 4: listing; 5–6: fill-in-the-blank and essay), *C* students (1: matching; 2: multiple-choice; 3: true/false; 4–5: fill-in-the-blank and listing;

Subsection: level-2 headings (36–37)

The summary correlates with tables or figures.

In-text reference to a figure (32–33)

STUDENTS' REACTIONS   7

6: essay), *D* students (1: true/false; 2: multiple-choice;
3: matching; 4: listing; 5: fill-in-the-blank; 6: essay),
and *F* students (1: true/false; 2: multiple-choice; 3:
matching; 4: listing; 5: fill-in-the-blank; 6: essay).

An average of the mean responses to all six question types for each grade category indicates an increasing degree of anxiety: for *A* students, the averaged mean response is 2.75; for *B* students, 3.08; for *C*
students, 3.57; for *D* students, 3.61; and for *F* students,
3.83. Although the increments are small, there is a
steady progression from one student group to the next;
however, none of the averaged means falls far from the
3–4 range *(no reaction),* suggesting that, generally, no
question format makes students as a group feel either
very secure or very anxious.

Discussion

The data indicate that, for students, question
types fall into two distinct groups: low-stress questions
(true/false, multiple-choice, matching) and high-stress
questions (listing, fill-in-the-blank, essay). However,
the data also indicate that, on average, students' anxiety levels related to question types do not vary greatly
(mean responses ranged from 2.75 for *A* students to
3.83 for *F* students), which suggests that although
question-related anxiety exists, it is not dramatic.

An analysis of the data further indicates that
low-anxiety questions (true/false, multiple-choice,
matching) are format based, providing information
and allowing students to select among options.

"Discussion" section: comments on the data, correlates with the hypothesis (29)

STUDENTS' REACTIONS　8

In contrast, high-anxiety questions (listing, fill-in-the-blank, essay) are open-ended, requiring students to recall and arrange information on their own.

A comment on the value of the study (29)

The results of this brief study are, of course, tentative and need to be reproduced with a larger, more comprehensive sample. However, the study does suggest the value of analyzing specific question formats because they can contribute in a small but significant way to overall test anxiety.

STUDENTS' REACTIONS

9 Consecutive page numbers (29, 63)

References

Hancock, D. R. (2001). Effects of test anxiety and evaluative threat on students' achievement and motivation. *The Journal of Educational Research, 94,* 284–290.

Nelson, J. S., Jayanthi, M., Epstein, M. H., & Bursuck, W. D. (2000). Student preferences for adaptations in classroom testing. *Remedial and Special Education, 21*(1), 41–52.

Schutz, P. A., Davis, H. A., & Schwanenflugel, P. J. (2002). Organization of concepts relevant to emotions and their regulation during test taking. *The Journal of Experimental Education, 70*(4), 316–342.

Spielberger, C. D., & Vagg, P. R. (Eds.). (1995). *Test anxiety: Theory, assessment and treatment.* Washington, DC: Taylor.

Swanson, S., & Howell, C. (1996). Test anxiety in adolescents with learning disabilities and behavior disorders. *Exceptional Children, 62,* 389–397.

Weiner, B. (1994). Integrating social and personal theories of achievement striving. *Review of Educational Research, 64,* 557–573.

Wigfield, A., & Eccles, J. S. (1989). Test anxiety in elementary and secondary school students. *Educational Psychologist, 24,* 159–183.

Zeidner, M. (1995a). Adaptive coping with test situations: A review of the literature. *Educational Psychologist, 30,* 123–133.

Zeidner, M. (1995b). Coping with examination stress: Resources, strategies, outcomes. *Anxiety, Stress, and Coping, 8,* 279–298.

Reference list: alphabetized, double-spaced (67, 68–70)

Italicized, not underlined (49)

First lines at the normal margin; subsequent lines indented (66)

Names repeated in subsequent entries (98–99)

Consecutive page numbers (33)

Numbered table on a separate page (31–32)

Table 1

Overall Responses (Security to Insecurity) to Question Types

Table title in italics (31)

Ruled lines to separate elements (31)

Column spacing is adjusted for easy reading. (31)

Question type	Rating					
	1	2	3	4	5	6
Matching	25.8	30.3	23.6	11.2	3.4	5.6
True/false	31.4	25.8	24.7	13.5	3.4	1.1
Fill-in-the-blank	2.2	10.1	22.5	13.5	27.0	24.6
Multiple-choice	25.8	32.6	25.9	6.7	6.7	2.2
Listing	4.5	5.6	24.7	21.4	22.5	21.4
Essay	6.8	13.5	7.9	10.1	12.4	49.4

Numbered figure on a separate page (32)

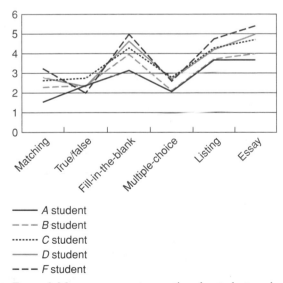

——— *A* student
— — — *B* student
········ *C* student
——— *D* student
— — — *F* student

Figure 1. Mean responses to questions by student grade categories.

STUDENTS' REACTIONS   12

Appendix

Test Anxiety Questionnaire

Survey: Test Anxiety—Reactions to Kinds of Test Questions

M   F

Grade Last Nine Weeks: A   B   C   D   F

Circle one response for each kind of test question: *1* means that you feel *comfortable/secure* with these kinds of questions (you won't worry about that part of the test); *6* means that you feel *uncomfortable/insecure* with these question types (you will worry about how you do on that part of the test). Consider tests for all classes, not just English.

	Secure		No reaction		Insecure	
1. Matching	1	2	3	4	5	6
2. True/false	1	2	3	4	5	6
3. Fill-in-the-blank	1	2	3	4	5	6
4. Multiple-choice	1	2	3	4	5	6
5. Listing	1	2	3	4	5	6
6. Essay	1	2	3	4	5	6

A   Poster Presentations

As alternatives to traditional documented papers, poster presentations provide opportunities for researchers to share the results of either text-based or experimental research in visually oriented and interactive ways.

Poster presentations were developed as part of professional meetings. Recognizing that traditional, speech-based sessions limited the scope of conferences, organizers searched for ways in which to involve a greater number of researchers in conference activities, as well as to provide opportunities for people to share preliminary findings or to solicit reactions to "work in progress." Because poster presentations are now a common way to share research, teachers have begun to incorporate the format into their classroom activities so that student–researchers can develop skills in presenting their findings in interactive ways.

Poster Presentations—An Overview

Poster presentations emphasize visual elements, supported with printed information, and allow researchers to discuss their work with interested people.

At conferences, presenters are allotted a predetermined amount of space (4-by-4 feet, 4-by-8 feet, or sometimes more) in an exhibit hall, and they display their posters for review for an allotted amount of time (one hour or sometimes longer). Presenters stay with their posters, elaborate on their work, answer questions, and solicit reactions. The visual presentation of research findings provides an exciting alternative to traditional speeches (which are often readings of papers), and the interactive format allows for more give-and-take among those who attend conferences.

In classes and seminars, poster presentations allow students to present their research to the entire class, as opposed to just the teacher, and to gather helpful reactions to their work.

Features of Poster Presentations

Whether given at a conference or in a classroom, poster presentations share a variety of features, which may be surprisingly simple or highly elaborate.

- *Display surface.* The simplest "poster" can be prepared on a standard 2-by-3-foot sheet of poster board, mounted for stability. Displayed on an easel for easy viewing, this kind of poster is most commonly presented in the classroom. More elaborate posters are prepared as freestanding displays, may include multiple display panels, and may be quite expensive to prepare. Such complex posters are more commonly presented at conferences.

- *Content.* To ensure that people focus properly on your work, create a clear and interesting title for the poster and provide identifying information about yourself (your name and affiliation). Because posters of all kinds must present content in concise, easily readable form, use headings judiciously. The standard divisions of a research paper—method, results, discussion, and others—provide familiar ways to divide the content of the poster, although other organizational patterns are also acceptable.

- *Visual elements.* Because posters emphasize the visual presentation of research findings, use graphic elements to your advantage. Arrange information for easy interpretation, remembering that readers scan visual documents in the same way they read: from left to right and from top to bottom. When possible, reduce material to bulleted lists for easy scanning. Select simple fonts in sizes that can be read from three to six feet away. Use tables, charts, graphs, and images to clarify ideas. Employ color, when possible, to create visual interest.

- *Supporting documents.* Provide a one-to-two-page supporting document that summarizes the information presented on your poster. Label it clearly with the presentation's title and your identifying information; also include key elements from the poster. Make copies for those attending the conference or for class members.

- *Presentation.* You must facilitate the review of the poster. Without simply reading or summarizing the material for your audience (after all, they can do that), highlight key features and direct their attention to the most salient points. Also, be prepared to answer questions and guide discussion.

Suggestions for Poster Presentations

Because poster presentations provide a unique opportunity to share research findings, a well-planned presentation takes time to prepare and requires unique kinds of effort. Consider these suggestions:

- *Allow yourself sufficient time.* Do not assume that a poster session is easy to prepare. Not only does it require initial research, but it also warrants specialized preparation that may be new to you if you are used to preparing only written documents. Also, because the presentation includes more kinds of elements—visual and speaking components, as well as written content—preparing the poster presentation should not be a rushed effort.

- *Experiment with design elements.* Explore alternative ways to design your poster. Prepare material in several formats (try different fonts and font sizes; use different color combinations; prepare tables *and* figures), and then decide which format creates the best visual effect.

- *Solicit reactions.* Seek responses to your work. Ask for overall reactions but also ask specific questions about presentational elements. If you have prepared alternative versions of your poster, ask which is most effective.

- *Practice your presentation.* Although a well-prepared poster should in some regards "speak for itself," consider the ways in which you can help an audience review your poster. Develop a set of "talking points," a brief list of comments to guide your explanations. When possible, practice your presentation to ensure that your expression is clear and helpful.

- *Anticipate questions.* Think critically and predict questions that your audience might pose; then practice responding to those questions.

Poster presentations provide a unique way to share the results of research. Their conciseness, visual clarity, and interactivity make them an effective means to share the results of your research work.

Students' Reactions to Kinds of Test Questions
A Piece in the Test-Anxiety Puzzle

Gabriel Stevenson

Indiana State University

Participants:	89 high school freshmen (44 females and 45 males), from three untracked English classes; students had completed one grading period, with grades ranging from *A* to *F*.
Materials:	A brief questionnaire: (a) gender, (b) grades in English, (c) a six-element questionnaire using a Likert-type scale to indicate their anxiety-related responses to six types of test questions, and (d) a section for additional comments about types of test questions.
Procedures:	The students' teacher distributed the questionnaire and read the instructions aloud; students were given 10 minutes to complete the questionnaire.

Overall Responses to Question Types (Security to Insecurity)

	Rating					
	Secure		No reaction		Insecure	
Question Type	1	2	3	4	5	6
Matching	25.8	30.3	23.6	11.2	3.4	5.6
True/false	31.4	25.8	24.7	13.5	3.4	1.1
Fill-in-the-blank	2.2	10.1	22.5	13.5	27.0	24.6
Multiple-choice	25.8	32.6	25.9	6.7	6.7	2.2
Listing	4.5	5.6	24.7	21.4	22.5	21.4
Essay	6.8	13.5	7.9	10.1	12.4	49.4

The data indicate that, for students, question types fall into two distinct groups: low-stress questions (true/false, multiple-choice, matching) and high-stress questions (listing, fill-in-the-blank, essay). Further analysis indicates that low-anxiety questions (true/false, multiple-choice, matching) are format based, providing information and allowing students to select among options. In contrast, high-anxiety questions (listing, fill-in-the-blank, essay) are open-ended, requiring students to recall and arrange information on their own.

Index

●

Format for APA Reference-List Entries

1. Begin the first line at the left margin and indent subsequent lines $^1/_2$ inch.
2. Invert the author's name so that the last name appears first; use first and middle initials.
3. When no author is named, list the source by title.
4. Place the publication date in parentheses, followed by a period.
5. Cite the complete title, including subtitles.
6. Use a period followed by one space to separate author, date, title, and publication information.

See Chapters 4–8 for additional information and examples.

Sample Reference-List Entries

Article in a Journal With Continuous Paging (5a)

Nuttman-Shwartz, O. (2007). Is there life without work? *The International Journal of Aging and Human Development, 64,* 129–147.

Article in a Journal With Separate Paging (5b)

McDonald, T. P., Poertner, J., & Jennings, M. A. (2007). Permanency for children in foster care: A competing risks analysis. *The Journal of Social Science Research, 33*(4), 45–56.

Article in a Monthly Magazine (5d)

Martinez-Conde, S., & Macknik, S. L. (2007, August). Windows on the mind. *Scientific American, 297*(2), 56–63.

Article in a Newspaper (5f)

Rodriguez, A. (2007, September 16). When health care does more harm than good. *The Chicago Tribune,* p. 1:18.

A Book by One Author (6a)

Thornicroft, G. (2006). *Shunned: Discrimination against people with mental illness.* New York, NY: Oxford University Press.

Book by Two or More Authors (6b)

Lazarus, R. S., & Lazarus, B. N. (2006). *Coping with aging.* New York, NY: Oxford University Press.

An Edition Other Than the First (6e)
Young, M. E., & Long, L. L. (2007). *Counseling and therapy for couples* (2nd ed.). Belmont, CA: Brooks/Cole.

An Original Selection in an Edited Collection (6g)
Drewes, A. A. (2005). Play in selected cultures: Diversity and universality. In E. Gil & A. A. Drewes (Eds.), *Cultural issues in play therapy* (pp. 26–71). New York, NY: Guilford Press.

An Article in an Encyclopedia or Other Reference Work (
Sullaway, F. J. (2007). Birth order and sibling competition. In R. I. M. Dunbar & L. Barrett (Eds.), *Oxford handbook of evolutionary psychology* (pp. 297–311). New York, N Oxford University Press.

A Motion Picture (7a)
Pakula, A. J., Barish, K., Gerrity, W. C., & Starger, M. (Producer & Pakula, A. J. (Director). (1982). *Sophie's choice* [Motion picture]. [With M. Streep, K. Kline, & P. MacNichol]. United States: Universal.

An Article in an Online Journal (8a)
Pachter, W. S., Fox, R. E., Zimbardo, P., & Antonuccio, D. O. (2007). Corporate funding and conflicts of interest: A primer for psychologists. *American Psychologist, 62*(9) 1005–1015. Retrieved from http://www.apa.org/ journals/

An Article in an Online Encyclopedia or Other Referer
Work (8h)
Sternberg, R. J. (2008). Intelligence, human. In *Encyclopaedi Britannica online.* Retrieved from http://search.eb.com/

An Online Scholarly Project, Information Database, or
Professional Website (8i)
American Library Association. (1986, July 1). Mission, priorit areas, goals. Retrieved from http://www.ala.org/ala

An Online Posting—Discussion Group or Blog (8p)
Nguyen, K. T. (2007, August 4). Re: Pre-teen body image issues. [Blog message]. Retrieved from http:// www.cnn.com/HEALTH/blogs/

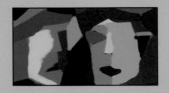

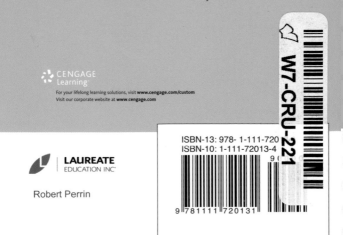

CENGAGE
Learning

For your lifelong learning solutions, visit www.cengage.com/custom
Visit our corporate website at www.cengage.com

ISBN-13: 978- 1-111-720
ISBN-10: 1-111-72013-4

9 781111 720131

LAUREATE
EDUCATION INC

Robert Perrin